Designing Materials for Medical Devices

Fundamentals

Designing Materials for Medical Devices

Fundamentals

Editor

Teoh Swee Hin

Hunan University, China

World Scientific

NEW JERSEY · LONDON · SINGAPORE · BEIJING · SHANGHAI · HONG KONG · TAIPEI · CHENNAI

Published by

World Scientific Publishing Co. Pte. Ltd.

5 Toh Tuck Link, Singapore 596224

USA office: 27 Warren Street, Suite 401-402, Hackensack, NJ 07601

UK office: 57 Shelton Street, Covent Garden, London WC2H 9HE

Library of Congress Control Number: 2024038429

British Library Cataloguing-in-Publication Data
A catalogue record for this book is available from the British Library.

DESIGNING MATERIALS FOR MEDICAL DEVICES
Fundamentals

ISBN 978-981-12-9588-1 (hardcover)
ISBN 978-981-12-9589-8 (ebook for institutions)
ISBN 978-981-12-9590-4 (ebook for individuals)

For any available supplementary material, please visit
https://www.worldscientific.com/worldscibooks/10.1142/13921#t=suppl

Desk Editors: Aanand Jayaraman/Joy Quek

Typeset by Stallion Press
Email: enquiries@stallionpress.com

Foreword

This book, *Designing Materials for Medical Devices: Fundamentals*, edited by Prof. Swee Hin Teoh, is a revised version of the highly successful book *Engineering Materials for Biomedical Applications*, which has sold more than 1000 copies and received good reviews. It is written in a simple manner for non-specialists to understand. The newly revised book will be a handy reference for those working with metals, polymers, ceramics, and composites fabricating many medical devices.

Most of the chapters of this book emphasize the compositions, processing techniques, and physical properties of the materials commonly used in applications such as orthopedic and dental implants. The book provides valuable information about durability, including fatigue, wear, and corrosion of metals, which is often lacking in other texts. It also includes detailed coverage of the surface treatments of metals and a special chapter on prosthetic appliances for the disabled, an important but often overlooked topic in biomaterials. Additionally, this book covers polymeric hydrogels, an important class of synthetic polymers, and chitin, one of the most abundant marine materials with excellent potential in biomaterials.

Last but not least, the inclusion of regulatory issues will help readers understand the importance of ensuring the safety and efficacy of materials used in medical devices before they are launched commercially. Disruptive technologies like lasers have mass-produced intricate medical devices like coronary stents at a fraction of the cost.

This highlights the need to integrate other disciplines into the design of medical device materials. This new version will be a valuable addition to the library of biomaterials engineering for scientists, clinicians, and engineers.

Luke P. Lee
Harvard Medical School
Boston USA

Dietmar W. Hutmacher
Centre of Regenerative Medicine
Queensland Univ of Technology
Brisbane, Australia

Preface

The success of any implant or medical device depends very much on the biomaterial used. Synthetic materials (such as metals, polymers, ceramics, and composites) have made significant contributions to many established medical devices. The aim of this publication is to provide a basic fundamental understanding of the engineering and processing aspects of the biomaterials used in medical applications from surface modification to corrosion and regulation. Of paramount importance is the tripartite relationship between material properties, processing methods, and design. As the target audience covers a wide interdisciplinary field of professions ranging from engineers, scientists, clinicians, and technologists to graduate students, the content of each chapter is written with a detailed background so that the audience of another discipline will be able to understand it. For the more knowledgeable reader, a detailed list of references is included.

In 2004, I embarked on the book *Engineering Materials for Biomedical Applications.* More than 1000 copies were sold. "It was very well received" (World Scientific Publishing Co.). A reviewer said, "I borrowed this book from the library, but after reading the first 2 chapters I realized that it is a book that I should have at home. Everything is explained in a very simple way" (Reviewed in the United Kingdom on September 5, 2013).

This book *Designing Materials for Medical Devices: Fundamentals* is a revision of the book *Engineering Materials for Biomedical Applications* with the addition of two more chapters — one on regulatory affairs and another on lasers in medical devices.

Chapter 1 gives a broad overview of biomaterials engineering and processing. Here, the requirements of biomaterials and the effects, such as grain size, composite layering, and molding conditions, on mechanical properties are discussed. It also endeavors to give a fore-taste of the newly emerging field of tissue engineering and the challenges ahead.

Chapter 2 deals with the durability of common metallic implant materials such as stainless steel and titanium. The host-tissue response to metallic debris, the effect of micro motion that leads to fretting fatigue, and the forecast of metallic biomaterials are discussed here.

Chapter 3 deals with the fundamentals of metallic corrosion, giving the audience a strong basic understanding of the thermodynamics and kinetics aspects of corrosion. The main disadvantage of metallic implant materials is that they corrode. This is an important topic that many students without a chemistry background will have difficulty understanding. The case examples cited will help the audience appreciate how these principles are applied.

Chapter 4 talks about an important aspect of surface modification of metallic implants: It attempts to describe the interactions of cells and proteins on metallic surfaces. This is an interesting chapter that helps the reader develop a greater appreciation of the basic science of surface chemistry and the adhesion mechanics of cells and proteins.

Chapter 5 is a good application chapter on dental restorative bio-materials and the technology advancements in this field. Here, one can see how ceramics, metals, and polymers have all been used in the early trials of biomaterials.

Chapter 6 introduces a significant topic — bioceramics — which has been a subject of intense research in the biomaterials field. Not only the inert but also the bioresorbable types are important nowadays.

Chapter 7 describes the polymeric hydrogels that have now earned a place in many useful applications — ranging from contact lenses to control of drug release devices. The structure of polymers is an important topic, especially in the quest to engineer and use polymers as biomaterials.

Chapters 8 and 9 are on composites: The former is on polymer–bioceramic composites, especially those materials used as implants, while the latter describes the textile composite which has found some useful applications, such as in vascular grafts. The mathematics and mechanics are expanded so that should anyone wish to do any design work, they may find the references cited helpful.

Chapter 10 may seem out of place. But with the latest prosthetic materials and the new technologies that have gone into this traditional field, this chapter sheds new light on what materials engineers have accomplished in the field of prosthetics: lightweight and intelligent lower-limb prostheses. The use of computers has indeed revolutionized the way we design materials. The evolution of osteointegration and advanced bionics has made this topic extremely interesting, especially for handicapped patients.

Chapter 11 describes a natural biomaterial — chitin. Chitin is fast becoming a useful material not only in wound dressings but also in tissue engineering scaffolds because of its special cell mediation properties.

Chapter 12 introduces regulatory issues in safety and efficacy, and the need for all designers of medical devices to adhere to strict regulatory standards be it FDA 510K, CE mark, or just understanding ISO13485 and ISO 109963.

Chapter 13 on lasers in medicine is included to emphasize the role of enabling technology such as lasers in many fabrication processes including engraving, which has made many micro implant devices commercially possible.

It is hoped that all the chapters written by many distinguished experts will provide a good start to a better understanding of designing materials for medical devices.

S. H. Teoh
Emeritus Prof,
Nanyang Technological University, Singapore
Distinguished Professor and Director,
Center for Advanced Medical Engineering (CAME)
College of Materials Science and Engineering,
Hunan University
7 June 2024

About the Editor

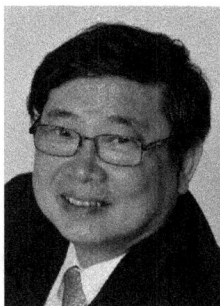

Teoh Swee Hin, Fellow of the Academy of Engineers Singapore, is Director and Distinguished Yuelu Chair Professor, Center for Advanced Medical Engineering (CAME), College of Materials Science and Engineering, Hunan University, China. He is also Emeritus Professor at Nanyang Technological University (NTU) and the recipient of the NTU President's Chair Award for his outstanding research and education leadership. He is well known for his excellence in teaching, research, and entrepreneurship. He is renowned for his contribution to the development, commercialization, and clinical translation of 3D bioresorbable scaffolds, due to which he received the prestigious "Golden Innovation Award" at the Far East Economic Review and the Institute of Engineers "Prestigious Engineering Achievement Award" in 2004. Majoring in Materials Engineering at Monash University, his research journey focused on translating materials research to biomedical benefits. To date, Osteopore International, his medical device company, has implanted medical devices in more than 120,000 patients globally. The company successfully achieved IPO status (ASX-Australia) in 2019. With more than 40 Ph.D.'s, 300 publications, and 22 patents, he is an excellent educator in the bioengineering field and a research scientist in translational regenerative medicine.

Acknowledgments

This book would not have come about without the dedication and active participation of all the authors who over time have become friends and collaborators. They are Adrian, U. J. Yap, Yu Na, B. Ben-Nissan, D. J. Blackwood, T. Hanawa, Z. M. Huang, E. Khor, J. Li, Peter, V. S. Lee, Hans A. Gray, G. Pezzotti, S. Ramakrishna, K. H. W. Seah, M. Sumita, M. Wang, Qilong Zhao, Jack Wong, Zhekun Chen, Xiaohan Xing, Yuchen Yang, and Minghui Hong. I thank them for their patience and for bearing with me.

To all my students at the College of Materials Science and Engineering, Hunan University, China; the Biomaterials Engineering and Advanced Biomaterials course, Mechanical Engineering Department, National University of Singapore; and the School of Chemical and Biomedical Engineering, the Renaissance Engineering Programme, and the School of Materials Science and Engineering, Nanyang Technological University, Singapore, over the last 25 years, it has been a joy to learn from your criticisms and the mistakes you have pointed out in my lectures. If not for your feedback, this revised book would not have been able to address your concerns. I thank you.

I want to thank two very old friends — Prof. Luke Lee, Harvard Medical School, USA, and Prof. Dietmar Hutmacher, Queensland University of Technology, Brisbane, Australia — for endorsing this book and writing the foreword. They have provided such encouragement in the midst of their very heavy schedules.

Last but the least is World Scientific Publishing (WSP), especially Prof. KK Phua, Founder of WSP, whom I have known since my days at the National University of Singapore (more than 20 years ago), and Ms. Joy Quek and Khoo YH, who endured my delayed response for a long time. Thank you for your patience and kind instructions while working on this second edition. I thank you for awarding me the Outstanding Publication Award for achieving sales of more than 1000 copies of the 1st edition.

Contents

Chapter 1

Introduction to Biomaterials Engineering

S. H. Teoh

*Center for Advanced Medical Engineering (CAME),
College of Materials Science and Engineering, Hunan University,
#2 South Lushan Road, Changsha 410082, China*
teohsh@hnu.edu.cn

The success of a material to be used as a biomaterial in medical devices, is related to biocompatibility, the ease of fabrication to form into complicated shapes and the sterilizability of the material used. This chapter provides an overview of biomaterials engineering, paying particular attention on the effect of processing methods on the mechanical properties of biomaterials. The effects of grain refinement in metals and ceramics, molding conditions on polymeric wear, and composite lamination are discussed. This is because the ability of a biomaterial to be formed into shape easily often determines its success as a medical device in the long run. When it comes to the manufacturability of a biomaterial, processing techniques will affect the final property of the biomaterial, which means affecting the durability of the device. On this note, engineers need to examine the various processing effects that stem from grain refinement of steel, surface modification to molding conditions and adoption of new manufacturing methods such as 3D printing technology. Future direction seems to lead us to nanolaminate composites, which give better properties such as fracture toughness and wear enhancement. The era of tissue engineering also paves the way for new biomaterial processes to be developed and invented. The integration of different modalities from cells, biomaterials to medical imaging has opened up new challenges in the healthcare industry.

1

1.1 Introduction

Biomaterials engineering is concerned with the application of biomaterials science in the design and engineering aspects of medical
device fabrication. Traditionally, the study of biomaterials focuses
on issues, such as biocompatibility, host-tissue reaction to implants,
cytotoxicity, and basic structure–property relationships [1–8]. These
issues are important. They provide a strong scientific basis for a clear
understanding of many successful medical devices such as the stent
and mechanical heart valve. However, in biomaterials engineering,
the manufacturing and processing aspects emerge as a primary concern. While it may be easy to make a one-off laboratory prototype,
it is extremely challenging to produce a thousand units of identical
devices with good quality control and consistent properties, packed
in a sterile manner for storage and easy transportation. Topics such
as fatigue, corrosion, and surface modification are some essential elements in engineering biomaterials for medical applications.

The stent (see, e.g., Figure 1.1) is the number one most successful
medical device. Sometimes, it is a wonder that near miracles can
spring from the simplest innovations. The stent's main aim is to keep
clogged arteries open. It is a laser-perforated metal tube no smaller
than a paper clip. It is inserted into arteries during angioplasty, in
which a balloon is threaded into a clogged artery. When inflated,
the balloon keeps the artery open. It is this stenting procedure that
saved the late Senior Minister Lee Kuan Yew on 16 March 1997
(Figure 1.2).

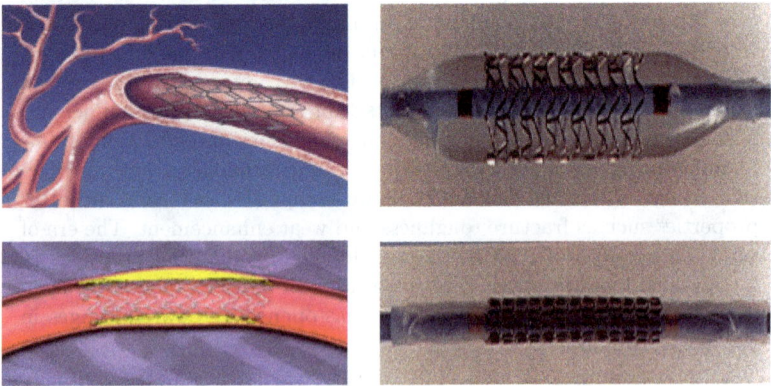

Figure 1.1. An example of a stainless steel stent in an artery.

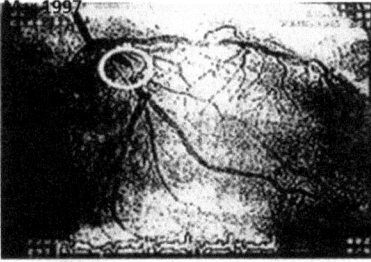

Before: X-ray angiogram showed obvious narrowing (circle) of the left circumflexed artery before stenting

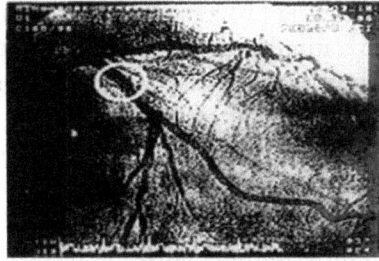

After: X-ray angiogram showed the restoration of flow at the left circumflexed artery after stenting procedure

Figure 1.2. Angiogram of the X-ray before and after stenting of the late Senior Minister Lee Kuan Yew on 16 March 1997.

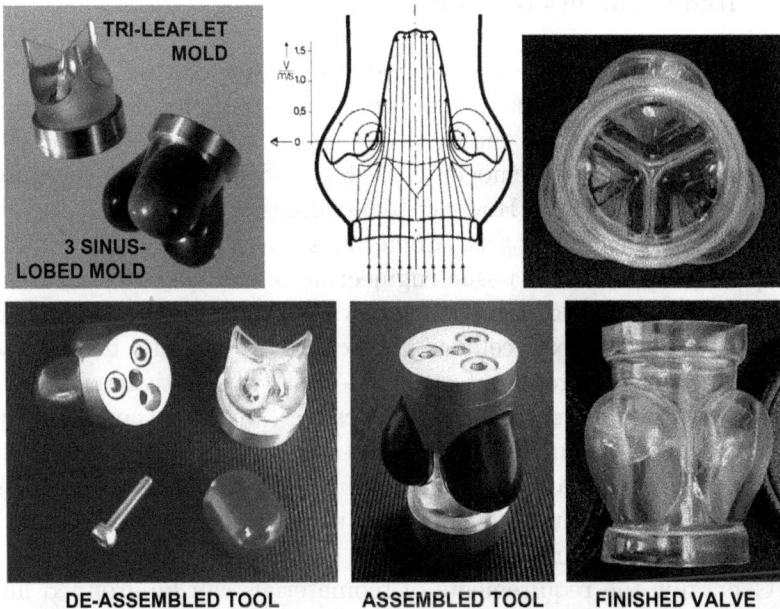

DE-ASSEMBLED TOOL   ASSEMBLED TOOL   FINISHED VALVE

Figure 1.3. Manufacturing steps in making a tri-leaflet polyurethane valve. Note the complex die assembly needed to produce a seamless polyurethane valve by thermoforming.

The intricate engineering design involving complex processing can be illustrated in the manufacture of the polymeric tri-leaflet valve. Figure 1.3 shows the intricate engineering mold design involved in the formation of a polyurethane (PU) tri-leaflet valve using a thermoforming process. The tri-leaflet heart valve is an interesting design which mimics the natural aortic valve with a central flow. First, a biocompatible PU sheet is thermoformed over the leaflet mold to yield the three-leaflet shape with a central flow. Next, the outer three sinus lobes need to be formed over the leaflet. The valve must be made without any parting lines which are often seen in two-part injection molds. The parting lines can be detrimental as they are lines of weakness and are subject to thrombus formation. An engineer developed a three-part mold that allows the PU sheet to be thermoformed over the assembled tool. The latter consists of three detachable lobes which can be unscrewed after the three-sinus-lobe mold is set.

1.2　Requirements of Biomaterials

Biomaterials must have special properties that can be tailored to meet the needs of a particular application — this is an important concept to bear in mind. For example, a biomaterial must be biocompatible, non-carcinogenic, corrosion-resistant, and have low toxicity and wear [1,2]. However, depending on the application, differing requirements may arise. Sometimes, these requirements can be completely opposite. In tissue engineering of the bone, for instance, the polymeric scaffold needs to be biodegradable so that as the cells generate their own extracellular matrices; the polymeric biomaterial will be completely replaced over time with the patient's own tissue. In the case of mechanical heart valves, on the other hand, we need materials that are biostable, wear-resistant, do not degrade with time, and are resistant to calcification. Materials such as pyrolytic carbon leaflet and titanium housing are used because they can last at least 20 years or more.

Generally, the requirements of biomaterials can be grouped into four broad categories:

1. **Biocompatibility:** The material must not disturb or induce unwelcoming response from the host, but rather promote harmony and good tissue-implant integration. An initial burst of inflammatory response is expected and is sometimes considered essential in the healing process. However, prolonged inflammation is not desirable as it may indicate tissue necrosis or incompatibility.

2. **Sterilizability:** The material must be able to undergo sterilization. Sterilization techniques include gamma, gas (ethylene oxide (ETO)) and steam autoclaving. Some polymers such as polyacetal will depolymerize and give off the toxic gas formaldehyde when subjected to high energy radiation by gamma. These polymers are thus best sterilized by ETO.

3. **Functionality:** The functionality of a medical device depends on the ability of the material to be shaped to suit a particular function. The material must therefore allow itself to be shaped economically using engineering fabrication processes. The success of the coronary artery stent — which has been considered the most widely used medical device — can be attributed to the efficient fabrication process of stainless steel from heat treatment to cold working to improve its durability.

4. **Manufacturability:** It is often said that there are many candidate materials that are biocompatible. However, it is often the last step, the manufacturability of the material, that hinders the actual production of the medical device. It is in this last step that engineers can contribute significantly.

1.3 Classification of Biomaterials

Biomaterials can broadly be classified as follows: (i) biological biomaterials; (ii) synthetic biomaterials. Table 1.1 shows the various classifications and some examples. Biological materials [3, 4] can be further classified into soft and hard tissue types. In the case of synthetic materials, it is further classified into the following: (a) metallic; (b) polymeric; (c) ceramic; (d) composite biomaterials.

1.4 Mechanical Properties of Biomaterials

The mechanical properties of a biomaterial can best be described by its modulus of elasticity, ultimate tensile strength, elongation to failure, and fracture toughness. These properties are often used for early screening of candidate materials for medical devices to match the tissue that will be replaced.

- Modulus of elasticity denotes the stiffness of the material and is usually obtained from the slope of a stress–strain diagram.

Table 1.1.   Classification of biomaterials.

I. Biological Materials	II. Synthetic Biomedical Materials

1. Soft Tissue
   Skin, Tendon,
   Pericardium, Cornea
	1. Polymeric
	   Ultra-High Molecular Weight
	   Polyethylene (UHMWPE),
	   Polymethylmethacrylate (PMMA),
	   Polyethyletherketone (PEEK),
	   Silicone, Polyurethane (PU),
	   Polytetrafluoroethylene (PTFE)

2. Hard Tissue
   Bone, Dentine, Cuticle
	2. Metallic
	   Stainless Steel, Cobalt-based Alloy
	   (Co–Cr–Mo), Titanium Alloy
	   (Ti–Al–V), Gold, Platinum
	3. Ceramic
	   Alumina (Al_2O_3), Zirconia (ZrO_2),
	   Carbon, Hydroxylapatite
	   [$Ca_{10}(PO_4)_6(OH)_2$], Tricalcium
	   Phosphate [$Ca_3(PO_4)_2$], Bioglass
	   [$Na_2O(CaO)(P_2O_3)(SiO_2)$], Calcium
	   Aluminate [$Ca(Al_2O_4)$]
	4. Composite
	   Carbon Fiber (CF)/PEEK,
	   CF/UHMWPE, CF/PMMA,
	   Zirconia/Silica/BIS–GMA

- Ultimate tensile strength denotes the ability of the material to withstand a load before it fails.
- Elongation to failure denotes how much strain the material can bear before it fails.
- Fracture toughness is an important measurement of the material's resistance to crack propagation.

The basic understanding of mechanical properties begins with the study of the mechanics of materials.

1.4.1   *Mechanics of Materials*

Mechanics refers to the study of the deformation of objects under forces. When a force is applied on a material, it is referred to as a "load". Such loads may be applied perpendicularly (often referred to as "normal") to a surface. Such normal loads may be acting to

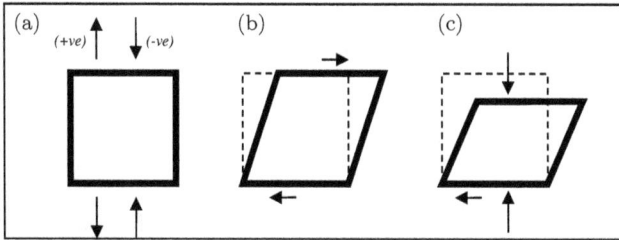

Figure 1.4. Schematic diagram to demonstrate (a) normal forces (b) shear force (c) compressive and shear force acting on a body.

compress ("compressive loads") or stretch ("tensile loads"). Force is a vector quantity, these forces are assigned directions. Accordingly, tensile forces are typically assigned positive values, and compressive forces are negative. Forces may also be applied in a direction parallel to a surface, whereby it is referred to as a "shear" force. A typical example of this is friction. In real situations, objects are likely to be subject to a combination of both. These are summarized in Figure 1.4. Typically, however, forces rarely act on a single point and are usually distributed over an area. Pressure is the measure of force per unit area applied on a surface. Similarly, in mechanics, stress is a measure of force per unit area acting on the surface of the object or on a plane within the object. As with forces, stresses are vector quantities and include normal and shear stresses.

1.4.2 *Stress-strain Behavior of Materials*

The characterization of the mechanical properties of materials is often done by performing a uniaxial tensile test where the stress (load/area) is plotted on the y-axis and the strain (extension/gauge length) on the x-axis, as shown in Figure 1.5. The slope of the stress–strain curve is the modulus of elasticity, the maximum load at failure is called the ultimate tensile stress and the elongation to failure is the maximum strain at failure. The behavior of materials can be brittle, ductile, or rubbery. Polymeric materials are viscoelastic, i.e., the deformation behavior is dependent on stress, temperature, and strain rate, and the last two parameters are inversely related. A decrease in temperature can be equivalent to an increase in the strain rate of testing.

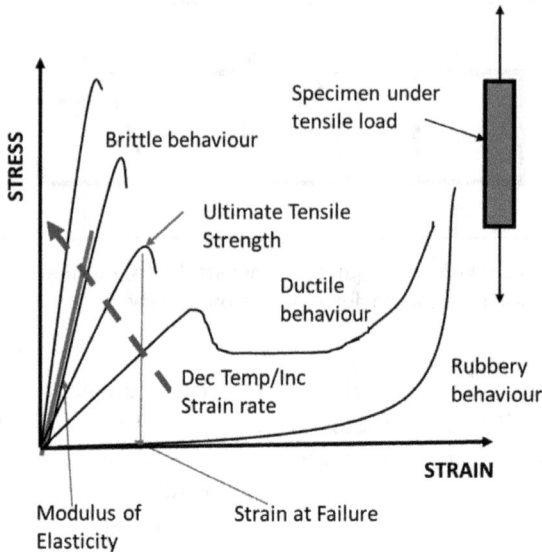

Figure 1.5. Stress–strain schematic of a uniaxial stretched material showing brittle, ductile and rubbery behavior.

1.4.3 *Fracture Toughness*

When materials are under tensile load, they will first elongate, as seen in Figure 1.6. As the load is increased, the object will continue stretching to a point at which it breaks. On an atomic scale, the breaking point can be visualized as the point at which all the forces holding the object intact on that plane are simultaneously broken, resulting in separation into two bodies, or "fracture". Thus, in a perfect object, the theoretical strength of a material should correspond to the sum of all atomic bonds within the plane of fracture. In real life, however, materials typically fail at conditions below this value. This is because of the presence of cracks on the surface.

The presence of pre-existing cracks results in alterations in the stress distribution and concentrates stresses at the crack tip. The crack will then progress and extend (crack propagation), leading ultimately to failure. It was deduced experimentally that the tensile strength varies inversely with the square root of the crack size, i.e., $\sigma_f \sqrt{a} = C$, where σ_f refers to the tensile strength and "a" refers to the crack size. This is commonly referred to as the Griffith Criterion. C is a constant, which may be theoretically derived from mechanical

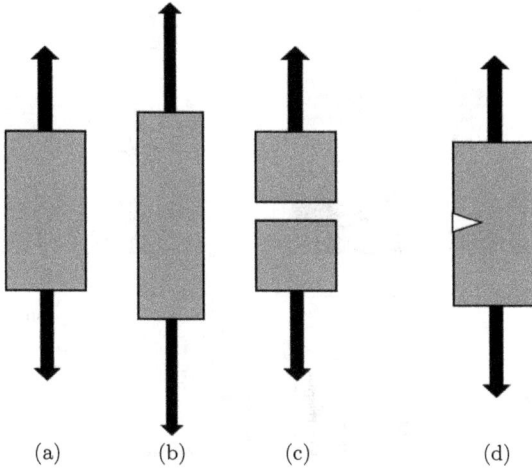

(a)　　　(b)　　　(c)　　　(d)

Figure 1.6. A body under tension (a) will elongate under tensile stress (b) and eventually fracture (c). All materials have surface cracks which weaken the material.

properties, such as stiffness and free surface energy. The Griffith criterion can also be rearranged to $a = \left(\frac{C}{\sigma_f}\right)^2$, which now suggests that for a fixed value of applied stress, there will exist a critical size for cracks, beyond which the material will fail under this load. Hence, this can be used as a design criterion in which existing cracks in the material cannot exceed this critical size.

To facilitate material selection and design, the parameter "fracture toughness" (denoted by K_{IC}), related to the constant C in Griffith's relation, has been developed. K_{IC} is a material property indicative of the ability of a material containing a crack to resist fractures and may be obtained from materials handbooks or data sheets. The fracture toughness is also often expressed as $K_{IC} = Y\sigma_f\sqrt{(\pi a)}$, where Y is a geometric factor. A material with K_{IC} less than $1\,\text{MPa}\sqrt{\text{m}}$ such as ceramic is considered brittle, while that above $100\,\text{MPa}\sqrt{\text{m}}$ such as steel is considered ductile and tough.

1.4.4 *Comparison of Mechanical Properties of Biomaterials*

Figures 1.7(a)–(d) show the comparisons among different classes of biomaterials with respect to the four properties mentioned above. It

(a) Modulus of Elasticity (GPa): Al₂O₃ 414, Co-Cr-Mo 234, Stainless Steel 193, Ti-Al-V 117, Ti 97, Hydroxyapatite, C-Si 62, Bone 21, Tri-Calcium Phosphate 21, Polymers 7, Soft Tissues 3, 0

(b) Ultimate Strength (MPa): Co-Cr-Mo (forged) 1241, Ti-Al-V 1172, Stainless Steel 1000, Co-Cr-Mo (cast) 620, C-Si 889, Hydroxyapatite 889, Titanium 483, Al₂O₃ 448, Bone 138, Polymers 69, Tri-Calcium Phosphate 21, Soft Tissues 7

(c) ELONGATION (%): Polymers 300, Soft Tissues 40, Titanium 40, Stainless Steel 40, Co-Cr-Mo (forged) 12, Ti-Al-V 10, Bone 1, Al₂-β₃ <0.2, C-Si <0.1, Hydroxyapatite <0.1, Tri-Calcium Phosphate <0.1

(d) Fracture Toughness [MPa√m] vs Relative Modulus (Bone = 1) Log scale — METALS: Stainless Steel, Cobalt Chrome, Ti; POLYMERS: PE, Bone; CERAMICS: Alumina

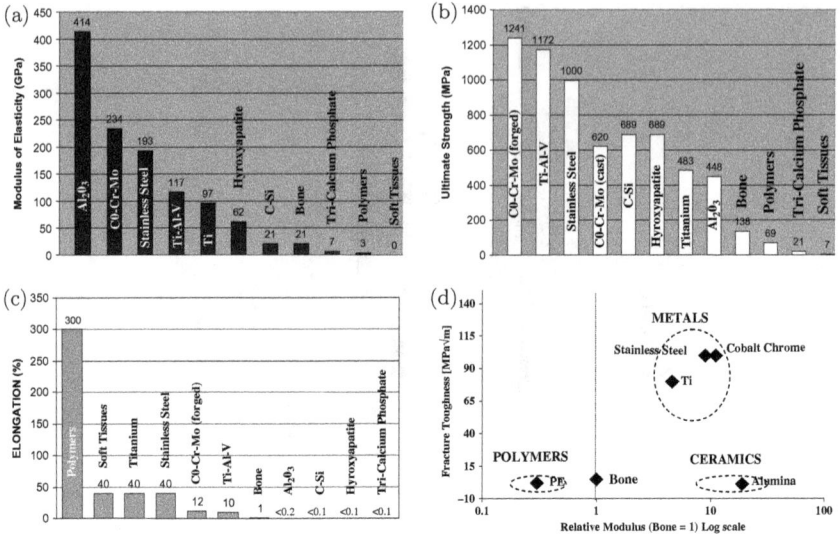

Figure 1.7. (a) Comparison of moduli of elasticity of biomaterials. Note the very high values for ceramics and metals. (b) Comparison of ultimate tensile strengths of biomaterials. Note the exceptionally high values for metals which make them the ideal choice for load-bearing applications. (c) Comparison of elongation at failure of biomaterials. Note that polymers have exceptional elongation as compared to other materials. This is a measure of their high ductility. (d) Comparison of fracture toughness of biomaterials relative to the log (Young's modulus) with bone as the reference. Note that the fracture toughness values of metals are generally several orders of magnitude higher than those of the other materials. Young's modulus is also much higher than that of bone, giving rise to stress shielding (PE = Polyethylene; Ti = Titanium).

can be seen that metals are generally very stiff and have high fracture toughness. In sharp contrast to the metals are the polymers, which have low stiffness and fracture toughness. However, the polymers have a high elongation to failure. The high stiffness of metals, on the other hand, can be a disadvantage since this can give rise to "stress shielding" in bone fracture repair. Stress shielding is a phenomenon where bone loss occurs when a stiffer material is placed over the bone. Bone responds to stresses during the healing process. Since the stress is practically shielded from the bone, the density of the bone underneath the stiffer material decreases as a result. Ceramics are very hard, with high elastic modulus, but are very brittle. Our bone consists primarily of hydroxyapatite and, although functionally osteoconductive, it is a brittle material. This is one reason why most ceramics are used as a coating for metallic medical devices.

1.5 Effects of Processing on Properties of Biomaterials

1.5.1 *Effect of Post-Processing and Grain Size*

Numerous properties of biomaterials can be improved by processing techniques. Figure 1.7 shows the fatigue strengths of some commonly used metals. It can be seen that the fatigue strengths of forged 316L stainless steel and cobalt-chromium are significantly higher than in their cast state. The increase in fatigue strength can be attributed to the large compressive force applied on the surface of the metal during the forging process as well as to grain refinement. How grain refinement leads to an increase in fatigue strength can be understood from the Hall–Petch equation. The equation states that the yield strength of a material (σ_{yd}) is inversely proportional to the square root of the grain size (d):

$$\sigma_{yd} = k/\sqrt{d}, \tag{1.1}$$

where k is a constant.

For many years in the steel industry, the subject of grain refinement has been intensely pursued to help improve the yield strength of steel. Nanograin structures have been produced via severe plastic deformation with remarkable success [9]. The other common route is to use powder metallurgy where ultra-fine particles are consolidated, compacted, and sintered at elevated temperatures. Figure 1.8 shows that after the cobalt-chromium alloy is subjected to hot isostatic pressing (H.I.P.), its fatigue strength is almost double that in the cast state [10]. The use of isostatic pressure also helps to reduce defects — such as voids — in the alloy.

Fast fracture occurs when the fracture toughness becomes larger than the critical fracture toughness, K_{IC}. Fracture strength, σ_S, can then be given by

$$\sigma_S = K_{\mathrm{IC}}/\{Y\sigma\sqrt{a}\}. \tag{1.2}$$

Composite processing by combining two or more phases is one method to produce enhanced properties of biomaterials. Another

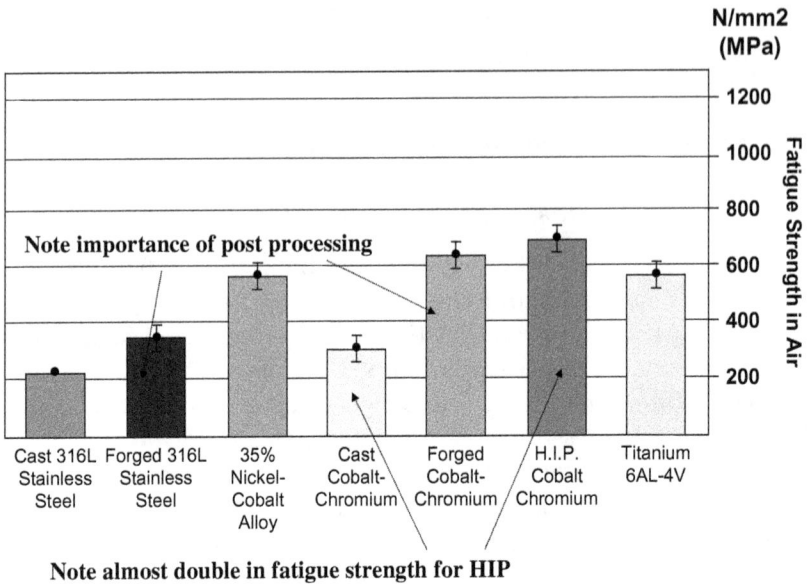

Figure 1.8. Fatigue strengths (in air) of common alloys used as implants. Note the effect of post-processing conditions to improve fatigue strength (after Teoh [12]).

approach to obtain improved strength and reliability is to refine ceramic processing to produce homogeneous components with a defect size as small as possible. This can be done by refining powder processing to eliminate microstructural flaws. Ceramics such as alumina have been used for femoral heads in total hip replacements (THR) as an alternative to metal. This is because the wear rate in a ceramic–polyethylene combination was shown to be reduced significantly. However, reports of *in vivo* brittle fractures of ceramics due to delayed slow crack growth brought about a new development in using composites of alumina and zirconia. The influence of processing conditions (such as those in colloidal processing) on the microstructure development of zirconia-toughened alumina composites and the effect of these microstructures on the mechanical properties of alumina–zirconia composites are discussed by De Aza *et al.* [11]. They have demonstrated that, by using colloidal processing, microstructure refinement has brought about a significant improvement in the fracture toughness of ceramics (see Table 1.2).

Table 1.2. Fracture threshold, toughness and hardness of alumina, zirconia, and alumina–zirconia composites (after De Aza *et al.* [11]).

Ceramic	Fracture Threshold, K_{I0} (MPa$\sqrt{m}$)	Fracture Toughness, K_{IC} (MPa$\sqrt{m}$)	Hardness (Vickers)
Alumina (Al_2O_3)	2.5 ± 0.2	4.2 ± 0.2	$1,600 \pm 50$
Zirconia (ZrO_2)	3.1 ± 0.2	5.5 ± 0.2	$1,290 \pm 50$
Al_2O_3–10vol%ZrO_2	4.0 ± 0.2	5.9 ± 0.2	$1,530 \pm 50$

1.5.2 *Effect of Molding Conditions and Irradiation on Polymeric Wear*

The wear of polymeric materials used in implants is perhaps the most difficult to understand [7]. As a result, numerous reports on polymeric wear have emerged over the years [12, 13]. In biomedical applications such as occluders in mechanical heart valves and joint prostheses, fatigue fracture and wear of the polymers have been considered to be important factors in determining the durability of the prostheses. In the case of UHMWPE, many factors influence its wear properties. For example, when UHMWPE was molded between 190°C and 200°C and some antioxidants were added during processing, its wear resistance appeared to improve. Molding at higher pressures and increasing the molecular weight, on the other hand, were reported to be detrimental. Nonetheless, there is a possibility that there could be an optimum processing condition and molecular weight distribution that could give the best wear characteristics. More recent work has shown that processing conditions play a vital role in the cyclic fatigue of UHMWPE. In particular, γ-radiation and oxidative aging are very detrimental to the fatigue threshold and crack propagation resistance (Table 1.3). Moreover, compression molding appears to render a better fatigue resistance when compared to extrusion.

1.5.3 *Effect of Composite Lamination*

Nanolaminates layer of interpenetrating-networked composites such as those found in nature have unique fracture resistance. Examples are seashells, which have been shown to yield improved fracture resistance with unique wear characteristics [15] (see Figure 1.9).

Table 1.3. Effect of processing conditions on the fatigue threshold (ΔKth) of UHMWPE (after Pruiit and Bailey [14]).

Condition	ΔKth
Compression-molded	1.8
Compression-molded γ-air	1.2
Extruded 90°	1.7
Extruded 0° non-sterilized	1.3
Extruded 0° γ-air	1.0
Extruded 0° γ-peroxide	1.1

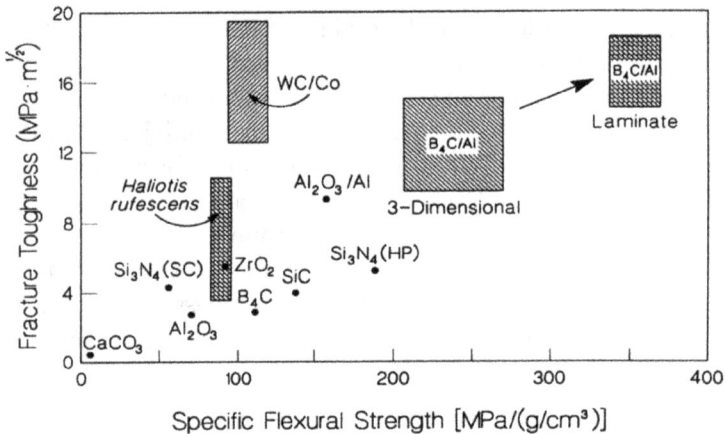

Figure 1.9. Fracture toughness versus specific flexural strength of some bioceramics and nanolaminates of metal matrix-ceramics composites. Note the effect of laminates in improving both fracture toughness and flexural strength (after Saikaya and Aksay [15]; reprinted with permission from Springer–Verlag, Berlin).

The microstructure is made of a nanobrick-type arrangement of a ceramic phase sandwiched by ultra-thin polymeric protein layers. Presumably, the small brick-like ceramic components (often biodegradable) allow easy removal/dissolution, a concept that needs to be mimicked in engineering a biomaterial with wear debris, which is eco-compatible. By using the laminate concept, fracture toughness reaching values as high as $16\,\text{MPa}\sqrt{\text{m}}$ can be achieved — as in the case of boron carbide/aluminum laminates. These laminates

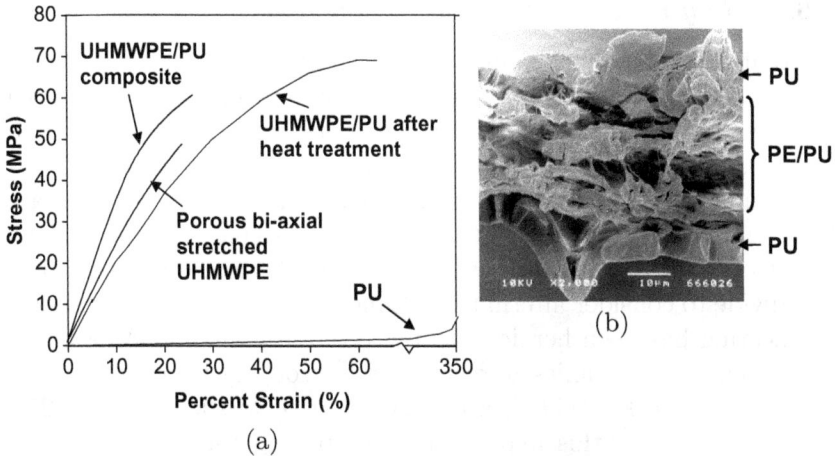

Figure 1.10. (a) Bi-axial stretching of UHMWPE and infiltrating with elastomeric polyurethane (PU) to produce microlaminates with significantly improved mechanical properties; (b) cross-sectional view of internal microstructure (after Teoh *et al.* [16]).

also have high flexural strength. Microlaminates of interpenetrating-networked composites (Figure 1.10) can be produced by bi-axial stretching of one crystalline phase (UHMWPE) or by infiltrating with elastomeric polyurethane (PU) [16]. These microlaminates show significant improvement in strength and fracture toughness, and are used for elastomeric composite membranes (less than $40\,\mu$m) in biomedical applications.

1.6 Tissue Engineering — New Wave in Biomaterials Engineering

1.6.1 *Need for Organ and Tissue Replacement*

Loss of human tissues or organs is a devastating problem for the individual patient. Each year in United States alone, it is estimated that organs failure and tissue loss cost an estimated US$400b. Incidentally, patients waiting for organ transplants are also on the rise. Moreover, as life span increases in developed countries, coupled with rising number of calamities ranging from earthquakes to diseases outbreak and war tragedies, the need for organ and tissue replacement is expected to reach astronomical numbers.

1.6.2 *Limitation of Current Technologies*

Current technology for organ and tissue replacement has limitations. These include donor scarcity, adverse immunological response from the host tissue, biocompatibility, infection, pathogen transfer, and high cost to patient. Then, there is the perennial deficiency of synthetic material to provide the multifunctional requirement of organ. For example, bone is not just a structural element but also a "factory to produce bone marrow". These limitations prompt scientists worldwide to consider alternative technologies, amongst which tissue engineering has been heralded as the promising answer. As a result more than 20 companies were founded, according to an 1998 issue in Business Week ("The Era of Regenerative Medicine", July 27). However, recently, this hype soon met up with the reality of business enterprises when a number of them had to close, merge, or be bought up by large conglomerates. Nevertheless, new technologies and processes need to be discovered and invented.

1.6.3 *Platform Technology Development in Tissue Engineering*

The aim of tissue engineering (TE) is to restore tissue and organ functions with minimal host rejection. This arose from the need to develop an alternative method of treating patients suffering from tissue loss or organ failure. TE has been heralded as the new wave to revolutionize the healthcare-biotechnology industry. It is a multidisciplinary field and involves the integration of engineering principles, basic life sciences, and molecular cell biology.

The success of tissue engineering lies in five key technologies (Figure 1.11). They are namely: (1) Biomaterials; (2) Cells; (3) Scaffolds; (4) Bioreactors; and (5) Medical Imaging technology. It may seem simple to produce a one-off, tissue-engineered product in the laboratory, but it is a completely different matter to produce hundreds of products of consistent quality for clinical use.

TE involves a scaffold which acts as a temporary extracellular matrix for the cells to adhere to, differentiate, and grow. Breakthrough has been made in the development of a platform technology which integrates medical imaging, computational mechanics, biomaterials, and advanced manufacturing to produce three-dimensional,

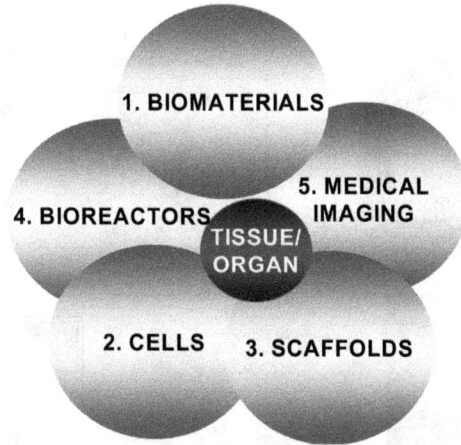

Figure 1.11. Five core technologies (biomaterials, cells, scaffolds, bioreactors, and medical imaging) required for tissue engineering.

porous load bearing scaffolds for tissue engineering of bone [17, 18]. The technology makes use of polycaprolactone (PCL) bioresorbable polymer and Fused Deposition Modeling (FDM) rapid prototyping advanced manufacturing fabrication process to produce the scaffolds without a mold [19] (Figure 1.12). Controlled three-dimensional architecture with interconnected pores enables good cells entrapment, facilitates easy flow path for nutrients and waste removal, and demonstrates long-term cell viability. Patient-specific scaffolds can now be made using this technology. More than 100,000 scaffolds made by 3D printing PCL have been used globally (Osteopore Intl Pte Ltd). This biomaterial processing technology has paved the way for patient-specific tissue engineering concepts not dreamed of a few years ago.

1.6.4 *Tissue Engineering Issues and Challenges*

In tissue engineering, there are certainly issues and challenges which are yet to be resolved. These issues range from cell-biomaterial interactions, stem cells technology to know-how in scaffolds manufacturing. For example, in the case of cell-biomaterial interactions, though we can grow single cell sheets such as cartilage, we hardly understand how the cells in composite tissues (such as the heart valve leaflets) recognize their own territories and hence do not cross and violate

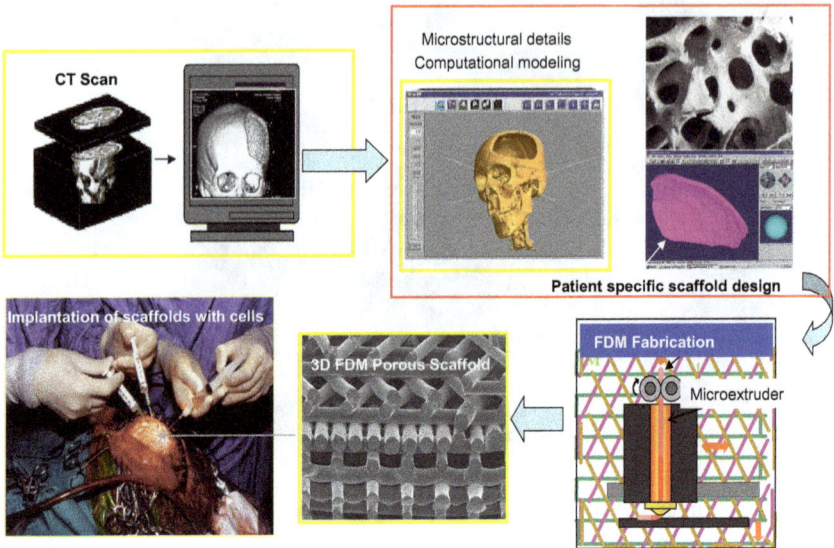

Figure 1.12. Platform technology for patient-specific scaffolds for bone tissue engineering.

each other. They seem to know how to live in harmony. Although we no longer need to focus on biochemical effects such as growth factors, we need to study the mechano-induction effects. This is because the manner in which cells differentiate, proliferate, and express their extracellular matrix (ECM) is also a function of the stress fields they experience.

Stem cells and scaffolds technologies also pose some challenges. Some work on human blood vessels was done by Auger's group [20] in Canada. They showed that by growing the cells in sheets and then rolling them into a tube helps to eliminate immunological mismatch. This is because smooth muscles cells (SMCs) re-expressed desmin, a differentiation marker known to be lost under culture conditions. As a result, large amounts of ECM were produced and the structural integrity maintained. However, the handling of the sheets is delicate and it is not clear if the material would survive the viscoelastic compliance mismatch in long-term *in vivo* physiological environment. Other major obstacles exist. One of them is over SMCs proliferation. This could be related to the presence of endothelial progenitor cells

(EPCs) in inhibiting SMCs, and EPCs are known to express nitric oxide. However, dipyridalmole is also a strong inhibitor of SMCs, and much work has been done to immobilize this chemical on porous scaffolds.

Okano's group [21] in Japan developed an interesting cell sheets technology where cells grew on culture surfaces grafted with temperature-responsive polymer, poly(N−isopropylacrylamide) (PIPAAm). By reducing temperature (instead of using enzymatic treatment which traumatizes cells), confluent cells simply detached from the polymer as a cell sheet. Layered cell sheets of cardiomyocytes then began to pulse simultaneously and morphological communication via connexin 43 was established between the sheets. When sheets were layered, engineered constructs were macroscopically observed to pulse spontaneously too.

The examples quoted above point to the fact that tissue engineering breakthroughs will further gravitate towards even greater challenges ahead.

1.7   Conclusions

For a material to be used as a biomaterial, and eventually, as a successful medical device, it must possess the mandatory properties of biocompatibility and sterilizability. In addition, a biomaterial must be manufacturable with ease to produce many products so that the cost is reasonable and affordable. Scalability in production should be considered early in the design process. This is because the ability of a biomaterial to be formed into shape easily often determines its success as a medical device in the long run. When it comes to the manufacturability of a biomaterial, processing techniques will affect the final property of the biomaterial, thus affecting the durability of the device. On this note, engineers need to examine the various processing effects that stem from grain refinement of steel, surface modification to molding conditions, and the adoption of new manufacturing methods, such as 3D printing technology. Future direction seems to lead us to nanolaminate composites, which give better properties such as fracture toughness and wear enhancement. The era of tissue engineering also paves the way for new biomaterial processes

S. H. Teoh

to be developed and invented. The integration of different modalities from cells, biomaterials to medical imaging has opened up new challenges in the healthcare industry [22].

References

[1] B. D. Ratner, A. S. Hoffman, F. J. Schoen, and J. E. Lemons (eds.), *Biomaterials Science: An Introduction to Materials in Medicine* (Elsevier Sci., New York, 1996).

[2] J. B. Park and R. S. Lakes, *Biomaterials — An introduction*, 2nd Edition (Plenum Press, New York, 1992).

[3] K. C. Dec, D. A. Puleo, and R. Bigirs (eds.), *An Introduction to Tissue-Biomaterial Interactions* (John Wiley & Sons, NY, 2002).

[4] J. Black, *Biological Performance of Materials*, 2nd Edition (Marcel & Dekker, New York, 1992).

[5] D. Hill, *Design Engineering of Biomaterials for Medical Devices* (John Wiley & Sons, New York, 1998).

[6] R. S. Greco, *Implantation Biology: The Host Response and Biomedical Devices* (CRC Press, London, 1994).

[7] K. R. St. John (ed.), *Particulate Debris from Medical Implants* (American Society of Testing and Materials, Philadelphia, USA, 1992) ASTM STP1144.

[8] R. D. Jamison and L. N. Gilbertson (eds.), *Composite Materials for Implant Applications in the Human Body* (American Society of Testing and Materials, Philadelphia, USA, 1993) ASTM STP1178.

[9] N. Tsuji, Y. Saito, S. H. Lee, and Y. Minamino, ARB (accumulative roll-bonding) and other new techniques to produce bulk ultra-fine grained materials, *Adv. Eng. Mat.*, 2003, 5:338–344.

[10] H. A. Luckey and L. J. Barnard, Improved properties of Co–Cr–Mo alloy by hot isostatic pressing of powder, in *Mechanical Properties of Biomaterials*, eds. G. W. Hastings and D. F. Williams, (John Wiley & Sons, 1980) Ch. 24.

[11] A. H. De Aza, J. Chevalier, G. Fantozzi, M. Schehl, and R. Torrecillas, Crack growth resistance of alumina, zirconia and zirconia toughened alumina ceramics for joint prostheses, *Biomaterials*, 2002, 23: 937–945.

[12] S. H. Teoh, Fatigue of biomaterials: A review, *Int. J. Fatigue*, (Special Issue on Biomaterials, 2000) 22:825–837.

[13] S. H. Teoh, Failure in biomaterials, in *Comprehensive Structural Integrity Series*, Vol. 9, eds. Y. W. Mai and S. H. Teoh, (Elsevier, London, UK, 2003) Ch. 1.

[14] L. Pruitt and L. Bailey, Factors affecting near-threshold fatigue crack propagation behavior of orthopedic grade ultra high molecular weight polyethylene, *Polymer*, 1998, 39:1545–1553.

[15] M. Saikaya and I. A. Aksay, Nacre of abalone shell: A natural multifunctional nanolaminate ceramic-polymer composite material, in *Structure, Cellular Synthesis and Assembly of Biopolymers*, ed. S. T. Case, (Springer–Verlag, Berlin 1992), Ch. 1, Fig. 1.

[16] S. H. Teoh, Z. G. Tang, and S Ramakrishna, Development of thin composite membranes for biomedical applications, *J. Mat Sci.: Mat Med.*, 1999, 10:343–352.

[17] S. H. Teoh, Tissue engineering challenges and issues — The Asian perspective, *Tissue Eng.*, 2003, 9(Sup 1):S1–S3.

[18] D. W. Hutmacher, J. T. Schantz, I. Zein, K. W. Ng, S. H. Teoh, and K. C. Tan, Mechanical properties and cell cultural response of polycaprolactone scaffolds designed and fabricated via fused deposition modeling, *J. Biomed. Mat. Res.*, 2001, 55:203–216.

[19] I. Zein, D. W. Hutmacher, K. C. Tan, and S. H. Teoh, Fused deposition modeling of novel scaffold architectures for tissue engineering applications, *Biomaterials*, 2002, 23:1169–1185.

[20] N. L'Heureux, S. Paquet, R. Labbe, L. Germain, and F. A. Auger, A completely biological tissue-engineered human blood vessel, *FASEB J.*, 1998, 12:47–56.

[21] T. Shimizu, M. Yamato, Y. Isoi, T. Akutsu, T. Setomaru, K. Abe, A. Kikuchi, M. Umezu, and T. Okano, Fabrication of pulsatile cardiac tissue grafts using a novel 3-dimensional cell sheet manipulation technique and temperature-responsive cell culture surfaces, *Circ. Res.*, 2002, 90:E40–E48.

[22] R. Lanza, R. Langer J. P. Vacanti and A. Atala, *Principles of Tissue Engineering* (Elsevier Science Publishing Co Inc, US, 2020).

Chapter 2

Durability of Metallic Implant Materials

M. Sumita[*,‡] and **S. H. Teoh**[†,§]

Biomaterials Center, National Institute for Materials Science,
1-2-1, Sengen, Tsukuba, Ibaraki, 305-0032, Japan
† *Center for Advanced Medical Engineering (CAME)*
College of Materials Science and Engineering, Hunan University,
#2 South Lushan Road, Changsha 410082, China
‡ *sumita.masae@nims.go.jp*
§ *teohsh@hnu.edu.cn*

Metallic implant materials such as stainless steel, titanium, and cobalt-based alloys have found many applications as medical devices. This is due to their excellent mechanical properties, such as fatigue strength and fracture toughness. Their durability however is dependent on their corrosion and wear resistance. The heat treatment and manufacturing method also affect these properties. The issues of adverse cellular response to wear debris from fretting fatigue and contact motion in artificial joints continue to present many challenges to the design of medical implants. The leaching of metallic ions such as nickel during the corrosion process has caused considerable concerns. This has paved way to the development of new nickel-free alloys and amorphous metals that are more biocompatible.

2.1 Introduction

Metallic materials are often used to replace musculoskeletal components of the human body because they surpass plastic or ceramic

23

materials in terms of tensile strength, fatigue strength, and fracture toughness. As such, they are used in medical devices, such as artificial joints, dental implants, housing for artificial hearts, bone plates, staples, wires, and stents. They also possess better electro conductivity qualities and hence are used for enclosing electronic devices, such as pacemaker electrodes and artificial inner ears. Figure 2.1(a) shows typical applications of metallic implant devices, and Figure 2.1(b) shows a stainless-steel stent used successfully in a coronary artery.

It was in Egypt and Phoenicia that teeth were tied with golden wires as a form of treatment [1]. Golden wires in prosthodontics were used in Egypt 2500 years ago. In Etruria, golden bridges and partial dentures were in use around 700 BC. It was during the ancient Greek period that metals were used in orthopedic procedures for the first time. Hippocrates (460–377 BC), who is known as the Father of Medicine, is believed to have used golden wires to treat fractures. Records of employing gold, iron, and bronze to suture lacerations in the 17th century were found. As iron and bronze corrode more easily than gold, they have been difficult to verify when they were first used as biomedical materials. The gold and unalloyed metals used then were weak and could not therefore be used for load-bearing applications. The unalloyed metals also corroded easily and did not promote osteointegration. They were also not wear-resistant.

2.2   Typical Metallic Biomaterials

With the advent of the Iron Age and industrial revolution, steel materials were used in the 19th century as bone plates and screws to fix fractures. Fixing fractures with screws allowed a stronger fixity than the earlier method of fixing with metallic wires. Steel made from nickel-plating steel and vanadium steel later replaced carbon steel materials as steel corrodes easily in the human body. However, these newer materials were not sufficiently corrosion-resistant. It also became clear that they become toxic inside the human body. Consequently, stainless steels, cobalt–chromium–molybdenum alloys (Vitallium), titanium, and titanium alloys gradually become the main biomedical materials used presently in orthopedic applications.

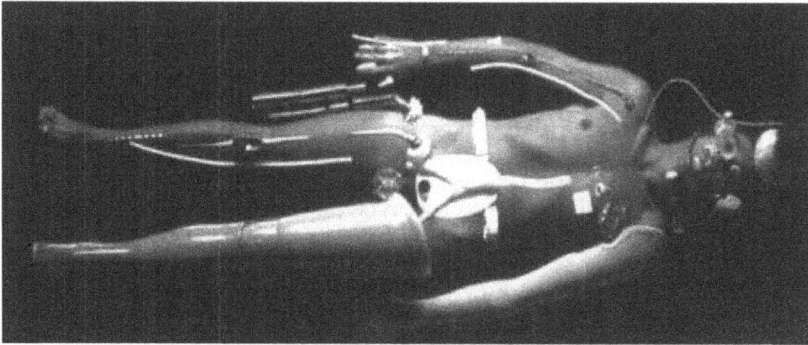

(a)

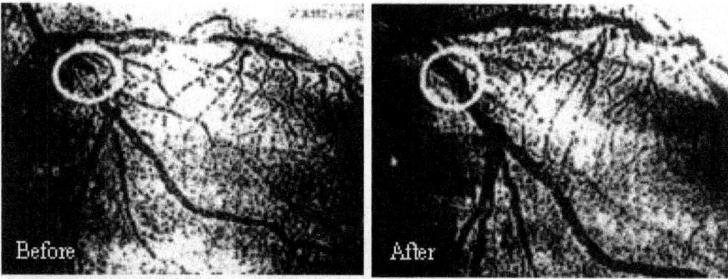

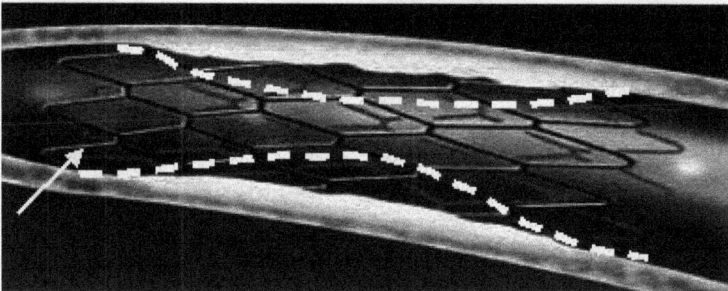

(b)

Figure 2.1. (a) Some examples of metallic implant devices in the body. (b) The first X-ray shows a severe narrowing (circle) of the coronary artery; the second X-ray shows that after the stainless steel stent (arrow) has been put in place, broadening of the artery occurred allowing blood to flow normally.

Presently, the typical metallic biomaterials used for implant devices are as follows:

- 316L stainless steels,
- cobalt–chromium alloys,

- CP (commercially pure) titanium,
- Ti–6Al–4V alloys,
- Ni–Ti alloys.

These materials were originally developed for industrial uses. They were subsequently used in many implant devices, as a biomaterial, due to their relatively high corrosion resistance. Unfortunately, when used as biomaterials, they pose several problems. These include the following:

- toxicity of corrosion products arising from wear and fretting debris,
- excessively high rigidity when compared to bone, giving rise to stress shielding which leads to bone loss,
- high specific gravity, adding extra weight and causing surrounding organs to be subjected to undue stresses,
- fracture due to corrosion fatigue and fretting corrosion fatigue,
- lack of biocompatibility with surrounding tissue,
- inadequate affinity for cells and tissues integration which resulted in the loosening of the metallic devices in time,
- shielding of X-rays which makes radiographic examination difficult.

2.2.1 *Stainless Steels*

Corrosion resistance of various steel types increases with increase in chromium content. Corrosion-resistant steels are made by adding more than 12% of chromium, which results in the formation of a thin, chemically stable, and passive oxide film. The oxide film forms and heals itself in the presence of oxygen. Steels containing more than 12% of chromium are known as stainless steels. Stainless steel itself does not generally corrode. However, pitting corrosion occurs in saline and chloride environments. Pitting corrosion, resulting from the abnormal progress of internal corrosion, causes deep pits on the metal surfaces. This pitting corrosion is further accelerated when dissolved oxygen reacts with chloride ions [2].

Apart from chromium, nickel and molybdenum are added to stainless steels to stabilize the carbide phase. Other elements such as silicone, manganese, and nitrogen are also added. Nickel and molybdenum increase corrosion resistance. Carbon, on the other hand, is detrimental to corrosion resistance in stainless steels. This is because chromium content is decreased when chromium carbides are formed during the manufacturing process like hot working and high-temperature heat treatment, and the carbides exist in the matrix as inhomogeneous microstructures.

The microstructures of steel can be classified into three categories based on their crystallographic structures: ferritic (α-body-centered cubic, BCC), martensitic (a distorted BCC obtained by rapid quenching), and austenitic (γ-face-centered cubic, FCC)

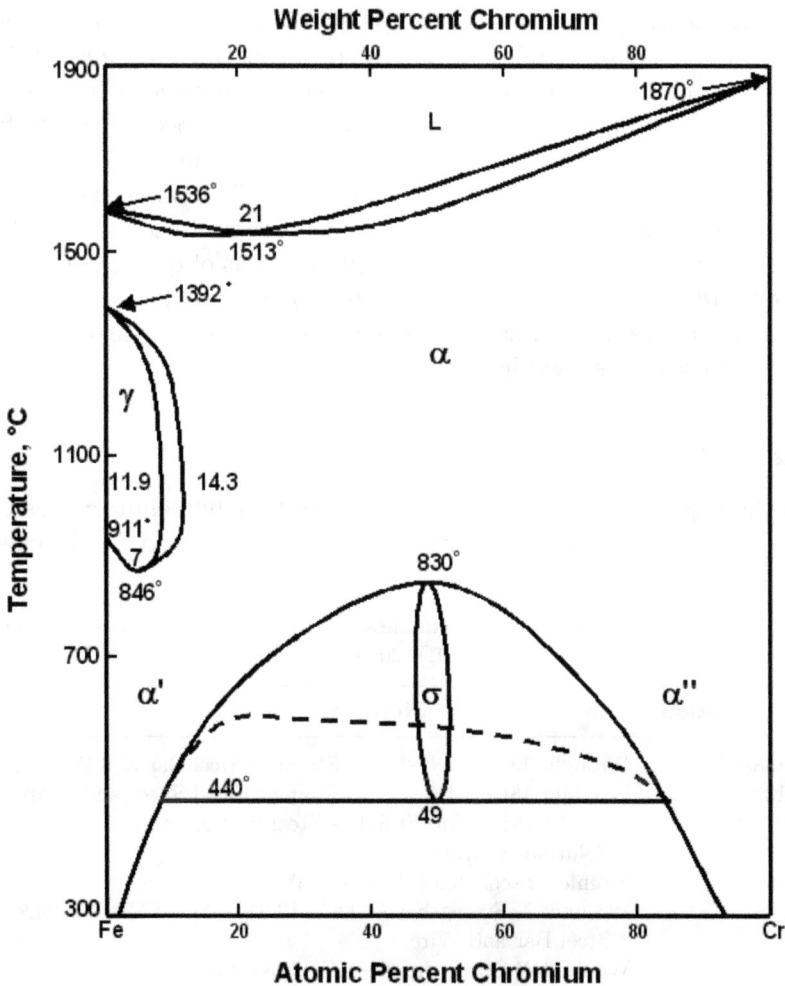

Figure 2.2. Fe–Cr phase diagram.

(see Figure 2.2) [3]. Only the austenitic type is non-magnetic. Austenitic stainless steels are more superior to ferritic and martensitic steels in terms of corrosion resistance, toughness, and workability. Nickel is the main alloying element that stabilizes the austenitic form of iron. There are many types of austenitic stainless steels, most of which originate from Type 302 (18Cr–8Ni) stainless steel. Type 316L has its corrosion resistance improved by adding molybdenum and reducing the carbon content.

The use of stainless steel is now confined to temporary devices for load-bearing applications because of nickel toxicity to the human body and its susceptibility to stress corrosion cracking and crevice corrosion [4]. However, for stents in the coronary artery where there is adequate supply of oxygen in the blood, it has been a successful permanent device for many years. The price of 316L stainless steels is one-tenth to one-fifth of other typical metallic biomaterials' price [5]. This is the reason why stainless steels are still used as metallic biomaterials in large quantities, though in terms of quality, stainless steels are inferior when compared to cobalt–chromium alloys and titanium alloys. ASTM standards of stainless steels for medical and surgical uses are shown in Table 2.1.

2.2.2   *Cobalt–Chromium Alloys*

At the beginning of 20th century, the cobalt–molybdenum–tungsten alloy — which was called Stellite — was developed by Haynes.

Table 2.1.   Standards related to stainless steels for surgical implants (*Annual Book of ASTM Standards*, Vol. 13(01), 2000).

Specification	Nominal Contents
F 138–97	Wrought 18Cr–14Ni–2.5Mo Stainless Steel Bar and Wire
F 139–96	Wrought 18Cr–14Ni–2.5Mo Stainless Steel Sheet and Strip
F 745–95	18Cr–12.5Ni–2.5Mo Stainless Steel for Cast and Solution-Annealed
F 899–95	Stainless Steel Billet, Bar, and Wire
F 1314–95	Wrought N Strengthened-22Cr–12.5Ni–5Mg–2.5Mo Stainless Steel Bar and Wire
F 1586–95	Wrought N Strengthened-21Cr–10Ni–3Mg–2.5Mo Stainless Steel Bar

It exhibited better strength at high temperatures as well as better corrosion resistance when compared to other superalloys. This alloy was used originally in aircraft engines. Then it was used for biomedical applications in the 1930s, during which it was called Vitallium. By modifying Vitallium, the following alloys have been developed: Co–Cr–Mo alloy, Co–Ni–Cr–Mo–W–Fe alloy, and Co–Ni–Cr–Mo alloy [2, 6].

Cobalt-based superalloys are superior to stainless steels in corrosion resistance. The Co–Cr–Mo alloy — presently used as a casting alloy — was developed by replacing tungsten with molybdenum. Casting alloys can give rise to course grains, grain boundary segregations, gas blow holes, and shrinkage cavities in the structure. Though inferior to non-cast alloys in terms of fatigue strength and fracture toughness, cast alloys excel in wear resistance, pitting resistance, and crevice corrosion resistance.

Molybdenum is added to refine grain size, enhance solid-solution strengthening, as well as increase corrosion resistance. Nickel is added to increase castability and workability; the amount, however, should be limited to less than 1% to ensure low toxicity in the body. Castability is then improved by adding 0.2–0.3% of carbon to the alloy to decrease the melting point by about 100°C. Distribution of Cr-rich carbides $M_{23}C_6$ and the work hardenability of this alloy help increase wear resistance. This alloy allows an artificial hip joint to be made totally of metal due to its excellent tribological properties, though sockets made of plastic materials are generally used presently. The lower the carbon content, the higher the ability to forge the alloy. Forged alloy is inferior to cast alloy in wear resistance but is superior in fatigue strength and corrosion resistance. ASTM standards of cobalt–chromium alloys for medical and surgical uses are shown in Table 2.2.

2.2.3 *Titanium and its Alloys*

Compared to stainless steels and cobalt–chromium alloys, titanium is superior in specific strength, corrosion resistance, and biocompatibility but inferior in tribological properties. Titanium is non-ferrous — its elastic modulus is about half of those of stainless steels and cobalt–chromium alloys. In addition, a very stable passive film is formed at room temperature due to rapid reaction with oxygen [2, 7, 8].

Table 2.2. Standards related to cobalt–chromium alloys for surgical implants (*Annual Book of ASTM Standards*, Vol. 13(01), 2000).

Specification	Nominal Contents
F 75–98	Co–28Cr–6Mo Casting Alloy and Cast Products
F 90–97	Wrought Co–20Cr–15W–10Ni Alloy
F 562–95	Wrought Co–35Ni–20Cr–10Mo Alloy
F 563–95	Wrought Co–Ni–Cr–Mo–W–Fe Alloy
F 799–99	Co–28Cr–6Mo Alloy Forgings
F 961–96	Co–35Ni–20Cr–10Mo Alloy Forgings
F 1058–97	Wrought Co–Cr–Ni–Mo–Fe Alloys
F 1537–94	Wrought Co–28Cr–6Mo Alloy

Titanium has an allotropic transformation temperature at 885°C, where we have the following:

- At a lower temperature than this, its structure is hexagonal close-packed (i.e., the alpha form). Elements that stabilize the alpha structure are aluminum, tin, carbon, oxygen, and nitrogen. They elevate the transformation temperature and expand the alpha phase area in the equilibrium diagram (see Figure 2.3).
- At a higher temperature than this, its structure is BCC (i.e., the beta form). Elements that stabilize the beta structure are molybdenum, niobium, vanadium, chromium, and iron. They decrease the transformation temperature and increase the beta phase area in the equilibrium diagram.

Addition of beta structure stabilizers makes it possible the existence of a two-phase structure of both alpha and beta structures, or only beta structure at room temperature. Commercially, pure titanium (called CP titanium) has an all-alpha structure. Four grades of CP titanium exist, with varying small amounts of iron, nitrogen, oxygen, and other elements. Total amount of other elements increases from Grade 1 to 4 (maximum of 0.7% at Grade 4). Tensile strength increases with increase in Grade number. Pure titanium has superior resistance to corrosion, compared to titanium alloys. Compared with beta titanium alloys, alpha titanium alloys are superior in heat resistance and weldability but inferior in strength and workability. Beta titanium alloys are alloys which are solution-strengthened by adding

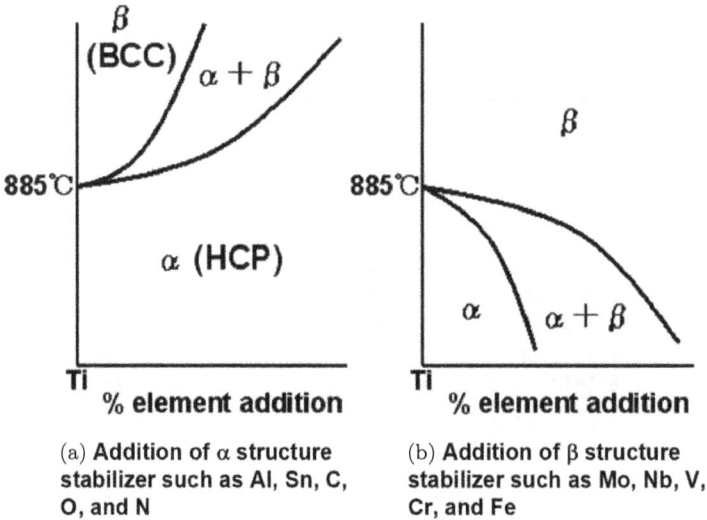

(a) **Addition of α structure stabilizer such as Al, Sn, C, O, and N**

(b) **Addition of β structure stabilizer such as Mo, Nb, V, Cr, and Fe**

Figure 2.3. Schematic explanation of Ti–X two-phase diagram; 885°C is the allotropic transformation temperature.

beta structure stabilizers. All-beta structure at room temperature can be obtained by solution treatment (i.e., rapid cooling). Alpha phase precipitates in all-beta structure by aging treatment. Beta structure with precipitated alpha phase has excellent strength.

Two-phase alloys with a dispersion of the beta form in the alpha phase have been developed with excellent properties of each phase. Ti–6Al–4V is a typical two-phase alloy which is used widely. The alloy structure strongly depends on the working and heat treatment. The alloy whose impurities are reduced to improve toughness at low temperature and crack extension resistance is called ELI Ti–6Al–4V alloy (extra low interstitial). ASTM standards of titanium and titanium alloys for medical and surgical uses are shown in Table 2.3.

2.2.4 *Nickel–Titanium Alloys*

Nickel–titanium (Ni–Ti) alloys are shape memory alloys. In terms of application, Ni–Ti alloys are used as metallic biomaterials for stent, catheter, orthodontic wire, the clip for aneurysm repair, as well as guide wire. The chemical composition range for Ni–Ti alloys is 49.5–57.5% Ni. Shape memory alloys are defined as alloys which

Table 2.3. Standards related to titanium and titanium alloys for surgical implants (*Annual Book of ASTM Standards*, Vol. 13(01), 2000).

Specification	Nominal Contents
F 67–95	Unalloyed Titanium
F 136–98	Wrought Ti–6Al–4V ELI Alloy
F 620–97	Ti–6Al–4V ELI Alloy Forgings
F 1108–97a	Ti–6Al–4V Alloy Castings
F 1295–97a	Wrought Ti–6Al–7Nb Alloy
F 1472–96	Wrought Ti–6Al–4V Alloy
F 1713–96	Wrought Ti–13Nb–13Zr Alloy
F 1813–97	Wrought Ti–12Mo–6Zr–2Fe Alloy

possess the function to return to the original shape from a plastically deformed shape due to a small amount of temperature change. The maximum strain is 5–6% in terms of shape recovery after plastic deformation. In the family of shape memory alloys, alloys in the Ni–Ti alloy system are the only ones employed as biomaterials, though alloys such as Ag–Cd, Al–Cd, Cu–Al, Cu–Sn, and Cu–Zn have shape memory function too.

In the alloy systems where the shape memory function is present, martensite transformation usually occurs. Shape memory is a phenomenon which is caused by crystallographically reversible phase transformation between the stable phase at high temperature and the stable martensite phase at low temperature. Under martensite transformation, the lattice is deformed by a small shearing-like shift of the atom arrangement while at the same time keeping adjourning relations to each other. Hence, martensite transformation is a lattice transformation, not a diffusion transformation. Martensite transformation does not accompany macroscopically plastic deformation.

The transformation starts at martensite transformation starting temperature (Ms) and grows gradually with decrease in temperature. The Ms of Ni–Ti alloys is between $-130°C$ and $60°C$. The temperature generally decreases with increase in nickel content. Martensite transformation also grows gradually by applying stress. To return a martensite-transformed structure to its original structure, heat is to be applied or stress be removed as the lattice reverse-shifts against that of martensite transformation.

Ni–Ti alloys exhibit superior ductility, fatigue strength, corrosion resistance, and biocompatibility [9]. For Ni–Ti alloys to be used as metallic biomaterials, there is the ASTM Standard which contains F2063-00 Standard Specification for Wrought Nickel–Titanium Shape Memory Medical Devices and Surgical Implants.

2.3   Body Environment to Metallic Materials

Under normal conditions, human body fluid contains 0.9% saline (NaCl) solution which contains amino acids and proteins. The human body fluid is composed of different fluid types, such as tissue fluids, lymph fluids, and blood. It includes cells, such as leukocytes, macrophages, and blood corpuscles (e.g., lymphocyte, thrombocytes, and erythrocytes). The pH of the fluid is normally 7 but may fall to 4 or 5 when there is inflammation caused by surgery or injury. The normal body temperature is 37°C and 1 atmosphere pressure (where internal partial pressure of oxygen is about one-quarter strength of atmospheric oxygen).

The biological environment of the human body described above is a strongly corrosive one for metallic materials since metals are ionic in nature. Many metallic implants rely on the formation of passive oxide films — such as chromium oxide in stainless steels and titanium dioxide in titanium alloys — for corrosion protection. When the partial pressure of oxygen is reduced inside the body, the corrosion process accelerates. This is because the lower partial pressure of oxygen reduces the recovering speed of the passive oxide film on the surface once it is broken or removed.

Another major concern arises from the adverse host tissue response to wear debris generated by the fatigue and wear process in joint prosthesis. This has been highlighted by Teoh [10] in a recent review on fatigue of biomaterials. This appears to be a natural defense mechanism of the body. The wear debris often invokes an inflammatory and immunological response. This in turn causes blood clotting processes, where leukocytes, macrophages, and, for severe cases, giant cells move in on the foreign wear particles resulting in interfacial problems between the implant and the host tissue. Numerous biochemical activities occur at this stage. These include change of the local environment to a highly acidic one (pH less than 3), where cells produce superoxides and peroxides, such as H_2O_2 [11] to degrade the implant faster. In general, assuming that the wear debris is non-toxic, there are four scenarios:

(i) The cells will try to digest the foreign debris by releasing chemicals and enzymes to dissolve and later, absorb them so that the by-products can be eliminated through the blood circulation and lymphatic system into various organs such as the kidney and liver.

(ii) If the foreign matter cannot be digested, the body will try to excrete them out of the body system (in the case of fatigue wear in the oral cavity such as wear products from dental biomaterials during the chewing process, the wear products are easily flushed out through the digestive system and are therefore less of a concern compared to other implant materials).

(iii) If the foreign matter cannot be digested or expelled, then cellular fibrous linings will engulf the foreign bodies to keep them away (isolate) from the surrounding host tissue. This scenario is of great concern as the interfacial strength between the implant and the host tissue will drop drastically, giving rise to micromotion and hence fretting-fatigue-corrosion failure.

(iv) Finally, if the amount of foreign matter keeps increasing in the body and none of the above mechanisms seems to work, the host will send signals to "give up". For example, in the case of a prolonged generation of large amount of wear debris, the host cannot cope and sends osteoclast cells — cells which are involved in the process of bone resorption — to demineralize the surrounding bone, thus causing the prosthesis to loosen.

The majority of tissue-implant activities occur in the surface and subsurface layers (see Figure 2.4), which may lead to the formation of an aqueous sandwich layer of biological components to establish a good bond between the host tissue and the biomaterial. It is here that the host tissue interacts with the implant, and if it is not biocompatible, then an avalanche of biochemical reactions occur. However, the molecular absorbed layer is dependent on the underlying passive oxide layer, which protects the base material from corrosion. If the deformed layer has a high compressive stress field (such as in the case of forged stainless steel), the incident of crack initiation is

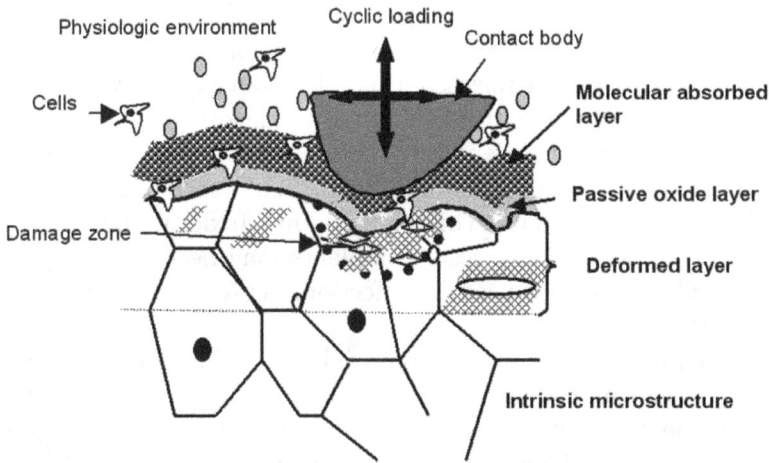

Figure 2.4. Schematic illustration of a cross-section of a deformed metallic biomaterial surface showing the complex interactions between the material's surface and the physiologic environment (after Teoh [10]).

reduced and hence the fatigue strength of the material is increased. One can readily see that the process of removal of these layers (by wear) can greatly affect the fatigue of biomaterials.

2.4 Life of Implanted Metallic Materials

Implanted metallic materials are expected to last the entire lifespan of the patient. Bone plates are an exception. They are implanted to fix failed bones and, in principle, are taken out when the failed bones recover. The life of implanted metallic biomaterials depends on the following two factors:

A. Degree of damages to implanted metallic materials due to the human body environment: This includes concerns for corrosion, corrosion fatigue, and fretting corrosion fatigue. Implanted devices made of metallic materials may fail due to corrosion fatigue and fretting corrosion fatigue [10, 12, 13], thereby leading to their replacement. They seldom fail due to mere corrosion because higher corrosion-resistant materials are used as metallic biomaterials.

B. Degree of damages to the human body caused by implanted metallic materials: It is inevitable that small amounts of metal ions and debris are released from implanted metallic materials inside the living body during their long-term use [14–16]. Metal ions and debris released from the materials may then trigger adverse reactions from cells and tissues, leading to tumor formation, allergy, and teratogenicity [2, 17]. In this light, corrosion and fretting/wear of metallic materials and their toxicity are inextricably linked to each other, which means that toxicity may influence the life of implants. As a result, implants may need to be replaced due to inflammation caused by infection, acute pain, necrosis, and complication.

Factors A and B are just two out of the many implant replacement causes. For example, an implanted artificial hip joint, one of the most frequently used biomedical devices, may be replaced due to the wearing out of its plastic-made socket, loosening and stress shielding caused by osteoclasis, or dislocation.

2.5 Corrosion, Wear/Fretting, and Fatigue

2.5.1 *Fatigue Testing Method*

Fatigue failure occurs under conditions of large number of cyclic loading. Fretting fatigue failure occurs under conditions of cyclic loading and cyclic friction loading.

A fretting fatigue test is shown in Figure 2.5. A contact normal load is applied to the pads on both flats of the fatigue specimen. When cyclic load is applied to the specimen, a small relative slip occurs between the specimen and the pads, and fretting damage is produced in the contact area. The relative slip between the specimen and the outer edges of the pads is measured using a calibrated extension meter. Frictional force between the fatigue specimen and a pad is measured using gauges bound to the outer edges of the central part of the pad. Fretting fatigue is contributed by friction stress to plain fatigue stress. Cracks can initiate at the contact sites, and one of them may propagate and eventually lead to breakage.

Basic methods of presenting engineering fatigue/fretting fatigue data are by means of the S–N curve and the da/dN–ΔK curve (Figure 2.6), where S is the maximum applied stress or stress amplitude, N is the number of cycles to failure, da/dN is the crack growth

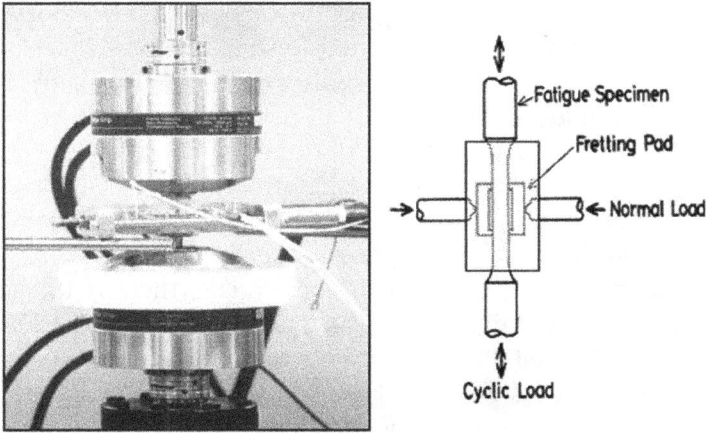

Figure 2.5.   Fretting fatigue test in a pseudo-body fluid.

Figure 2.6.   Fatigue testing based on (i) stress-life (S/N) approach and (ii) fracture mechanics approach.

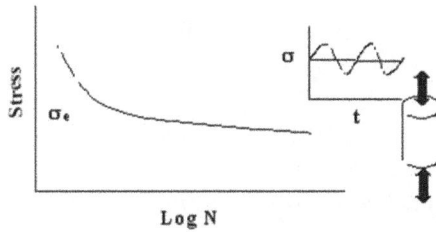

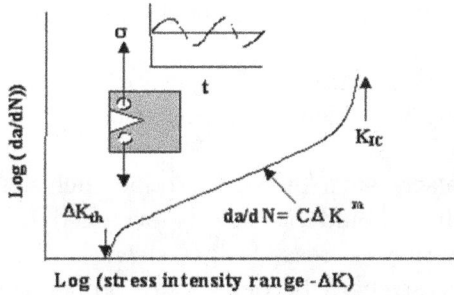

rate, and ΔK is the stress intensity factor range. It is important to collect data on fatigue strengths and fretting fatigue strengths (i.e., S–N curves) of metallic biomaterials even in pseudo-body fluids. They are useful for material selection, device design, material development, and fracture analysis. On the other hand, da/dN–ΔK curves of materials are used when designing structures such as passenger planes because their designs are carried out based on the fail-safe concept, following the fracture mechanics approach.

For fatigue testing of metallic biomaterials, there is the ASTM standard which contains ASTM designations F1801-97, F1717-96, F1612-95, and F1440-92. For fretting corrosion testing of metallic biomaterials, there is F897-84. However, no standards are available for fretting fatigue testing of metallic biomaterials, except for a test procedure described by Nakazawa [18].

2.5.2   *Notes for Fatigue/Fretting Fatigue Tests*

(a) Fatigue strength and fretting fatigue strength depend on the following testing conditions:

- type of cyclic loading (such as uniaxial loading, bending, rotating bending, and reversed torsion),
- stress ratio (i.e., the ratio of minimum stress to maximum stress in a cyclic stress),
- testing environment,
- stress frequency (under corrosive environment).

Fatigue strength and fretting fatigue strength cannot contend for superiority among specimens if testing conditions described above were not uniformly applied.

(b) Stress raisers such as non-metallic inclusions, blow holes, flaws, and notches should be strictly excluded from the implant material because they decrease fatigue strength. The effect of stress raisers on fatigue strength becomes more pronounced as the work-hardening coefficient of metallic material decreases. The effect on fatigue strength is induced using a work hardening model which assumes that when the stress that has been increasing under a given cyclic stress amplitude attains the material's fracture stress, a crack will be initiated at a stress raiser [19]. The fatigue limit with defect,

σ_w, can be expressed by the following expression:

$$\sigma_w = 1/10(10/K_s + ((1 - K_s)/K_s)1/n)\sigma'_y \qquad (2.1)$$

where K_s is the stress concentration factor of the defect, n is the work-hardening coefficient, and σ'_y is the yield strength. n is defined by $n = (\varepsilon/\sigma)(d\sigma/d\varepsilon)$, where ε is strain and σ is stress.

Metallic biomaterials have relatively lower work hardening coefficients. This means that their fatigue strengths are sensitive to stress raisers. Flaws on an implant's surface, accidentally scratched by surgical knife during operation, may therefore decrease the fatigue strength substantially. Existence of stress raisers such as non-metallic inclusions in metallic biomaterials is also detrimental to their corrosion resistance because inclusions easily become the starting site of corrosion.

(c) Fretting fatigue strength depends on the contact pressure. The case of a Ti–6Al–4V alloy is shown in Figure 2.7 [18].

The fretting fatigue life exhibits a minimum at low contact pressure and becomes constant at high contact pressures. The initiation site of the main crack depends on contact pressure (see Figure 2.8):

- When the contact pressure is high and the stick region is wide, the main crack initiation occurs near the outer edge of the fretting pad.
- When the contact pressure is low and the stick region narrow, the main crack initiation occurs at the middle portion of the fretted area.

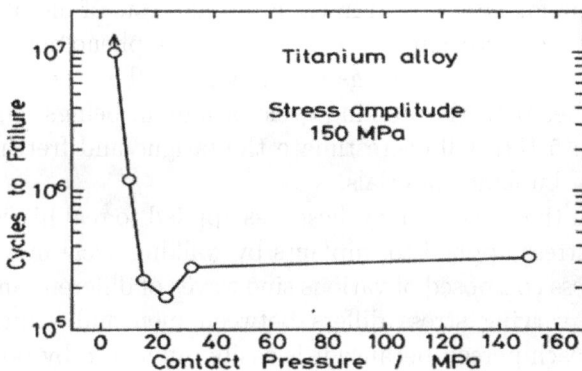

Figure 2.7. Effect of contact pressure on fretting fatigue life in air for a Ti–6Al–4V alloy.

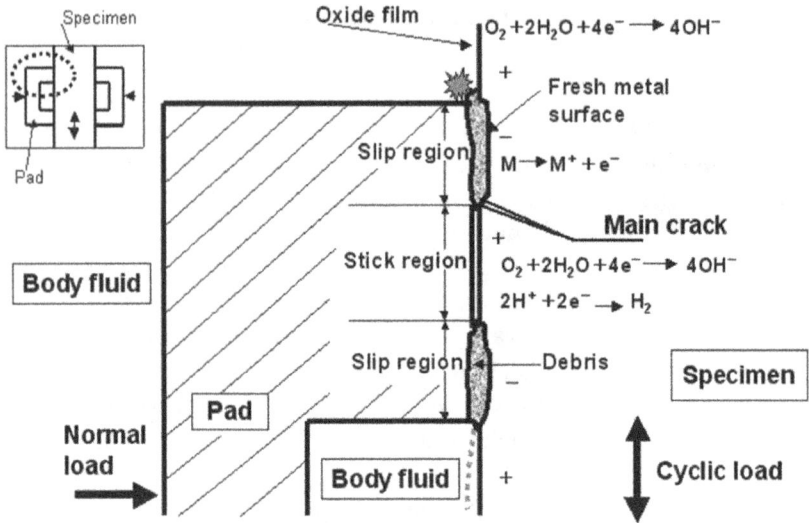

Figure 2.8. Schematic explanation of fretting and corrosion damages on the contacting surfaces of implants in the living body (the part of the circle with broken line in the small figure at the upper left corner is enlarged).

Based on the above observations, the minimum life is probably caused by this high concentration of friction stress amplitude.

(d) Fatigue strength and fretting fatigue strength of metallic materials may depend on the stress frequency in the human body. Fatigue lives decrease as stress frequency decreases in a pseudo-body fluid for CP titanium [20]. It is important to use a stress frequency of roughly 1 Hz for fatigue and fretting fatigue tests of metallic biomaterials because corrosion is a time-dependent phenomenon and the walking cycle of human beings is about 1 Hz. The use of stress frequency higher than the walking cycle of human beings (such as one higher than 5 Hz) will overestimate the fatigue and fretting fatigue strengths of implant materials.

(e) From the analogy of cyclic stress applied to real hip joints [21], the cyclic stress applied to implants by walking cycle may be cyclic varying stress composed of various sine waves of different amplitudes. The cyclic varying stress differs between men and women and is unique for each person because it is easily influenced by body weight and walking habits. However, the corrosion fatigue strength under cyclic varying stress is almost equivalent to the value obtained under constant cyclic stress for smooth specimens in air and under a corrosive environment [22]. This implies that Miner's rule (the liner damage addition rule) can be applied. Equivalent stress amplitude, $\sigma_{a,\text{eq}}$, and equivalent number of cycles, N_{eq}, are defined respectively by the following expressions (2.2) and (2.3):

$$\sigma_{a.\text{eq}.} = \alpha\sqrt{\ } \{\Sigma(\sigma_{a.i}^{\alpha} \cdot n_i)/\Sigma n_i\} \tag{2.2}$$

$$N_{\text{eq}} = \Sigma n_i \tag{2.3}$$

where $\sigma_{a.i}$ and n_i are stress amplitude and number of cycles for each stage, and α is the exponent of the S–N curve under a constant stress amplitude, which is expressed by

$$\sigma_a^{\alpha} \cdot N_f = C \tag{2.4}$$

where σ_a is the stress amplitude, N_f is the cycles to failure, and C is a constant.

Therefore, constant stress amplitude can be used in corrosion fatigue and fretting corrosion fatigue tests for metallic biomaterials.

2.5.3   *Corrosion Fatigue*

In the body, mechanical and chemical effects act simultaneously. Fatigue evaluations of biomaterials use simulated body fluid environment with electrochemical and fretting mechanisms incorporated. When fatigue occurs alongside corrosion, it is known as corrosion fatigue. Metallic materials implanted into human bodies are often damaged by corrosion fatigue or fretting corrosion fatigue [12]. The living body is a chemically and mechanically harsh environment for metallic materials. Moreover, flaws on an implant's surface — which can be caused by an accidental scratch of the surgical knife during operation — also decrease fatigue strength. The combined mechanical and chemical processes play a vital role in crack initiation. The inability to repassivate quickly causes the electrochemical breakdown of the surface layers. It is interesting to note the work of Taira and Lautenschlager (1992) — who studied the *in vitro* corrosion fatigue of 316L cold-worked stainless steel — which found that the monitoring of corrosion current could give a clear indication of crack initiation which otherwise would have been missed. They have also shown that by applying 200 mV to the metal surface to suppress passivation of the oxide layers, a significant drop in fatigue strength (in the order of 150 MPa) is observed.

Human beings normally walk several thousands of steps a day at a rate of 1 Hz. Artificial hip joints, knee joints, spinal fixations, bone plates, and wires — which have been implanted into a human body — suffer from alternate stresses which correspond to the walking cycle. In the case of artificial hip joints, the stress level is several times higher than that of the body weight. As hip joint is located out of the perpendicular line of the body weight, the balance between body weight and muscular strength pivots on only one leg. As for the pacemaker electrode, the alternate stress corresponds to the myocardium activity. And as for dental implants, the alternate stress corresponds to the chewing cycle.

Inside the living body, surface fretting of metallic materials causes wear, which leads to successive release of metal ions, metallic compounds, and debris. The release of these products into the tissues surrounding an implant may provoke toxicity on local tissue or the affected organ. For example, the black-coloring of the tissue surrounding an implant — a phenomenon called metallosis in clinical orthopedics [23, 24] — is due to the release of large amount of debris.

2.5.4 *Fretting Corrosion Fatigue*

2.5.4.1 *Fretting fatigue*

Fatigue failure is a mechanical phenomenon where under cyclic load, an initiated crack propagates to failure. If a crack is not initiated by stress raisers such as non-metallic inclusions and notches, it is usually initiated at the root of the intrusion — where shallow channels are formed. The crack initially propagates along the slip line at an angle of about 45° to the tensile stress — because maximum shearing stress lies on a 45° plane, followed by change of the propagation direction to an angle of about 90° to it (as schematically shown in Figure 2.9).

Corrosion usually accelerates crack initiation and its propagation. However, as metallic biomaterials in practical uses have higher corrosion resistance, the effect of corrosion on the acceleration of fatigue crack initiation and propagation is very low. Metallic ions release is hardly accelerated by fatigue in PBS(−) (see Table 2.4).

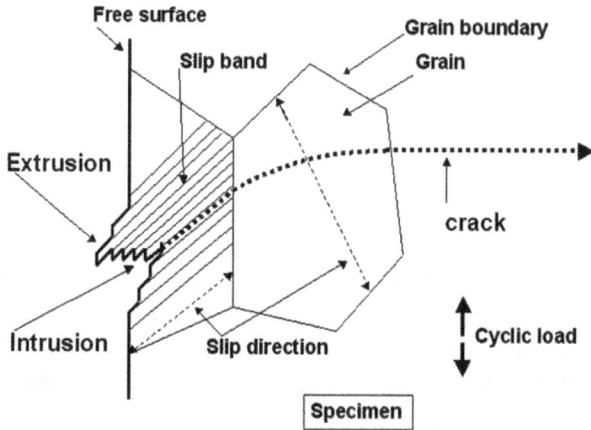

Figure 2.9. Schematic explanation of fatigue crack initiation.

Table 2.4. Concentration of metallic elements of a Ti–6Al–4V in test solutions (μg/l).

		Ti	Al	V	Fe	Cr	Ni	Mn
Unused PBS(s)		<5	<2	<5	<2	<2	<1	<1
PBS(−) after	Filtered	<5	2	<5	2	<2	3	<1
Immersion for 30d	Unfiltered	6	3	<5	3	<2	3	<1
Fatigue	Filtered	<5	3	<5	5	<2	<2	1
$N_f = 3.69 \times 10^6 (21d)$	Unfiltered	9	8	<5	12	4	<2	1
Fretting fatigue 1	Filtered	<5	3	11	7	<2	7	3
$N_f = 1.08 \times 10^5 (0.6d)$	Unfiltered	2420	1150	130	42	970	130	110
Fretting fatigue 2	Filtered	<5	3	<5	4	<2	25	2
$N_f = 4.10 \times 10^6 (24d)$	Unfiltered	23	6	8	18	<2	26	4

Note: N_f – Cycles to failure; stress frequency – 2 Hz.

Fretting damage occurs on the contacting surfaces of components which are clamped together and subjected to cyclic loads (see Figure 2.8). Fretting occurs as a result of relative movement with a small amplitude (10–20 micron), which may occur between contacting surfaces of components [25].

From mechanical viewpoint, cyclic shear stress on the surface is a major factor that initiates fretting fatigue cracks. The cyclic shear stress arises from the frictional force induced occasionally by the oscillatory movements. The maximum cyclic stress amplitude, σ_f, at the edge of the fretted area on the surface is calculated as follows:

$$\sigma_f = \sigma_a = 2f_a \tag{2.5}$$

$$F_a = \mu p \tag{2.6}$$

where σ_a is the plain fatigue stress amplitude, f_a is the friction stress amplitude, μ is the friction coefficient, and p is the contact pressure.

The areas affected by fretting are limited to the shallow surface layers. Fretting fatigue strength is almost mechanically equivalent to the fatigue strength of a specimen with short cracks [26]. Fretting fatigue behavior is very much related to notch sensitivity. Nonpropagating cracks, which occur easily near the specimen's surface at the fretted areas, are like those that appear easily at the root of a shallow notch [12].

The effect of body fluids on fretting fatigue strength is related to friction coefficient change, pits formation on fretted sites, and hydrogen generation due to electrochemical reaction. Under a certain in-air or in-PBS(–) fretting fatigue testing condition, there exists a stick region at the middle portion of the fretted area and slip regions on either side of it (see Figure 2.8). The relative slip changes — with increase in contact pressure caused by applied normal load — in the following modes: only slip region, narrow stick region plus wide slip region, and wide stick region plus narrow slip region:

- In the slip region, the contact surface is heavily damaged and wear debris is produced. Part of the wear debris is displaced out of the fretted area.

  Net contact pressure acting in the slip region is probably lower than the average contact pressure since the normal load is given through the medium of wear debris.
- On the other hand, in the stick region, the net contact pressure is probably higher than the average contact pressure since the normal load is increased by a decrease in normal load in the slip region. Hence, net contact pressure and net frictional stress amplitude acting in the stick region are higher, while those in the slip region are lower than the average values.

Therefore, stress concentration occurs near the boundaries between the stick and slip regions. The main crack initiation at the boundaries between the slip and stick regions is confirmed by the observation of fracture surfaces using optical microscope [18].

The amount of produced metal debris depends not only on cycles but also strongly on the relative slip amplitude between the specimen and the pad. The relative slip amplitude is proportional to the stress amplitude. Large relative slip amplitude easily causes a gross slip between the specimen and the pad, producing a large amount of metal debris. The difference in debris amount (concentration of unfiltered metallic elements) between Fretting Fatigue 1 and Fretting Fatigue 2 in Table 2.4 can be explained by the gross slip difference between them.

In the filtered solution recovered after the fretting fatigue test for a Ti–6Al–4V alloy, trace impurities such as nickel, manganese, and iron were detected in relatively high concentrations compared to the chemical composition of the alloy [27]. Preferential release of certain elements such as chromium and molybdenum was also detected in the fretting fatigue test solutions of a Co–Cr–Mo alloy [28].

2.5.4.2 *Metallic ions release from fretted side*

Metallic ions release is accelerated easily under fretting fatigue tests in PBS(–). This occurred not only for a 316L stainless steel [29] and a nickel-free Co–Cr alloy [28] but also for a Ti–6Al–4V alloy [27] though the metallic materials hardly dissolved due to immersion or fatigue tests in PBS(–) (see Tables 2.4 and 2.5).

Under fretting fatigue tests in PBS(–), fresh metal surfaces are produced on the slip region of the fretted site between the specimen and the pads. This production alternates with the formation of very thin oxide films on the fresh metal surfaces during every load cycle. Oxygen near the fresh metal surfaces is consumed to form oxide films. As its supply between the specimen and the pads is delayed due to the crevice, the oxygen concentration under the pads may become lower than that on the area not covered with the pads (see Figure 2.8). Therefore, oxygen concentration cells are formed and electrical potential difference arises between them to accelerate metallic ions release.

However, in the case of titanium, the material is insensitive to oxygen concentration. This means that anodic current density seldom changes correspondingly with electrical potential difference.

Table 2.5. Concentration of metallic elements of metallic materials in the immersion test solutions in PBS(−) for 30d at 37°C without load (μg/l).

		Ti	Al	V	Cr	Mn	Fe	Ni
Unused PBS(s)		*	*	*	*	1	2	G
316L	Filtered	*	2	*	*	*	3	3
	Unfiltered	6	5	*	*	*	3	3
CP Ti	Filtered	*	2	*	*	*	3	3
	Unfiltered	6	5	*	*	*	3	3
Ti–6Al–4V	Filtered	*	2	*	*	*	2	3
	Unfiltered	6	3	*	*	*	3	3

Note: * The element analyzed is not detected. The detective limits are shown as follows: 1ppb (μg/l) for Mn; 2ppb for Al, Cr, and Fe; 3ppb for Ni; 5ppb for Ti and V.

Therefore, the metallic ions release mechanism due to oxygen concentration will not be applicable for titanium.

At the same time, passive–active cells are produced at the fretted area [30]. These cells are produced in the presence of a cathode (which is the surface covered with oxide film) and an anode (which is the fresh metal surface). At the anode, metallic ions release can be accelerated according to the following formula:

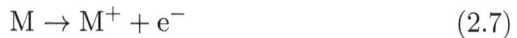

$$M \rightarrow M^+ + e^- \tag{2.7}$$

At the cathode, the following takes place:

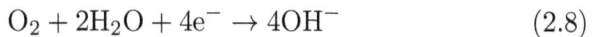

$$O_2 + 2H_2O + 4e^- \rightarrow 4OH^- \tag{2.8}$$

As the supply of consumable oxygen is delayed at the area covered with pads, the generation of OH^- decreases. As a result, Cl^- invades the crevice to keep the electric balance and metallic salts (M^+Cl^-) are formed as follows:

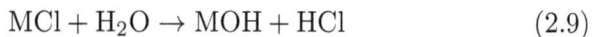

$$MCl + H_2O \rightarrow MOH + HCl \tag{2.9}$$

Due to the above hydrolysis, the pH of the fresh metal surface decreases and corrosion accelerates to form a deep pitting.

At the cathode, hydrogen is generated on the stick region by the following formula when oxygen is not supplied:

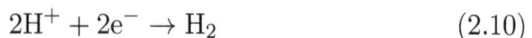

$$2H^+ + 2e^- \rightarrow H_2 \tag{2.10}$$

Table 2.6. Fatigue and fretting fatigue strengths at 10^7 cycles.

		Stainless steel				Ti–6Al–4V	
		316L	**447J1**	**Co–Cr**	**Pure Ti**	**Anneal**	**STA**
UTS (MPa)		602	591	956	440	930	1,104
0.2%P.S. (MPa)		328	525	432	306	861	1,006
Fatigue	Air	205	210	240	150	290	270
Strength (MPa)	PBS	200	200	240	140	290	270
Fretting fatigue	Air	140	150	210	100	120	142
Strength (MPa)	PBS	110	150	210	85	100	105

Note: Fatigue strengths and fretting fatigue strengths are the failure stress amplitudes at 10^7 cycles, respectively.

2.5.4.3 *Fatigue and fretting fatigue strengths at high cycle for typical metallic biomaterials in pseudo-body fluid*

Table 2.6 shows fatigue strengths and fretting fatigue strengths at 10^7 cycles in air and in PBS(–) for the following typical metallic biomaterials:

- 316L stainless steel (which contained 12.10%Ni) and 447J1 stainless steel (which contained 0.20%Ni impurity) [31],
- cobalt–chromium alloy [28],
- commercially pure titanium [20],
- annealed Ti–6Al–4V alloy [27],
- STA-treated Ti–6Al–4V alloy [27].

S–N curves for the commercially pure titanium are shown in Figure 2.10 as an example of an *S–N* curve.

Tests were carried out at tension to tension mode with a stress ratio of 0.1 under constant stress amplitude using a sine wave. Stress frequency was 20 Hz in air and 2 Hz in PBS(–) at 37°C.

The following trends are derived from the test results:

(1) Both in air and in PBS(–), the fretting fatigue strength at 10^7 cycles is lower than the fatigue strength at 10^7 cycles for each material tested.

- The annealed Ti–6Al–4V alloy in PBS(–) presented the largest difference. The fretting fatigue strength at 10^7 cycles was three times lower than the plain fatigue strength at 10^7 cycles.

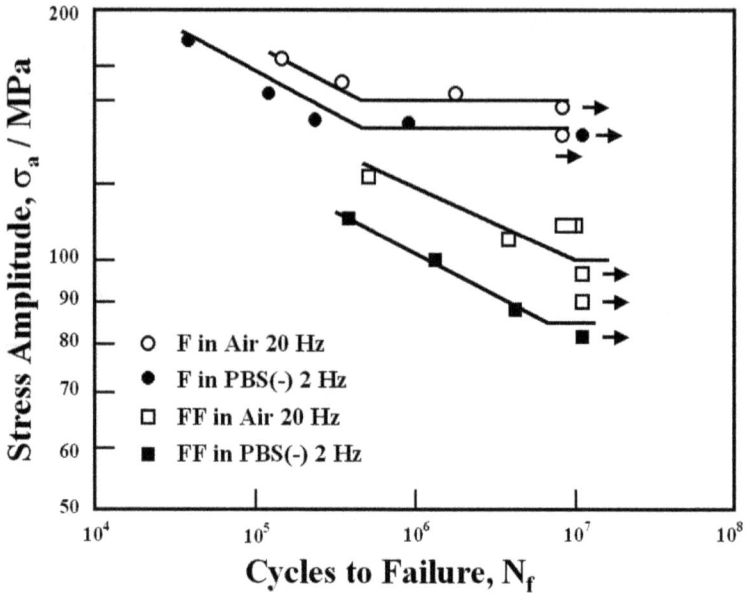

Figure 2.10. *S–N* curves of CP Ti (JIS grade 3) in air and PBS(−).
Note: (F: fatigue and FF: fretting fatigue).

- The cobalt–chromium alloy in air and PBS(−) presented the smallest difference. The fretting fatigue strength at 10^7 cycles was about 10% lower than the plain fatigue strength at 10^7 cycles.

(2) The fatigue strengths at 10^7 cycles increase with the increase in ultimate tensile strength; this trend is consistent with the results obtained in air for 15 metallic materials by Waterhouse (1981) [12].

(3) The fretting fatigue strengths at 10^7 cycles do not depend on the ultimate tensile strength; this trend is consistent with the results obtained in air for 15 metallic materials by Waterhouse (1981) [12].

(4) The fatigue strengths at 10^7 cycles in air are almost the same as those in PBS(−).

(5) The fretting fatigue strengths at 10^7 cycles in PBS(−) are lower than those in air for the 316L stainless steel, the commercially pure titanium, and the two kinds of Ti–6Al–4V alloys but are

Table 2.7. Friction coefficient at fretting fatigue limit.

| | Stainless Steel | | Co–Cr | Ti–6Al–4V |
	316L	447J1		STA
Air	1.0	0.8	0.7	0.6
PBS(–)	0.5	0.5	0.3	0.3

almost the same as those in air for the 447J1 stainless steel and the cobalt–chromium alloy.

The following factors in a quasi-biological environment may influence the fretting fatigue life of metallic biomaterials:

(a) **Friction coefficient between the specimen and the pad:** The friction coefficient in PBS(–) is about half of that in air at the endurance limit of each material (see Table 2.7). The friction stress amplitude is proportional to the friction coefficient. Therefore, the friction stress amplitude applied to a specimen in PBS(–) is about half of that in air.

(b) **Relative site of the boundary between stick and slip regions at the fretted area of the specimen:** It is not clear how the relative site of the boundary is displaced by the existence of PBS(–) (see Figure 2.8).

(c) **Corrosion pits formed on the fresh metal surface of the fretted area:** Corrosion pits may act as stress raisers to accelerate crack initiation.

(d) **Hydrogen generated on the stick regions:** If hydrogen is generated on the stick regions, it may accelerate crack initiation and its propagation, which then causes the decrease in fretting fatigue strength. The fretting fatigue strength in PBS(–) is lower than that in air for the 316L stainless steel (Table 2.6). Grain boundary cracking is observed at the crack initiation site as shown in Figure 2.11 [31]. The grain boundary cracking suggests cracking due to hydrogen.

(e) **Paring off the micro cracks initiated at the fretted areas:** Damages on the fretted surfaces of the cobalt–chromium alloy and the Ti–6Al–4V alloy are shown in Figures 2.12(a)–2.12(c) [28]. The damage in PBS(–) is more outstanding than that in air.

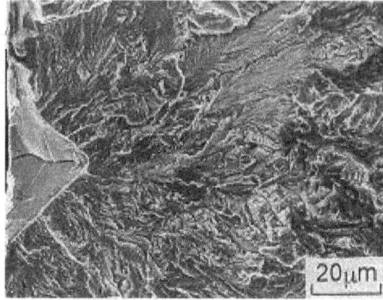

Figure 2.11. Crack initiation site in 316L stainless steel fretting fatigued in PBS(−); $\sigma_a = 178\,\text{MPa}$, $N_f = 2.1 \times 10^5$.

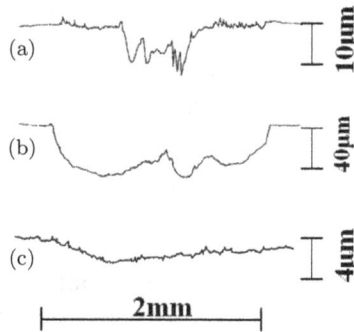

Figure 2.12. Cross-sectional profile on fretted surface: (a) Co–Cr, Air, $\sigma_a = 200\,\text{MPa}$, $N_f = 2.97 \times 10^7$; (b) Co–Cr, PBS(−), $\sigma_a = 202\,\text{MPa}$, $N_f = 1.32 \times 10^7$; (c) Ti–6Al–4V, PBS(−), $\sigma_a = 107\,\text{MPa}$, $N_f = 4.98 \times 10^6$.

The damage for the cobalt–chromium alloy is greater than that for the Ti–6Al–4V alloy. The large amount of debris produced due to intense paring off may cause delayed crack initiation and crack propagation at its early stage.

(f) **Temperature rise on the fretted areas in PBS(−):** The increase in temperature on the surface of a mild steel due to fretting is about 500°C [32]. No experimental findings are available about the increase in temperature on the fretted surface of metallic biomaterials.

Among these factors, (a) and (e) may increase the fretting fatigue life of a material in PBS(−). Factors (c) and (d) may decrease the fretting fatigue life in PBS(−) compared to their effects in air.

The effects of (b) and (f) on the fretting fatigue life in PBS(–) are not clear. The cancelation and involvement of these factors depend on the stress amplitude, appearing as the difference in the S–N curve under the fretting fatigue load in air and PBS(–).

2.5.4.4 *Some failures of implants*

For a bone plate made of pure titanium with the ultimate tensile strength of 450 MPa, the fracture stress after one year of implantation is estimated to be about 50 MPa. For a stem made of a cobalt–chromium alloy with an ultimate tensile strength of 900 MPa, the fracture stress after nine years of implantation is also estimated to be about 50 MPa. These fractures are assumed to be caused by fretting corrosion fatigue [13]. Strengthening methods which can be applied to increase fretting corrosion fatigue strength are not available except the addition of compressive residual stress to the surface of metallic materials, while corrosion fatigue strength can be strengthened by heightening the material's UTS with high corrosion resistance.

2.6 Toxicity Reaction to Metallic Implants

The most critically indispensable property of biomaterials is low toxicity. Adverse effects of metallic implants on the human body are classified into two categories: chemical and mechanical. When metallic materials are implanted inside the human body, they may corrode and wear out, releasing ions and debris which have toxic effects on tissues and organs. From the chemical perspective, toxicity of a metallic biomaterial depends on the kind, amount, and chemical state of metallic elements released from the metallic material [2,33–35,37]. As for toxicity from the mechanical perspective, mechanical stress is applied upon bones because Young's moduli of metallic biomaterials are 5 to 10 times higher than that of the bone. As a result, bone density is decreased due to stress shielding [38].

Metal ions and debris released from implants in the human body not only accumulate in the tissues surrounding the implants but are also carried to the whole body by the body fluid. Some of them are then discharged out of the body. Toxicity of a chemical to the human body is classified into two types: local and whole. Acute toxicity and chronic toxicity exist for both. Acute toxicity includes inflammation, ocular and skin irritations, clot formation, necrosis, and allergy. Chronic toxicity includes carcinogenicity, calcification, granulation, teratogenicity, and immunotoxicity.

In toxicity, a preceding stage exists prior to the final stage which can be organ disorder or death due to the released metal ions and debris. For example, cancer progresses as follows: metal ions released inside a living body, absorption, distribution, metabolism, molecular initiation, cancerous cells, cancerous organ, and organism response. The abnormal proliferation of cancerous cells exists as the preceding stage of a cancerous property. Cell proliferation is a critical characteristic. This is the reason why cells are used as a significant means to quantitatively estimate metal ions toxicity [39].

Toxicity testing is required for any new biomaterial introduced into the marketplace. Reactions of animals such as rats, rabbits, and mice to chemicals are the best available predictors of potential toxicity. However, the use of animals in evaluating chemical safety is costly, time-consuming, and increasingly criticized by animal welfare groups [39]. Toxicity of metallic compounds and chemicals has been evaluated using cultured cells increasingly in detail because of lower cost, shorter term, higher reproducibility, and greater reliability than *in vivo* evaluation. As a result, toxicity evaluation has been carried out *in vitro* using tissue culture techniques on metal plates, metal ions, metal salts, particulate metals, and wear debris [33–36, 40].

Metal ions toxicity is described in terms of the relationship between concentration and biological response, such as growth rate or death (see Figure 2.13). The relative cytotoxicity of a metal ion is ranked by its concentration. One that produces 50% relative plating efficiency (RPE) is known as IC_{50} ("IC" stands for inhibitive concentration). ED_{50} ("ED" stands for effective dose) is also shown in the figure. Note that if a poisonous metal ion is administered in small concentration, it renders no toxic effects. Conversely, if a nutritious metal ion is administered in excessive amount, it triggers adverse responses.

The C_{50} of metal salts for murine fibroblasts (L929) are shown in Table 2.8. In practical applications, these relatively high-toxic salts such as $K_2Cr_2O_7$, VCl_3, $CuCl_3$, $CoCl_2$, and $NiCl_2$ are included in metallic biomaterials. The toxicity of a metallic compound depends

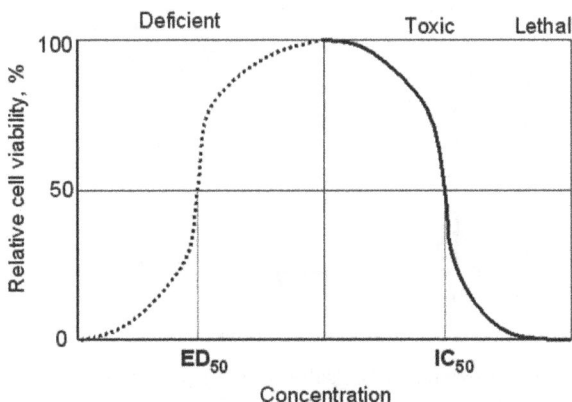

Figure 2.13. Dose-response curve.

Table 2.8. IC_{50} of metal salts for L929.

Metal Salt	$IC_{50}(\text{mol } l^{-1})$	Metal Salt	$IC_{50}(\text{mol } l^{-1})$
$K_2Cr_2O_7$	1.58×10^{-6}	$TiCl_4$	1.09×10^{-3}
VCl_3	2.82×10^{-6}	$MoCl_5$	1.19×10^{-3}
$CuCl_2$	4.15×10^{-5}	$ZrCl_4$	1.64×10^{-3}
$CoCl_2$	8.12×10^{-5}	$NbCl_5$	3.63×10^{-3}
$NiCl_2$	1.06×10^{-4}	$Al(NO_3)_3$	4.18×10^{-3}
WCl_6	6.22×10^{-4}	$FeCl_3$	4.42×10^{-3}
$Cr(NO_3)_3$	7.43×10^{-4}	$FeSO_4$	6.95×10^{-3}

on its chemical species. For example, the IC_{50} of $Cr(NO_3)_3$ is about 500 times larger than that of $K_2Cr_2O_7$ for L929 (see Figure 2.14). This reading indicates that chromium toxicity differs depending on whether it releases hexavalent or trivalent chromium ions (or compounds) in the body. The IC_{50}s of metal salts have a close correlation (correlation coefficient $r = 0.69$–0.94, which are calculated based on metal salts' IC_{50}s in logarithm) among six cell lines (L929, MC3T3-E1, J774.1, HeLa S3, IMR-32, and IMR-90), suggesting the existence of generic tendency in metal salts' cytotoxicity. Note also that cytotoxicity may be correlated to the strength of inflammation, ocular and skin irritations, or acute toxicity [34–36].

Mutagenicity is a very fundamental and important toxicity trait related to carcinogenicity and reproductive/developmental toxicity.

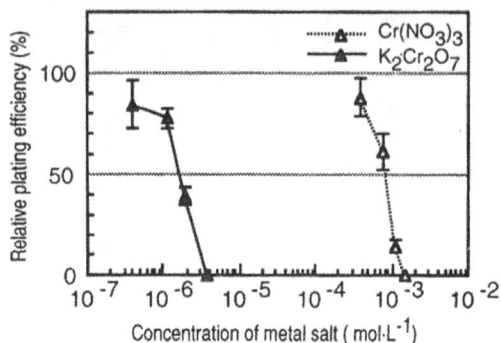

Figure 2.14. Cytotoxicity of the salts of oxo acids of chromium for L929; the error bar in the graph shows the standard deviation.

This is because the damage to genes or DNA can be caused by carcinogenesis and developmental abnormalities. The *umu* test can evaluate the genotoxicity of tested substances by measuring the induction of the bacterial SOS response which is induced by single-strand DNA gaps or DNA fragments produced as a result of damage to DNA. Cu^{2+}, V^{3+}, Cu^+, Rh^{3+}, CrO^{4-}, Ir^{4+}, and Mg^{2+} were tested positive in the *umu* test [37].

2.7   Metallic Biomaterials for the Future

The safety of metallic biomaterials to the human body has the highest priority among their essential characteristics. It is definitely preferable that metallic biomaterials be constructed without the metallic elements that may produce toxic compounds in the human body. However, for a large number of metallic elements and for a wide range of toxicity such as acute toxicity, carcinogenicity, and hypersensitivity, their toxicity data of metallic ions and compounds are not widely available.

To date, toxicity of metallic elements to the human body is not systematically understood. For example, the International Agency for Research on Cancer (IARC) of World Health Organization (WHO) speculates that Be, Cd, Cr(VI), and Ni compounds are carcinogenic, while Co, Pb, and Hg compounds, metal Ni, and Ni alloys are probably carcinogenic too [2]. However, there is no reported professional literature on the carcinogenicity of metallic materials implanted into the human body [41]. Newly developed metallic bio-materials do not contain metallic elements which have highly suspicious toxicity to the human body, such as nickel and vanadium. Some of these new developments are, namely:

- nickel-free stainless steels [42],
- nickel-free cobalt–chromium alloys [28],
- vanadium-free titanium alloys (ASTM F 1813),
- amorphous alloys [43] — amorphous alloys usually exhibit higher tensile strength, lower Young's modulus, and higher corrosion resistance than crystalline alloys.

Devices such as hip stem, bone plate, artificial knee joint, spinal fixator, sensor, and ventricular assist system need to be downsized as there is no spare space in the human body to accommodate these foreign bodies. Leveraging on this concern, there is a pressing need to develop new materials or a new system to break the present impasse on structural biomaterials. With 3D printing technology becoming a viable manufacturing process, new formulation is now available [44, 45].

References

[1] K. Okuno, The history of metallic biomaterials, in *Metallic Biomaterials — Fundamentals and Applications*, eds. M. Sumita, Y. Ikada, and T. Tateishi (ICP, Tokyo, 2000), pp. 11–18.

[2] IARC Monographs on the Evaluation of carcinogenic risks to humans: surgical implants and other foreign bodies, *Lyon*, 1999, 74:65–84.

[3] V. Raghavan, *Phase Diagrams of Ternary Iron Alloys — Part 1*, Monograph series on alloys phase diagrams (ASM International, 1988), p. 29.

[4] D. H. Kohn and P. Ducheyne, Materials science and technology — a comprehensive treatment, medical and dental materials, *Weinheim*, 1998, 14:39–41.

[5] M. Sumita, Present status and future trend of metallic materials used in orthopedics, *Ortho. Surg.*, 1997, 48:927–934.

[6] N. S. Stoloff, *Metals Handbook*, 10th Edition, Vol. 1 (ASM International, 1996), pp. 960–968.

[7] J. D. Destefani, *Metals Handbook*, 10th Edition, Vol. 2 (International, 1996), pp. 586–605.

[8]   Y. Nakayama, T. Yamamura, Y. Kotoura, and M. Oka, *In vivo* measurement of orthopedic implant alloys: comparative study of *in vivo* and *in vitro* experiments, *Biomaterials*, 1989, 10:420–424.

[9]   H. Hosoda and S. Miyazaki, Shape memory alloys, in *Metallic Biomaterials — Fundamentals and Applications*, eds. M. Sumita, Y. Ikada, and T. Tateishi (ICP, Tokyo, 2000), pp. 133–149.

[10] S. H. Teoh, Fatique of biomaterials: a review, *Int. J. Fatigue*, 2000, 22:825–837.

[11] S. C. Silverstein, R. M. Steinman, and Z. A. Cohn, Endocytosis, *Annu. Rev. Biochem.*, 1977, 46:669–722.

[12] R. B. Waterhouse, Fretting fatigue in aqueous electrolytes, in *Fretting Fatigue*, ed. Waterhouse (Applied Science Publishers, London, 1981), pp. 159–175, 221–240.

[13] M. Sumita, Corrosion fatigue and fretting corrosion fatigue, in *Metallic Biomaterials — Fundamentals and Applications*, eds. M. Sumita, Y. Ikada, and T. Tateishi, (ICP, Tokyo, 2000), pp. 233–270.

[14] P. D. Bianco, P. Ducheyne, and J. M. Cuckler, Local accumulation of titanium released from a titanium implant in the absence of wear, *J. Biomed. Mater. Res.*, 1996, 31:227–234.

[15] Y. Mu, T. Kobayashi, M. Sumita, A. Yamamoto, and T. Hanawa, Metal ion release from titanium with active oxygen species generated by rat macrophages *in vitro*, *J. Biomed. Mater. Res.*, 2000, 49:238–245.

[16] Y. Mu, T. Kobayashi, K. Tsuji, M. Sumita, and T. Hanawa, Causes of titanium release from plate and screws implanted in rabbits, *J. Mater. Sci.: Mater. Med.*, 2000, 13:583–588.

[17] A. Sato, Biological safety of metallic materials, *Zairyo–Kagaku*, 1982, 19:193–199.

[18] K. Nakazawa, M. Sumita, and N. Maruyama, Effect of contact pressure on fretting fatigue of high strength steel and titanium alloy, in *Standardization of Fretting Fatigue Test Methods and Equipment* (ASTM STP 1159, 1192), pp. 115–125.

[19] M. Sumita, I. Uchiyama, and T. Araki, Relationship between effect of inclusions on the endurance limits and the work hardening behaviors of carbon steels, *Trans. ISIJ*, 1974, 14:275–284.

[20] N. Maruyama, K. Nakazawa, M. Sumita, and S. Sato, Effect of stress frequency on fatigue and fretting fatigue lives for commercially pure Ti and Ti–6Al–4V alloy in pseudo-body fluid, *J. Jpn. Soc. Biomater.*, 2000, 18:17–23.

[21] T. Satoh, *Biomechanics* (The Japan Society of Mechanical Engineers, Ohm–sha, 1991), p. 257.

[22] Maruyama and M. Sumita, Effect of stress amplitude transient on fatigue crack initiation and propagation of high strength steel in synthetic sea water under cathodic protection, *Tetsu-to-hagane*, 1992, 78:640–647.

[23] H. F. Hildebrand and J. C. Hornez, Biological response and biocompatibility, in *Metals as Biomaterials*, eds. J. A. Helsen and H. J. Breme (John Wiley & Sons, New York, 1998), pp. 265–290.

[24] R. S. Petrie, A. D. Hanssen, D. R. Osmon, and D. Il Strup, Metal-blacked patellar component failure in total knee arthroplasty: a possible risk for late infection, *The Am. J. Ortho.*, 1998, 172–176.

[25] O'Connor, The role of elastic stress analysis in the interpretation of fretting fatigue failures, in *Fretting Fatigue*, ed. R. B. Waterhouse (Applied Science Publishers, London, 1981), pp. 23–66.

[26] I. Nishioka and K. Hirakawa, Fundamental investigations of fretting fatigue, Part 5: The effect of relative slip amplitude, *Bull. JSME*, 1969, 52:692–697.

[27] A. Yamamoto, T. Kobayashi, N. Maruyama, K. Nakazawa, and M. Sumita, Fretting fatigue properties of Ti–6AL–4V alloy in pseudo-body fluid and evaluation of biocompatibility by cell culture method, *J. Japan Inst. Metals*, 1995, 59:463–470.

[28] N. Maruyama, T. Kobayashi, K. Nakazawa, M. Sumita, and M. Sato, Fatigue and fretting fatigue behavior of Ni-free Co–Cr alloy in a pseudo-body fluid, *J. Jpn. Soc. Biomater.*, 1999, 17:172–179.

[29] A. Yamamoto, T. Kobayashi, N. Maruyama, and M. Sumita, Quantitative analysis and cytotoxicity evaluation of metallic elements in pseudo-body fluids used as environment of fretting fatigue test of metallic biomaterials, *J. Jpn. Soc. Biomater.*, 1996, 14:158–166.

[30] H. H. Uhlig, *Corrosion and Corrosion Control*, 3rd Edition (John Wiley & Sons, New York, 1989).

[31] K. Nakazawa, M. Sumita, and N. Maruyama, Fatigue and fretting fatigue of austenitic and ferritic stainless steels in pseudo-body fluid, *J. Japan Inst. Metals*, 1999, 63:1600–1608.

[32] R. B. Waterhouse, *Fretting Corrosion* (Pergamon Press, Oxford, 1972) (translated into Japanese by J. Satoh, 83, in 1984).

[33] J. C. Wataha, C. T. Hanks, and R. G. Craig, The *in vitro* effects of metal cations on eukaryotic cell metabolism, *J. Biomed. Mater. Res.*, 1991, 25:1133–1149.

[34] A. Yamamoto, R. Honma, and M. Sumita, Cytotoxicity evaluation of 43 metal salts using murine fibroblasts and osteoblastic cells, *J. Biomed. Mater. Res.*, 1998-a, 39:331–340.

[35]   A. Yamamoto, Biocompatibility evaluation of metallic biomaterials
       in vitro, Doctoral dissertation at Kyoto University, 1998-b, 59–134.
[36]   A. Yamamoto, R. Honma, A. Tanaka, and M. Sumita, Genetic ten-
       dency of metal salt cytotoxicity for six cell lines, J. Biomed. Mater.
       Res., 1999, 47:396–403.
[37]   A. Yamamoto, Y. Kohyama, and T. Hanawa, Mutagenicity evaluation
       of forty-one metal salts by the umu test, J. Biomed. Mater. Res., 2002,
       59:176–183.
[38]   W. H. Harris, The osteolysis phenomena in total hip and total knee
       replacement surgery, in World Tribology Forum in Arthroplasty, eds.
       C. Rieker, S. Oberholzer, and U. Wyss (Hans Huber, Bern, 2001),
       pp. 17–23.
[39]   A. M. Goldberg and J. M. Frazier, Alternatives to animals in toxicity
       testing, Scientific American, 1989, 261:16–22.
[40]   ISO 10993-5 Biological evaluation of medical devices — Part 5: Test
       for cytotoxicity — in vitro methods.
[41]   Y. Tabata, Foreign body reaction, in Metallic Biomaterials Funda-
       mentals and Applications, eds. M. Sumita, Y. Ikada, and T. Tateishi
       (ICP, Tokyo, 2000), pp. 335–346.
[42]   J. Menzel, W. Kirschner, and G. Stein, High nitrogen containing Ni-
       free austenitic steels for medical applications, ISIJ Int., 1996, 36:893–
       900.
[43]   S. Hiromoto, A. P. Tsai, M. Sumita, and T. Hanawa, Corrosion
       behavior of zirconium based amorphous alloys for biomedical use,
       Mater. Trans., 2001, 42:656–659.
[44]   O.K Radchenko and K.O. Gogaev, Requirements for metal and alloy
       powders for 3D printing (review). Powder Metall Met Ceram., 2022,
       61:135–154. https://doi.org/10.1007/s11106-022-00301-0
[45]   T. S. Tshephe S.O. Akinwamide and E. Olevsky, Additive manu-
       facturing of titanium-based alloys- A review of methods, properties,
       challenges, and prospects, Heliyon, 2022, 8: e09041. https://doi.org/
       10.1016/j.heliyon.2022.e09041

Chapter 3

Corrosion of Metallic Implants

D. J. Blackwood[*§], **K. H. W. Seah**[†], **and S. H. Teoh**[‡,¶]

*Department of Materials Science and Engineering, National University
of Singapore, Lower Kent Ridge Road, Singapore 119260, Singapore
†Department of Mechanical Engineering, National University of
Singapore, Lower Kent Ridge Road, Singapore 119260, Singapore
‡Center for Advanced Medical Engineering (CAME), School of Materials
Science and Engineering, Hunan University, #2 South Lushan Road,
Changsha 410082, China
§masdjb@nus.edu.sg
¶teohsh@hnu.edu.cn*

The practice of using metals and alloys to repair or replace human body
parts is now well established. Two of the most important parameters in
determining the suitability of a material for biomedical applications are
its biocompatibility and corrosion resistance. This chapter gives a basic
introduction to the thermodynamic and electrochemical aspects behind
corrosion, concentrating on the various forms of localized corrosion that
are responsible for most *in-vivo* failures. This will be followed by a brief
review of the successes and, in reality, the remarkably few failures of
the traditional materials: mainly titanium alloys, cobalt–chrome alloys,
amalgams and stainless steels. The desire to make use of a number of
advanced materials, such as memory-shaped alloys, porous materials and
rare earth magnets will then be discussed. Unfortunately, nearly all of
these materials have inadequate corrosion resistance to be used directly
in vivo without some form of protection. The chapter ends with some
case histories of surgical implant failures.

3.1 Introduction

The practice of using metal materials to repair or replace bones in the human body is now well established. An important parameter in determining the suitability of a material for use in surgical implants is corrosion. In many industrial applications, metal corrosion is controlled by the following: altering the local environment; changing the pH; lowering the temperature; or adding chemical inhibitors. Unfortunately, these techniques cannot be used to reduce the corrosion rate of surgical implants since the environment within the human body is fixed. Coatings (e.g., paints) are also widely used to control corrosion, however, these are limited to protecting implants since many of these (especially orthopedic devices) are subjected to wearing and abrasion processes that will damage most coatings [1]. The only generally successful method of reducing corrosion within the human body is to fabricate the implants from a corrosion-resistant alloy.

This approach has been extremely successful, at least with respect to extending the lifetime of biomedical devices, for although the corrosion of surgical implants was a major concern up to the late 1970s, the development of a range of corrosion-resistant alloys, such as Ti6Al4V and high nitrogen stainless steels, have reduced the number of failures to extremely low levels. Most of the few failures that still occur are often traced either to poor quality control, for example, the use of a 304L screw instead of one from 316L or to an unexpected and unusually aggressive local environment around the implant due to pathological changes in the surrounding tissue as it reacts to the surgical procedure. Most of the other earlier failures of implants tend to be due to either fatigue or fretting, which may or may not be accelerated by corrosion.

Nevertheless, the concern that extended exposure to even very low levels of corrosion products could result in medical complications remains. One major problem in this respect is that there is no consensus over what the safe levels are or even which metals are toxic. For example, a few years ago, aluminum was being linked with Alzheimer's disease. This has recently been disproved, but iron is now linked to Parkinson's disease [2]. To date, fortunately, titanium, the mainstay of biomaterials, has not been linked to any disease. However, there is no guarantee that it will not be in the future, especially as the average age of patients receiving implants is decreasing due, in part, to the modern popularity of physical sports which place a large strain on joints. Thus, the required life expectancy of the implant is increasing, and this in turn increases the risk of a high accumulation of toxic ions as well as the likelihood of failure due to fatigue and fretting. As a result, there will be a continued need to develop for surgical use alloys that have increasingly lower corrosion rates.

Corrosion problems in dental applications are more common, mainly due to the high acidity and chloride contents of many food-stuffs. Although fixtures in the oral cavity are readily accessible for repair, there exists the concern about the toxicity of the metals leaching out, and even more alarmingly, the potentials that can develop within galvanic cells have been linked with oral cancer [3, 4].

3.2 Corrosion Theory

3.2.1 *Basic Thermodynamics of Corrosion*

3.2.1.1 *The Nernst equation*

For a typical chemical reaction with non-charged species,

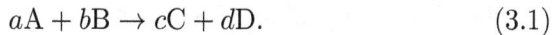

$$a\text{A} + b\text{B} \rightarrow c\text{C} + d\text{D}. \tag{3.1}$$

The free energy of the reaction is simply the difference between the chemical potentials of the products and reactants:

$$\Delta G = (\text{chemical potential of products} - \text{chemical potential}$$
$$\text{of reactants}) = (c\mu_{\text{C}} + d\mu_{\text{D}}) - (a\mu_{\text{A}} + b\mu_{\text{B}}). \tag{3.2}$$

At equilibrium, $\Delta G = 0$, and since the chemical potential of any species can be defined by

$$\mu = \mu^{\theta} + RT \ln(M), \tag{3.3}$$

where μ^{θ} is the standard chemical potential, R the gas constant, T the temperature and M either the fugacity or activity of the substance. Equation (3.2) can be expressed as

$$(c\mu^{\theta} + d\mu^{\theta}) - (a\mu^{\theta} + b\mu^{\theta}) + RT(c \ln M_{\text{C}} + d \ln M_{\text{D}})$$
$$- RT(a \ln M_{\text{A}} + b \ln M_{\text{B}}) = 0,$$

which can be rearranged as

$$(c\mu^{\theta} + d\mu^{\theta}) - (a\mu^{\theta} + b^{\theta}) = RT \ln \left(\frac{[M_C]^c [M_D]^d}{[M_A]^a [M_B]^b} \right)$$

or

$$\Delta G^{\theta} = -RT \ln K, \tag{3.4}$$

where ΔG^{θ} is the standard Gibbs free energy of the reaction and K is the equilibrium constant.

However, in electrochemical reactions, at least one of the species will carry a charge, in which case it is necessary to add an additional term to the chemical potential to represent the electrical free energy (the interaction of the charge with its environment). This yields the electrochemical potential which is defined as

$$\bar{\mu} = \mu + zF\Phi, \tag{3.5}$$

where z is the charge number (including sign, i.e., -1 for an electron), F is Faraday's constant ($96485 \, \text{C mol}^{-1}$), and Φ is the Galvani potential.

Now, consider the typical electrochemical reaction in which an electron is transferred from a metal electrode into a solution where it reduces an oxidized species (O) to a reduced species (R), one (or both) of which must be charged:

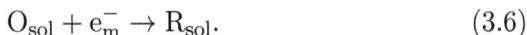

$$O_{\text{sol}} + e_{\text{m}}^{-} \rightarrow R_{\text{sol}}. \tag{3.6}$$

Once again ΔG must be zero at equilibrium so the electrochemical potentials of the products and the reactions must be equal:

$$\bar{\mu}_O + \bar{\mu}_{e,m} = \bar{\mu}_R \tag{3.7}$$

or in terms of chemical potentials and Galvani potentials

$$\mu_O + z_O F \Phi_{\text{sol}} + \mu_{e,m} - F \Phi_{\text{m}} = \mu_R + z_R F \Phi_{\text{sol}}.$$

Rearrangement yields

$$\Phi_{\text{m}} - \Phi_{\text{sol}} = (\mu_O - \mu_R + \mu_{e,m})/nF,$$

where n is the number of electrons transferred (i.e., $z_O - z_R$). Expanding the chemical potential terms as in Equation (3.3) yields

$$\Delta\Phi_{\text{m,sol}} = \Delta\Phi_{\text{m,sol}}^{\theta} + RT/nF \ln(M_O/M_R). \tag{3.8}$$

Unfortunately, this Galvani potential difference cannot be measured. However, if we place a second electrode into the solution, we can measure the cell electromotive force (emf), i.e., the difference between two Galvani potentials:

$$E_{emf} = \Delta\Phi_{m2,sol} - \Delta\Phi_{m1,sol} = E_{emf}^{\theta} + RT/nF \ln(M_O/M_R). \quad (3.9)$$

This expression is known as the *Nernst equation*. Fortunately, in practice, most solutions are sufficiently dilute to allow the activities to be replaced by concentrations and the emf subscript is normally neglected so that the Nernst equation is usually written as

$$E = E^{\theta} + RT/nF \ln([O]/[R]). \quad (3.10)$$

Furthermore, at equilibrium $E = 0$, the concentration terms in Equation (3.10) can also be replaced by the equilibrium constant yielding

$$E^{\theta} = -RT/nF \ln K \quad (3.11)$$

Inserting Equation (3.4) provides the link between an electrochemical reaction's standard potential and its standard Gibbs free energy change:

$$\Delta G^{\circ} = -nFE^{\circ}. \quad (3.12)$$

3.2.1.2 Standard potentials (E^{θ}) and the electrochemical series

As stated earlier, we can only measure the emf potentials between two electrodes (and not the Galvani potential of a single electrode). However, in order to relate this measured potential to any practical energy scale, it is necessary to have some reference point. By convention, the standard potential for the reversible hydrogen reaction in a solution with a proton activity of unity and at a partial pressure of hydrogen of one atmosphere is taken to be zero at all temperatures (i.e., chemical potentials for proton and hydrogen at unit activity and fugacity are zero):

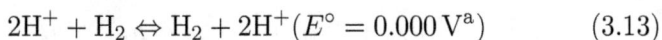

$$2H^+ + H_2 \Leftrightarrow H_2 + 2H^+ (E^{\circ} = 0.000\,V^a) \quad (3.13)$$

---

[a]The standard hydrogen electrode potential is in the region of 4.5 eV on the vacuum scale.

That is, the reaction at one electrode is

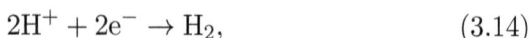

$$2H^+ + 2e^- \rightarrow H_2, \tag{3.14}$$

while that at the other is

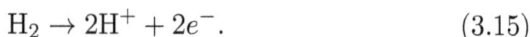

$$H_2 \rightarrow 2H^+ + 2e^-. \tag{3.15}$$

In practice, both these reactions will proceed on the same electrode since they occur at the same potential and no net current is required.

Reactions that involve the production or consumption of electrons are called *half-cell* reactions; these cannot exist independently. The standard potential for any other half-cell reaction is defined as being the potential that would be measured when the oxidation of molecular hydrogen to solvated protons acts as the second half of the cell with all species being in their standard states with activities and fugacities being unity.

For example, for a piece of zinc, the standard potential is determined from the equilibrium reaction:

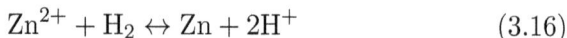

$$Zn^{2+} + H_2 \leftrightarrow Zn + 2H^+ \tag{3.16}$$

and the conditions required to induce unit activities and fugacities would be a solution that contains $1\,\mathrm{mol\,dm^{-3}}$ of Zn^{2+} ions at pH 1 subjected to one atmosphere of hydrogen gas. Under such conditions, the measured standard potential is $-0.76\,\mathrm{V}$. Note that solids always behave with unit activity and can thus be eliminated from the Nernst equation. It is normal to abbreviate Reaction (3.16) to the form

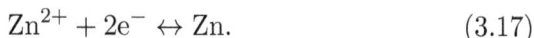

$$Zn^{2+} + 2e^- \leftrightarrow Zn. \tag{3.17}$$

Alternatively, in the event that the chemical potentials of all the species involved are already known, the standard potential can be calculated directly from Equation (3.12):

$$E^\theta = -\Delta G/nF$$

$$E^\theta = -(\text{chemical potential products} - \text{chemical potential reactants})$$

$$/nF = -[(\mu_{Zn} + 2\mu_{H^+}) - (\mu_{Zn}^{2+} + \mu_{H2})]/nF$$

$$= -(-\mu_{Zn}^{2+})/nF \quad \text{(all the other terms being zero by convention)}$$

$$= -0.76\,\mathrm{V}.$$

Table 3.1. Electrochemical series for the more common metals.

Half cell reaction	Standard potential (volts)
$Au^+ + e^- \leftrightarrow Au$	+1.68
$Pt^{2+} + 2e^- \leftrightarrow Pt$	+1.20
$Hg^{2+} + 2e^- \leftrightarrow Hg$	+0.85
$Ag^+ + e^- \leftrightarrow Ag$	+0.80
$Cu^{2+} + 2e^- \leftrightarrow Cu$	+0.34
$2H^+ + 2e^- \leftrightarrow H_2$	0.00
$Pb^{2+} + 2e^- \leftrightarrow Pb$	−0.13
$Sn^{2+} + 2e^- \leftrightarrow Sn$	−0.14
$Ni^{2+} + 2e^- \leftrightarrow Ni$	−0.25
$Cd^{2+} + 2e^- \leftrightarrow Cd$	−0.40
$Fe^{2+} + 2e^- \leftrightarrow Fe$	−0.44
$Cr^{3+} + 3e^- \leftrightarrow Cr$	−0.71
$Zn^{2+} + 2e^- \leftrightarrow Zn$	−0.76
$Ti^{2+} + 2e^- \leftrightarrow Ti$	−1.63
$Al^{3+} + 3e^- \leftrightarrow Al$	−1.67
$Mg^{2+} + 2e^- \leftrightarrow Mg$	−2.34
$Na^+ + e^- \leftrightarrow Na$	−2.71
$Ca^{2+} + 2e^- \leftrightarrow Ca$	−2.87
$K^+ + e^- \leftrightarrow K$	−2.92

The electrochemical series (Table 3.1) lists half-cell reactions in order of their standard potentials. A metal with a high standard potential (e.g., gold) is sometimes referred to as being noble, whereas those with low standard potentials (e.g., magnesium) are termed base.

Placing a base metal in a solution containing more noble ions should cause the noble metal to plate out at the expense of corrosion to the base metal:

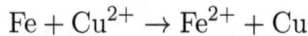

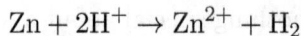

$$Fe + Cu^{2+} \rightarrow Fe^{2+} + Cu$$

$$Zn + 2H^+ \rightarrow Zn^{2+} + H_2$$

The second of these two examples reveals that all the metals that have negative standard potential can be expected to corrode in aqueous (or at least acidic) solutions. However, in practice, the presence of oxide films and complex ions can greatly influence the measured potentials, and thus, the above series should only be used as a guide.

3.2.1.3 Potential–pH equilibrium diagrams (Pourbaix diagrams)

In addition to calculating the standard potentials for solids in equilibrium with solutions of their ions, chemical potentials, when combined with solubility constants, can also be used to calculate the conditions of equilibrium for any system consisting of the following: two solid substances; one solid substance and one dissolved species; or two dissolved species. Pourbaix [5] used this technique to calculate the stable phases at equilibrium for most metal/water systems at 25°C. The data are displayed in the form of a diagram with pH as the X-axis and potential as the Y-axis.

Figures 3.1(a)–(i) show examples of Pourbaix diagrams for a number of important materials. Each diagram is divided into three different domains, labeled immunity, corrosion (which has been shaded for ease of reference) and passivation. The meanings of these three terms can be explained by considering the following:

When a piece of metal is placed in solution, it will corrode until the activity (effectively concentration) reaches that required to obtain thermodynamic equilibrium as demanded by the Nernst equation. That is, the driving force for corrosion is exactly matched by the driving force for electroplating.

- **Immunity:** The activity of metal ions required to obtain equilibrium is less than $10^{-6}\,\mathrm{mol\,dm^{-3}}$.
- **Corrosion:** The activity of metal ions required to obtain equilibrium is greater than $10^{-6}\,\mathrm{mol\,dm^{-3}}$.
- **Passivity:** The activity of metal ions required for an oxide/hydroxide film to form is less than $10^{-6}\,\mathrm{mol\,dm^{-3}}$. In this last case, equilibrium is established between the oxide film and the ions in the solution.

Note that there is nothing special about a level of $10^{-6}\,\mathrm{mol\,dm^{-3}}$; it was just chosen on the basis that it represents a very dilute solution. Also, under these definitions, immunity does not mean no corrosion, only that the amount of corrosion required to raise the concentration of ions to equilibrium levels is very low, and thus, one would expect that equilibrium is rapidly established and that the corrosion rate falls to a negligible level. However, at this point, it is worth

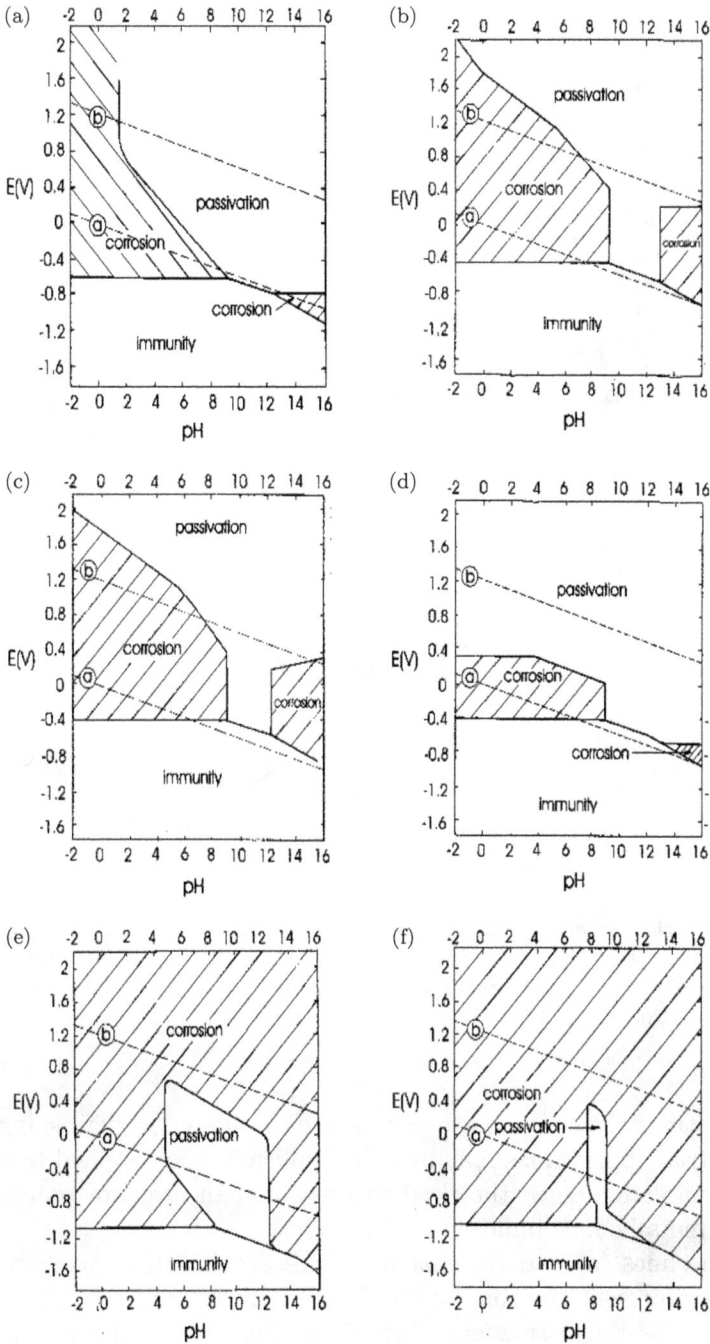

Figure 3.1. (*Continued*)

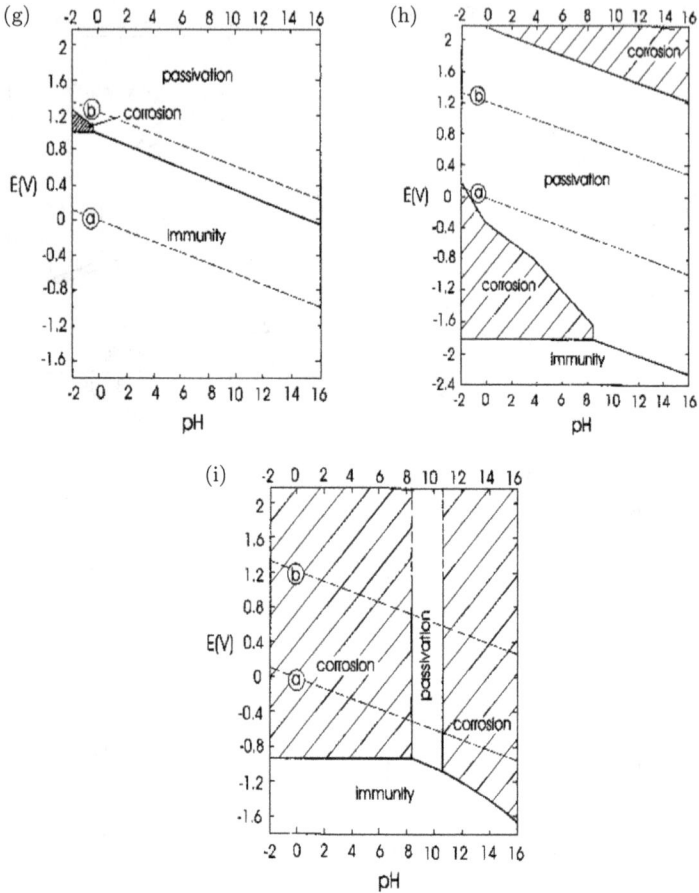

Figure 3.1. Potential against pH Pourbaix diagrams: (a) iron; (b) cobalt; (c) nickel (theoretical); (d) nickel (experimental); (e) chromium (absence of chloride); (f) chromium (presence of chloride); (g) platinum and (h) titanium; and (i) zinc. (Adapted from Ref. [5]).

reiterating that corrosion rates that are considered negligible in most industrial applications may be still significant when applied to a surgical implant due to the need to prevent high levels of potentially toxic metallic ions building up in the body.

The lines (a) and (b) that are marked on all the Pourbaix diagrams represent the zone of stability for water, and thus, it is only within this range that equilibrium can be obtained in an aqueous system. Below line (a), water is reduced to hydrogen:

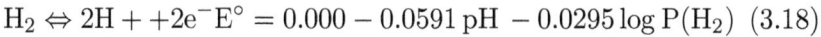

$$H_2 \Leftrightarrow 2H + +2e^- \, E^\circ = 0.000 - 0.0591 \, pH - 0.0295 \log P(H_2) \quad (3.18)$$

Above line (b), water is oxidized to produce oxygen:

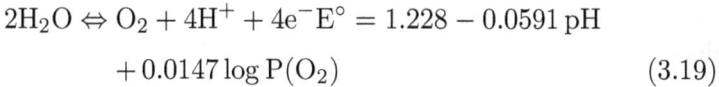

$$2H_2O \Leftrightarrow O_2 + 4H^+ + 4e^- \, E^\circ = 1.228 - 0.0591 \, pH$$

$$+ 0.0147 \log P(O_2) \quad (3.19)$$

Naturally, line (b) is also the limit below which any oxygen dissolved in the solution can be reduced. However, as we will see later, kinetic and mass transport limitations play an important role in the reduction of dissolved oxygen.

From an industrial perspective, the Pourbaix diagram for iron is the most important, it being the basis of all steels and stainless steels. It can be seen from Figure 3.1(a) that iron is classified as being immune at very negative potentials (strongly reducing conditions), but as the potential is increased, there is a tendency for the iron to become oxidized. Under either acidic or highly alkaline conditions, oxidation of iron results in active corrosion, however, in neutral environments, it results in passivation. It can also be seen from the Pourbaix diagram that increasing the potential tends to favor passivation over corrosion.

Examination of the other Pourbaix diagrams of the other metals shown in Figures 3.1(b)–(i) reveals that these have basically the same general pattern as seen for iron: immunity at very negative potential, corrosion under acidic or basic conditions and passivity in neutral environments. However, a closer examination of the diagrams reveals that for noble metals, such as platinum, the immunity domain extends across nearly the entire zone of water stability and this explains their excellent corrosion resistance. On the other hand, the immunity domains of active metals, such as zinc and titanium, are located well below the water stability zone, which means that they can be expected to be rapidly oxidized in an aqueous solution. In the case of zinc, the Pourbaix diagram shows that active corrosion occurs throughout almost the whole of the water stability zone, except for a small band around pH 12; hence, this is clearly not a suitable material for biomedical applications.

Fortunately, the oxides and hydroxides of titanium have extremely low solubilities, so a passive oxide film readily forms over the titanium's surface. Furthermore, this film is continuous and coherent, so it provides excellent protection to the underlying metal. It is the presence of this oxide film that is responsible for titanium's excellent corrosion resistance which enables it to be used in surgical applications. However, it is important to note that the Pourbaix diagram still shows two sets of conditions where titanium does undergo rapid corrosion: the first is in neutral or acidic conditions that are under extremely reducing conditions (negative potentials) where titanium fails to form a passive oxide; the second is under extremely oxidizing conditions where the solubility of titanium hydroxides starts to increase.[b] Although both of these regions fall outside of the water stability zone, it turns out that the kinetics for both the reduction and the oxidation of water at a titanium electrode are slow, and thus, it may be possible to enter the negative corrosion regions in anoxic environments or the positive region in the presence of a strong oxidizing agent such as hydrogen peroxide.

Although Pourbaix diagrams form a good basis for the study of corrosion reactions, these have limitations when applied to practical problems that should be appreciated. The lack of kinetic data is best illustrated by the case of nickel and cobalt. Figures 3.1(b) and 3.1(c) show that the Pourbaix diagrams for Ni and Co are very similar, with the theoretical domains for corrosion being quite extensive. However, experimentally, it is found that nickel passivates much more readily than predicted from thermodynamics and that corrosion is restricted to a much smaller range of conditions (Figure 3.1(d)). The explanation for this behavior is believed to be mainly due to the slow kinetics of the nickel dissolution reaction. In the case of cobalt, there is reasonably good agreement between theory and practice except in non-oxidizing acids, which thermodynamically should be very corrosive toward cobalt. However, in practice, cobalt is one of the metals least attacked by non-oxidizing acids as the kinetics of the hydrogen evolution reaction are very slow on its surface [5].

---

[b]The corrosion region at positive potentials is often marked with "question marks" due to the difficulty in obtaining reliable fundamental thermodynamic data under these conditions.

It is important to remember that Pourbaix diagrams are for the simple metal/water system. The presence of complex ions (chloride, cyanide, citrate, etc.) can greatly expand the zone of corrosion. This is particularly true for the case of chromium, for which the size of the passive domain can be severely reduced in the presence of chloride (Figures 3.1(e) and 3.1(f)). Given that chromium plays a dominant role in the formation of the oxide films that protect stainless steels, the importance of this phenomenon with respect to the performance of stainless steel implants is obvious.

3.2.2 *Basic Electrochemistry*

3.2.2.1 *Electrode reactions*

Definition: The transfer of electrons between chemical species and an electrode.

(a) Chemical species are **oxidized** if electrons are transferred to the electrode

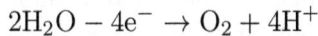

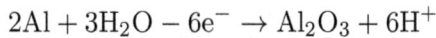

$$2H_2O - 4e^- \rightarrow O_2 + 4H^+$$

$$2Al + 3H_2O - 6e^- \rightarrow Al_2O_3 + 6H^+$$

Oxidizing reactions are also referred to as anodic processes and the electrode at which they occur is the anode. The more positive the applied potential, the faster these oxidizing reactions will proceed. By convention, currents arising due to anodic processes (oxidizing) are considered to be positive.

(b) Chemical species are **reduced** if electrons are transferred from the electrode

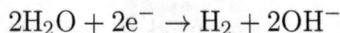

$$Fe^{3+} + e^- \rightarrow Fe^{2+}$$

$$2H_2O + 2e^- \rightarrow H_2 + 2OH^-$$

These are also referred to as cathodic processes and the electrode at which they occur is the cathode.

Overall charge balance must always be maintained. Therefore, for every electron transferred at the anode, another must be transferred at the cathode. The magnitude of the current flowing is directly proportional to the rate of the reaction and the total charge (q) passed yields the amount of chemical reaction that has taken place via Faraday's law:

$$q = mnF, \tag{3.20}$$

where m is the number of moles of reactant consumed, n is the number of electrons transferred per reactant, and F is Faraday's constant.

3.2.2.2 *Electron transfer*

Consider an inert electrode (e.g., platinum or gold) placed in a solution containing solution species O and R. A dynamic equilibrium will be established at the surface of this electrode which can be expressed as

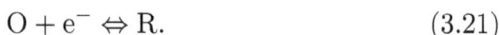

$$O + e^- \Leftrightarrow R. \tag{3.21}$$

It is very important to understand that equilibriums are dynamic. That is to say, both the reduction of O and the oxidation of R are still occurring, but at an equal rate, there is no net change. In terms of current flowing, this can be expressed as

$$-\overrightarrow{I} = \overleftarrow{I} = I_0, \tag{3.22}$$

where $\overrightarrow{I}$ and $\overleftarrow{I}$ are the partial current densities of the forward and back reactions and I_0 is the exchange current density. *No net current flows.*

The potential at which this equilibrium occurs is defined by the Nernst equation:

$$E_e = E_e^\theta + \frac{RT}{nF} Ln \frac{c_O^\sigma}{c_R^\sigma}. \tag{3.23}$$

The superscript σ has been used to indicate that it is the concentration at the surface of the electrode that determines the potential, which may be different from the bulk concentration.

Now, make the potential of our inert electrode more negative, i.e., apply an external voltage using a second electrode. Equilibrium can now only be re-established when the ratio between the surface concentrations of O and R has taken up the new value demanded by the Nernst equation. Therefore, a current must flow across the electrode/solution interface to convert O into R. Likewise, if a positive potential is applied a current will flow in the opposite direction to convert R to O. However, the magnitude of these currents will depend on kinetics rather than thermodynamics.

3.2.2.3 *Kinetics of electron transfer*

At any potential, the net current flowing is given by

$$I = \overrightarrow{I} + \overleftarrow{I} \quad (\text{where } \overrightarrow{I} \text{ is negative}) \tag{3.24}$$

with

$$\overrightarrow{I} = -nF\overrightarrow{k}c_O^\sigma \quad \text{and} \quad \overrightarrow{I} = nF\overrightarrow{k}c_R^\sigma$$

The k's are rate constants that vary with applied potential (i.e., the potential difference at the electrode's surface during the electron transfer) and usually have the form

$$\overrightarrow{k} = \overrightarrow{k}_0 \, Exp\left(\frac{-\alpha_C nF}{RT}E\right) \quad \text{and} \quad \overleftarrow{k} = \overrightarrow{k}_0 \, Exp\left(\frac{\alpha_A nF}{RT}E\right)$$

where α_A and α_C are constants (usually ≈ 0.5) and for simple electron transfer reactions,

$$\alpha_A + \alpha_C = 1. \tag{3.25}$$

Noting that overpotential (η) is defined as

$$\eta = E - E_e \tag{3.26}$$

and by definition, at $\eta = 0$,

$$I_o = -\overrightarrow{I} = \overleftarrow{I}$$

the *Butler–Volmer equation* can be derived as

$$I = I_0 \left[Exp\left(\frac{\alpha_A nF}{RT}\eta\right) - Exp\left(-\frac{\alpha_c nF}{RT}\eta\right) \right] \tag{3.27}$$

This is the fundamental equation of electrokinetics, with three limiting forms:

1. At high positive overpotentials, the second term can be ignored:

$$\log I = \log I_0 + \frac{\alpha_A nF}{2.3RT}\eta \tag{3.28}$$

2. At high negative overpotentials, the first term can be ignored:

$$\log -I = \log I_0 - \frac{\alpha_C nF}{2.3RT}\eta \tag{3.29}$$

3. At very low overpotentials where $\eta \ll (RT/\alpha_A nF)$ and $\eta \ll (RT/\alpha_C nF)$,

$$I = I_0\frac{nF}{RT}\eta \tag{3.30}$$

usually only valid for $|\eta| < 10\,\text{mV}$.

These three equations are known as the Tafel equations and are used to determine both I_0 and the α values.

3.2.2.4 *Mixed potential theory*

Corrosion processes differ from the simple case represented by Reaction (3.21) in that the forward and back reactions are not identical. For example, the reactions that occur when a piece of iron is placed into an acidic solution are as follows:

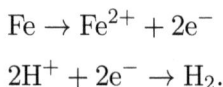

$$\text{Fe} \rightarrow \text{Fe}^{2+} + 2e^-$$

$$2\text{H}^+ + 2e^- \rightarrow \text{H}_2.$$

However, the iron is at an open circuit, so still, no net current can flow. Therefore, the corrosion potential is defined as the potential at which the forward and back reactions occur at the same rate and the corrosion current density can be defined as

$$-\overrightarrow{I} = \overleftarrow{I} = I_{Corr} \tag{3.31}$$

As long as both the forward and back reactions continue to obey the Butler–Volmer equation, the corrosion current density (I_{corr}) and corrosion potential (E_{corr}) can be obtained by plotting the log

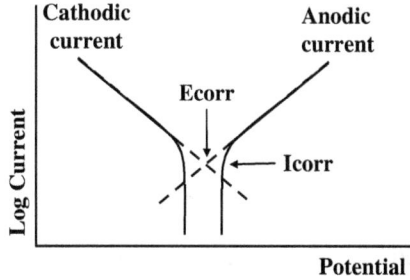

Figure 3.2. Plot of log current versus potential (polarization curve or Tafel plot) for the case where both the corrosion and cathodic reaction are under electron transfer control. The corrosion current and corrosion potential can be determined from the intercept of the anodic and cathodic regions.

of the current density against applied potential, as shown by the schematic diagram in Figure 3.2, which is sometimes referred to as a Tafel plot or Evans diagram. Note that the slopes of such a plot are often referred to as beta values, and from the Tafel equations (Equations (3.28) and (3.29)), it can be seen that

$$\beta = RT/\alpha nF \qquad (3.32)$$

3.2.2.5 *Cathodic reactions*

Under open-circuit conditions, that is, when the metal is freely corroding, there can be no net current flow. Thus, reducible species are required in the solution to act as a sink for the electrons produced during metal oxidation. It is clear from Figure 3.2 that the rate at which a metal corrodes depends not only on the kinetics of this anodic reaction but also on the rate at which the electrons are consumed by this supporting cathodic reaction. In an aqueous environment, the two most important cathodic reactions are the reduction of dissolved oxygen and the reduction of water (the hydrogen evolution reaction). It is worth mentioning at this point that Equations (3.18) and (3.19) reveal that both common cathodic supporting reactions lead to a localized decrease in pH at the metal's surface. In seawater, this can lead to the deposition of protective calcium carbonate scales [6], and in the case of surgical implants, this phenomenon may be helpful in encouraging the formation of hydroxyapatite films [7].

3.2.2.5.1 Oxygen reduction

Under aerobic conditions, the cathodic current is usually provided by the reduction of dissolved oxygen at the metal's surface, as represented by Equation (3.19). Unfortunately, the mechanism for the reduction of oxygen in aqueous media is complicated with hydrogen peroxide being a possible intermediate product of reaction:

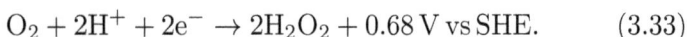

$$O_2 + 2H^+ + 2e^- \rightarrow 2H_2O_2 + 0.68\,V\,vs\,SHE. \qquad (3.33)$$

Figure 3.3 shows typical polarization curves for the reduction of dissolved oxygen. At very positive potentials, the oxygen reduction reaction is purely under electron transfer control, illustrated by a straight "Tafel" line.

However, as the solubility of oxygen in aqueous solutions is very low, the rate of its mass transport, mainly via diffusion, toward the metal's surface is slow. Therefore, oxygen reduction can only supply a limited amount of cathodic current before its surface concentration begins to fall and the rate of its reduction is partially under mass transport control. This causes the potential dependence of the cathodic current to curve below the Tafel line. In the extreme limit, the dissolved oxygen concentration at the metal's surface drops to zero, at which point the rate of its reduction becomes mass transport limited and therefore independent of potential. In the case where

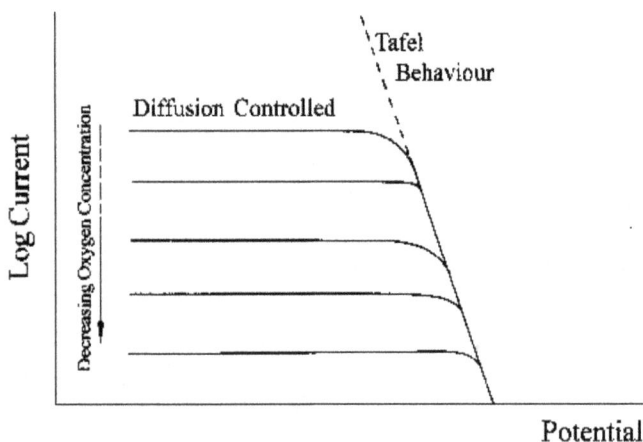

Figure 3.3. Polarization curve for oxygen reduction showing regions under electron transfer and mass transport control.

the only available form of mass transport is diffusion, the maximum cathodic current density, $I_{\lim}$, that can be supplied by the reduction of dissolved oxygen is given by [8]

$$I_{\lim} = \frac{4FDC_o}{\delta}, \tag{3.34}$$

where F is Faraday's constant, D is the diffusion coefficient of the dissolved oxygen ($\sim 10^{-5}\,\mathrm{cm^2\,s^{-1}}$), C_o is the concentration of dissolved oxygen in the bulk of the solution and is the diffusion layer thickness ($\sim 10^{-2}\,\mathrm{cm}$). As illustrated in Figure 3.3, the value of the limiting current depends directly on the dissolved oxygen concentration. In addition, in the presence of convection, such as fluid flowing through a pipe, the thickness of the diffusion layer reduces, such that for a given dissolved oxygen concentration, $I_{\lim}$ increases.

Since no net current can flow under open-circuit conditions, the corrosion potential adopted by a metal in aerobic conditions is that at which the demand for anodic current from the corrosion reaction is balanced by the available supply of cathodic current from the reduction of dissolved oxygen. Figure 3.4 shows that this decrease in dissolved oxygen concentration will cause the metal's corrosion potential to shift in the negative direction from intercept (d) to intercept (a).

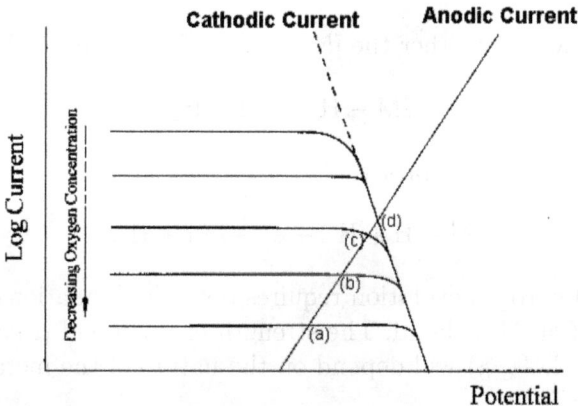

Figure 3.4. Combined polarization curves for an active metal and oxygen reduction. The corrosion potential will be at the intercept between the anodic and cathodic currents, i.e., at (a), (b), (c), or (d), depending on the level of the oxygen concentration.

3.2.2.5.2 The hydrogen evolution reaction

If the cathodic current available from dissolved oxygen is insufficient to balance the anodic corrosion current, the system will search for a fresh source of cathodic current. Although there may be a number of reducible species in the body that could potentially supply some of the required additional cathodic current, the only one in abundance is water, the reduction of which leads to the evolution of hydrogen. However, as indicated by Equations (3.18) and (3.19), the reduction of water occurs at a much more negative potential than the reduction of oxygen, hence it is only able to support the corrosion of the more active metals. In practice, this usually means metals with negative standard potentials (Table 3.1). However, the local chemical environment can reduce the potential at which some of the more noble metals corrode.

Water is nearly always in excess at the electrode interface, hence its reduction to hydrogen can be expected to be dominated by the kinetics of the charge transfer reaction rather than by mass transport processes. The electrochemistry behind the hydrogen evolution reaction has been studied in great detail over the years and its mechanism is now well understood [8]. The first step is the adsorption of hydrogen atoms

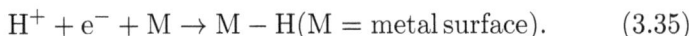

$$H^+ + e^- + M \rightarrow M - H (M = metal\, surface). \qquad (3.35)$$

This is followed by either the desorption of hydrogen molecules

$$2M - H \rightarrow 2M + H_2 \qquad (3.36)$$

or the reaction with a proton

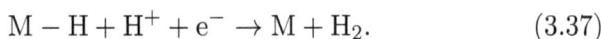

$$M - H + H^+ + e^- \rightarrow M + H_2. \qquad (3.37)$$

Note that hydrogen evolution requires both the formation of and the breaking of an M–H bond. The strength of this bond (free energy of adsorption ΔG_{ADS}) will depend on the nature of the metal.

- The greater the ΔG_{ADS}, the faster the rate of Reaction (3.35), but the slower the rates of Reactions (3.36) and (3.37).
- The lower the ΔG_{ADS}, the slower the rate of Reaction (3.35), but the faster the rates of Reactions (3.36) and (3.37).

Table 3.2. Exchange current densities for the hydrogen evolution reaction at various metal surfaces.

Metal	$-\log(I_o/\text{A cm}^{-2})$	Metal	$-\log(I_o/\text{A cm}^{-2})$
Ag	5.4	Ni	5.2
Au	5.5	Pb	12.2
Cd	11.0	Pd	2.3
Co	5.2	Pt	3.6
Cr	7.4	Ru	2.1
Cu	6.7	Ti	11.3
Fe	6.0	W	7.0
Hg	12.5	Zn	10.5

This effect is extremely significant as it can lead to reaction rates that vary by as much as 10 orders of magnitude on different metals (Table 3.2). Therefore, minor alloying elements or impurities can control the hydrogen evolution rate and with it the corrosion behavior of the parent metal. At times, this can be put to good use. For example, the hydrogen evolution reaction occurs very slowly on titanium. As a result, there is a danger that the protective passive oxide film does not form in reducing environments, however, this problem can be solved if as little as 0.25% palladium is alloyed to titanium, thereby increasing the hydrogen evolution rate and shifting the corrosion potential into the passive regime (see the Pourbaix diagram in Figure 3.1(h)).

3.2.2.5.3 Definition of anaerobic corrosion

From the perspective of corrosion, a condition is defined as being "anaerobic" if it is necessary for the reduction of water to occur in order to supply the cathodic current required to support the corrosion of the implant material in the body. Likewise, a condition is defined as being "aerobic" when the concentration of dissolved oxygen, plus any other reducible species, is sufficiently high to support the corrosion process without the need for the reduction of water. It should be noted that the corrosion behaviors of the various implant metals are different and, furthermore, depend on factors, such as local pH and salinity levels. These definitions for anaerobic and aerobic conditions are very metal specific, i.e., a single environment can appear as aerobic to one metal, yet anaerobic to another.

3.2.2.6   *Nature of electrode reactions*

Consider the following reaction:

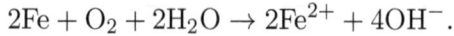

$$2Fe + O_2 + 2H_2O \rightarrow 2Fe^{2+} + 4OH^-.$$

In its simplest form, this must involve three steps:

(1) **Mass Transport:** The dissolved oxygen moves from the bulk solution to the surface of the iron (water is in excess, so it does not have to travel to the iron's surface)

$$O_{2(bulk)} \rightarrow O_{2(surface)}$$

(2) **Electron Transfer:** The electrons are transferred from the iron to the dissolved oxygen, which then steals protons from the surrounding water

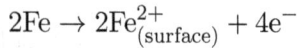

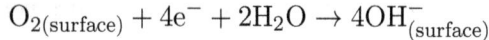

$$2Fe \rightarrow 2Fe^{2+}_{(surface)} + 4e^-$$

$$O_{2(surface)} + 4e^- + 2H_2O \rightarrow 4OH^-_{(surface)}$$

(3) **Removal of Products:** The products created by step 2 move away from the surface of the iron into the bulk solution

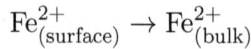

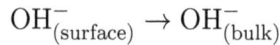

$$Fe^{2+}_{(surface)} \rightarrow Fe^{2+}_{(bulk)}$$

$$OH^-_{(surface)} \rightarrow OH^-_{(bulk)}$$

Any one of these three steps can be rate-limiting. Step 3, the removal of the products, deserves further consideration: if the hydroxide ions are not efficiently removed, there will be a localized increase in pH, which as seen from the Pourbaix diagram may favor passivation (Figure 3.1(a)); if the metal cations are not efficiently removed, their localized concentration may exceed their solubility limit and thus a solid corrosion product will form, which may or may not take the form of a protective passive film.

In practice, the real situation is likely to be further complicated as follows:

- The four electrons in step 2 are likely to be transferred one at a time with the creation of a number of intermediate species.

as localized corrosion, which will be discussed in more detail in Section 3.2. Therefore, an awareness of the mechanisms of the formation and destruction of passive oxide films is central to understanding the corrosion behavior of medical implants.

3.2.3.2 *Nature of passive films*

A film will develop on the surface of a corroding metal if the local concentration of ions exceeds that of the solubility product of the least soluble salt in the solution (Equation (3.39)). In practice, under the environments encountered in biomedical applications, the first films to develop are nearly always oxides or hydroxides, the one common exception being the black sulfide films that are responsible for tarnishing on dental amalgams. However, the formation of a film does not automatically imply passivation of the underlying metal, as this requires the film to be continuous, non-porous and well adhered. The Pilling–Bedworth ratio, which is the ratio of the oxide volume to the volume of the metal it replaces, can be used as a guide to predict whether an oxide film will provide protection [12]. If this ratio is less than 1, the oxide is too porous or discontinuous to protect the underlying metal. If the ratio is greater than 2, the stress resulting from the necessary volume expansion causes the oxide to spall off and so again it provides poor protection. Values between 1 and 2 predict an adherent non-porous protective coating. Although the Pilling–Bedworth prediction is followed by many metals when the oxide film is formed thermally, i.e., produced by heating a metal in air, it is less useful in aqueous solutions, where the film is likely to contain hydrated oxides and hydroxides. Another complicating factor in alloys is that the composition of the oxide film is usually not representative of that of the parent alloy. For example, the passive oxide on stainless steel consists of mainly chromium oxide, although there is typically only 18% chromium in stainless steel.

The thickness of a passive oxide film results from a balance between its rate of growth and its rate of chemical dissolution. On the one hand, the rate of growth is governed by the size of the electric field across the metal/solution interface which controls the migration rates of the charged species through the oxide to the position of growth. This may be either at the metal/oxide interface or at the oxide/solution interface. Since the electric field is approximately given by the potential drop across the metal/solution interface divided by the thickness of the oxide itself, it is clear that the rate of growth decreases as the oxide thickens [13]. On the other hand, the rate of chemical dissolution of the passive oxide film is a function of its solubility, which by definition is very small, and the rate at which the metal ions are transported away from the oxide/solution interface.

Although a full discussion of the processes controlling the thickness of passive films is beyond the scope of this chapter, suffice it to say that passive oxide films are very thin, typically only 5–10 nm. Hence, the presence of soluble foreign particles within the film that may have dimensions of the order of microns can lead to a serious breach of the protective barrier. In the case of the metals and alloys used in biomedical applications, the foreign particles are usually either contaminants from the production process or inclusions of sulfides and phosphides, which may be deliberately added to the alloy to obtain the required mechanical properties or may simply be present as impurities. Acid pickling is usually performed to control the former problem [14], while additional alloying elements, such as molybdenum, can be used to reduce the problems associated with sulfide and phosphide inclusions [15].

In addition to making alloying additions, the degree of protection afforded by passive films can also be increased by either increasing its thickness by anodization, that is, the passage of an electrical current in a benign solution such as sodium borate [16], or by sealing, a process that improves the oxide's crystallinity and blocks pores and can often be achieved by simply heating to about 80°C in distilled water [17].

Once formed, a passive film's main role can be envisaged as providing an impermeable barrier separating the metal from the surrounding environment. However, there are two important differences between passive films and other barrier coatings such as paints, one of which is an advantage whereas the other a disadvantage. The advantage is that, unlike a coating of paint, the oxide has some potential to repair itself if it is mechanically damaged. The disadvantage arises from the fact that passive films are normally n-type semiconductors rather than insulators. As such, electrochemical reactions can still occur on their surfaces. In particular, if a damaged film is unable to repair itself, the cathodic reactions necessary to support corrosion can take place on the undamaged parts of the passive film, leading to a rapid acceleration of the corrosion at the damaged site.

Finally, it is also important to remember that a passive film does not reduce the corrosion rate to zero, since all oxides do have some solubility in aqueous media, albeit extremely small. Although the rate is reduced to levels that are considered insignificant for most industrial applications, this may not be the case for biomedical applications. This is because the structural integrity of the metallic implant itself is not the only concern. It is also necessary to consider what happens to the corrosion products once these leave the medical device as care needs to be taken to guard against the build-up of metallic ion concentrations to potentially hazardous levels.

3.2.3.3 *Influence of the cathodic supporting reactions*

Figure 3.6 shows that if the dissolved oxygen concentration is very low, the limiting cathodic current it can supply can fall below that required to maintain anodic the passive current. At this point, a fresh source of cathodic current is required and this is most likely to be the reduction of water, which leads to the evolution of hydrogen. However, as indicated in Figure 3.6, the reduction of water occurs at a much more negative potential than the reduction of oxygen, therefore the corrosion potential of the active–passive metal will shift

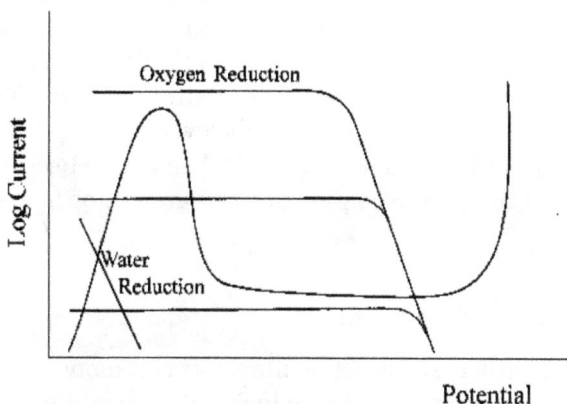

Figure 3.6. Combined polarization curves for an active–passive metal and oxygen/water reduction.

dramatically negative. In some metals, this negative potential shift can be sufficient to prevent the formation of the passive oxide film such that rapid active corrosion occurs. This is the case for titanium in highly reducing environments (more reducing than expected to be found in biomedical applications), where it is necessary to add a small quantity of palladium (typically 0.25%) to catalyze the hydrogen evolution reaction in order to shift the titanium's corrosion potential back into the passive regime [18].

3.3 Types of Corrosion

3.3.1 *General Corrosion*

When metal loss occurs at a uniform rate across the entire exposed surface, the metal is considered to be undergoing general or uniform corrosion. For metals capable of forming passive films, Figure 3.6 shows that general corrosion can occur in both the active and passive regions of the polarization curve, that is to say, the anodic and cathodic currents can cross in either of these regions. However, corrosion rates found within the active region are normally too high for the metal to be of interest in medical applications. In the passive region, the general corrosion is sometimes referred to as passive corrosion, and in the long term, its rate depends on a balance between the rates of growth and dissolution of the passive film. For a successful implant material, the long-term general corrosion rate should fall to less than $1\,\mu$m per year. For almost any other application, such low corrosion rates would be considered insignificant. However, even at these rates, it has been reported that after eight years of implantation, the nickel, chromium and cobalt levels in surrounding tissues can be five times the normal values [19]. It has also been shown that the presence of metal ions suppresses cell growth of human gingival fibroblasts [20].

3.3.2 *Localized Corrosion*

As mentioned earlier, stable oxide films form on many metals in neutral and alkaline environments, reducing the corrosion rate to very low levels. Although in the long term, even these very low corrosion rates could lead to high levels of metallic ions within the body, usually of more pressing concern is what happens if these very thin protective passive films are damaged or chemically breakdown. This results in the small areas of metal at the breakdown points in the oxide film being exposed to a potentially aggressive environment leading to very high corrosion rates. The localized corrosion rate is further aggravated by the fact that the driving cathodic reaction (Equation (3.3)) can occur on the much larger intact oxide surface. Breakdown of the passive film tends to occur under a number of different circumstances.

3.3.2.1 *Pitting corrosion*

In the presence of aggressive ions, particularly chloride, the rate of chemical dissolution of the passive film at flaws, such as sulfide inclusions, can be increased. This leads to the initiation of pitting corrosion. Once formed, a pit is analogous to a tiny crevice, and propagation is believed to proceed via the acidification process described in Section 3.2.2. The likelihood of pitting corrosion increases with increased aggressive ion concentration, higher temperature and oxidizing potential and lower pH, while increased solution flow rates and higher dissolved oxygen concentrations decrease the probability of pitting. Environments that are not quite aggressive enough to cause active pitting corrosion may still lead to the development of metastable pits. These are pits that initiate but are unable to obtain the required degree of acidity within their occluded cells to propagate and thus repassivate. A number of papers have been published on this so-called "birth and death" of pits [15, 21], a phenomenon that has important implications for stress corrosion cracking. (Section 3.2.3).

Pitting corrosion was a common problem with the early stainless steel implants that were mainly of grade 304. However, the addition of Mo (2–3%) to form the 316L grade stainless steel has greatly reduced the number of failures due to pitting corrosion, although the mechanism by which Mo reduces the pitting process is still uncertain [15, 22]. From a review of failures during 1980–1989, Zitter [23] has suggested that a pitting resistance equivalent (%Cr + 3x%Mo + 16x%N) greater than 26 is required to prevent *in-vivo* pitting corrosion. This is above the pitting resistance equivalent of 316L stainless steels which range between 23 and 26. However, if nitrogen additions are made, the value should exceed the threshold of 26.

Concerns that pitting corrosion of implants based on cobalt-based alloys could lead to carcinogens being released into the body have resulted in numerous *in-vitro* studies [24–29]. All of these reported that under static conditions, these alloys were resistant to pitting. Nevertheless, pitting corrosion of CoCr alloys has been detected when these were either subjected to cyclic loads or previously been severely cold-worked [30, 31].

Pure titanium can be considered immune to pitting corrosion in any *in-vivo* environment likely to be encountered. Titanium alloys are less resistant, as the alloying elements represent discontinuities in the protective oxide film. However, to date, no *in-vivo* pitting-related failures have been reported. Nevertheless, *in-vitro* experiments have shown that the Ti6Al4V alloy suffers superficial pitting corrosion at high potentials (> 1500 mV vs. SCE) in 1% NaCl solutions [32].

The resistance of nickel–titanium memory shape alloys has yet to be fully investigated. Results from *in-vitro* experiments are pessimistic with the NiTi alloy appearing to be less resistant than 316L stainless steel [33]. However, the results from the *in-vivo* test are more encouraging with the NiTi alloy outperforming 316L stainless steel [34].

3.3.2.2   *Crevice corrosion*

Crevices are formed whenever two surfaces come together, trapping a stagnant layer of solution. The width of a crevice needs to be sufficiently small so that natural convection no longer allows the trapped solution to mix with the bulk solution outside, such that diffusion is the only form of mass transport by which dissolved oxygen can enter the occluded region. Typically, this restricts crevices to widths less than 3 mm. In such crevices, the supply of dissolved oxygen within the trapped solution can be depleted such that the location of the anodic and cathodic reactions become separated, that is, the anodic corrosion reaction occurs in the crevice and the supporting cathodic reduction reaction on the much larger surface outside the crevice. Therefore, inside the crevice, the reaction is of the following type:

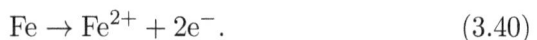

$$Fe \rightarrow Fe^{2+} + 2e^-. \tag{3.40}$$

To maintain charge neutrality, anions need to migrate into, and cations out of, the crevice (Figure 3.7). In the event that the salts of

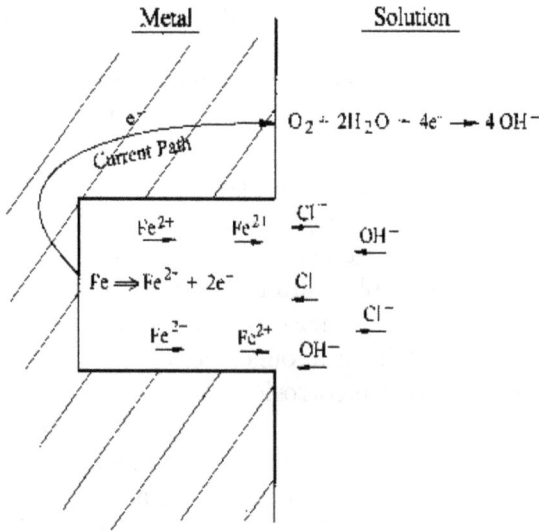

Figure 3.7. Schematic representation of corrosion within a crevice.

the anions moving into the crevice are more soluble than the corresponding oxide/hydroxide, the local pH value will fall. For example, if the incoming cation is chloride, the following reaction may occur:

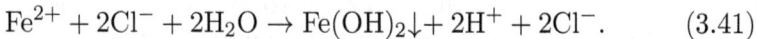

$$Fe^{2+} + 2Cl^- + 2H_2O \rightarrow Fe(OH)_2\downarrow + 2H^+ + 2Cl^-. \tag{3.41}$$

This increased acidity within the crevice causes the corrosion rate to accelerate yet further, increasing the need for yet more anions to migrate into the trapped solution, resulting in a lower pH value. Hence, the crevice corrosion mechanism is autocatalytic in nature. The final pH value within the crevice is only restricted by the solubility of the salt, i.e., in the case of Equation (3.41) by the solubility of $FeCl_2$. The environmental factors that influence the likelihood of crevice corrosion are the same as those mentioned above for pitting corrosion.

Typical examples of crevices that might be found in biomedical applications are beneath the heads of fixing screws and within the pores of some of the porous materials currently being proposed for use in surgical implants [35].

Crevice corrosion of stainless steel implants is a very serious problem even in the molybdenum-containing 316L grade. In 1959, Scales *et al.* [36] reported that 24% of type 316 stainless steel bone plates and screws removed from patients showed evidence of crevice corrosion. Reducing the non-metallic inclusion content by vacuum melting to form 316LVM stainless steel and an austenitic microstructure that is free of delta ferrite [37] has been shown to reduce the extent of, but not eliminate, crevice corrosion.

Syrett et al. [26] found no crevice corrosion on CoCrMo specimens that had been implanted in dogs and rhesus monkeys for two years. Likewise, Galante and Rostoker [38] found no crevice corrosion on implants removed from rabbits after one year. However, these authors did find single pits in the crevice regions. It is possible that if the experiments had been left for a longer period of time, these pits may have developed into crevice corrosion.

Crevice corrosion of titanium in neutral chloride environments has only been reported at temperatures exceeding 70°C [18]. However, Blackwood et al. [17] have shown that at a temperature of only 45°C, the protective oxide film on titanium will slowly dissolve if the environment is anaerobic and pH < 2. Although such conditions are theoretically possible within a crevice, they would probably take several years for such to develop. Nevertheless, Galante and Rostoker reported single pits in the crevice regions of Ti6Al4V specimens, again after implanting in rabbits for one year, but no actual crevice corrosion. As with pitting, corrosion titanium alloys will be less resistant to crevice corrosion than pure titanium. Crevice corrosion has also been proposed as the reason why porous titanium [39] and porous CoCrMo alloys [40] have much poorer corrosion resistances than their solid counterpart, the porous matrix itself providing ready-made crevices.

3.3.2.3   Stress corrosion cracking

Stress corrosion cracking (SCC) is a general term used to describe stressed metals and alloys that fail due to the propagation of cracks in corrosive environments [41]. SCC can initiate and propagate with little external evidence. Failure due to SCC is therefore insidious and fracture can occur without visible warning. SCC frequently initiates at surface discontinuities which have resulted from fabrication processes or as a consequence of poor design or workmanship. Features such as burrs, groves, laps and joints, provide potential sites for the initiation of crevice corrosion from which crack initiation may be favored [42]. In solutions containing chloride, SCC is known to initiate from localized corrosion sites, such as pits or crevices [43–46]. The transition between localized corrosion and cracking is dependent on the same parameters that control SCC, i.e., the electrochemistry occurring at the base of the pit, and the presence of a stress/strain system.

One of the essential requirements for cracks to propagate is a sharp tip at which the stress can be concentrated. Hence, SCC tends not to occur on specimens undergoing either active general corrosion or localized pitting corrosion. This is because these other forms of corrosion tend to blunt the crack tips. In the case of the metals and alloys commonly used in medical devices, this means that SCC usually occurs in conditions slightly less aggressive than those required for active pitting corrosion, that is, in the "metastable" pitting region mentioned in Section 3.2.1. Furthermore, since passive films are essentially ceramic materials, they are not as ductile as the underlying metal. Hence, any elongation of the metal by the applied tensile stress cannot be matched by the brittle films, which thus have to break. Similarly, anything in the local environment that can cause embrittlement of the metal's surface increases the likelihood of the occurrence of SCC.

Paradoxically, metals and alloys that are highly resistant to general corrosion due to their ability to readily form passive films are at greater risk of SCC failures than nominally less corrosion-resistant materials. This is because rapid reformation of the passive film helps keep the crack tip sharp and thus concentrates the stress, which leads to rapid crack propagation (Figure 3.8).

Another stress-related corrosion phenomenon is hydrogen embrittlement. This is very similar to SCC, except that it occurs at negative rather than positive potentials. If the potential is sufficiently negative for hydrogen to form, then hydrogen atoms can enter the metal's lattice and form metal hydrides at the surface. These tend to be brittle and thus crack when subjected to stress.

To the best of the authors' knowledge, SCC has not been observed on recovered surgical implants. Although implants may exhibit cracks, these do not show the physical characteristics associated with SCC and thus are believed to be due to mechanical damage that occurred during either manufacture or the recovery process [47]. Laboratory experiments appear to confirm that the common implant

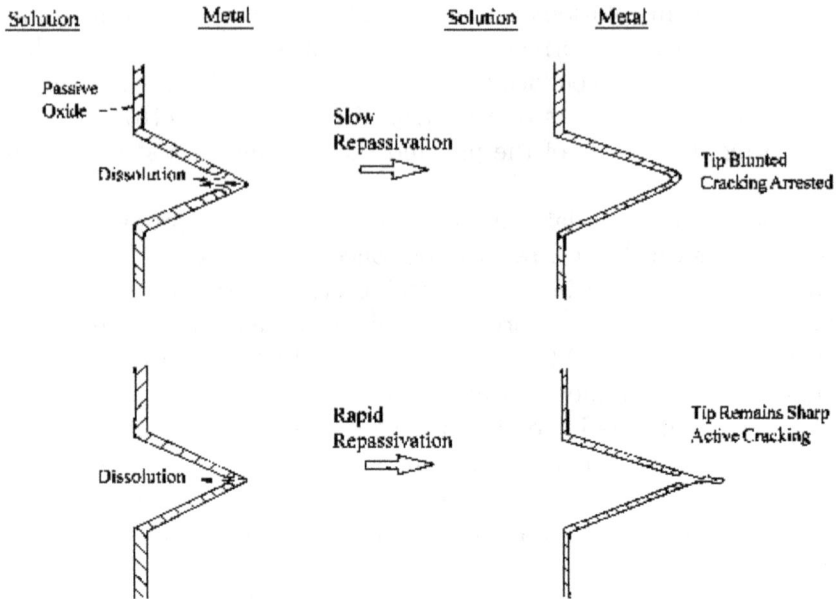

Figure 3.8. Schematic representation of how the repassivation rate influences stress corrosion cracking.

alloys are not susceptible to SCC in *in-vivo* environments [48]. However, Edwards *et al.* [49] have shown that CoCrMo alloys may be susceptible to hydrogen embrittlement in Ringer's solution if polarized at negative potentials such that significant amounts of hydrogen evolution occur on their surfaces. In practice, such a situation is only likely to occur *in vivo* if the CoCrMo was galvanically coupled to a more active material, such as stainless steel.

Bundy *et al.* [50] have shown that crack propagation continues in 316L stainless steel that has been pre-cracked in acidic $MgCl_2$ solutions before being transferred to Ringer's solution and subjected to a positive applied potential. Although these authors concluded that SCC of 316L stainless steel could occur *in vivo*, it is unlikely that their experimental conditions would ever exist in reality.

An excellent review of the advances in the theory and practice of SCC, including a discussion of the various SCC mechanisms, was published in 1990 by Newman and Procter [51].

3.3.2.4 *Corrosion fatigue*

Corrosion fatigue is very similar to stress corrosion cracking, the difference being that the load is now applied in a cyclic manner, and just as with mechanical failures, cyclic loads tend to cause corrosion failures at lower stresses than static loads. However, unlike normal mechanical fatigue, where there is a fatigue limit and the number of cycles required for failure to occur is independent of frequency, corrosion fatigue shows no fatigue limit (i.e., no safe loading) and it is worse at low frequencies. This makes laboratory testing of corrosion fatigue extremely time-consuming, (e.g., it takes almost a year to complete one million cycles at 1 Hz). It is believed that the frequency dependence of corrosion fatigue is due to the stressed metal being in contact with the aggressive solution for longer periods at low frequencies. Unfortunately, many medical devices are subjected to these low-frequency loads that are so conducive to causing corrosion fatigue. For instance, simply walking would result in a hip implant being subjected to cyclic loading at about 1 Hz.

Nevertheless, when, in 1982, Leclerc [52] reviewed the extensive literature related to corrosion fatigue of prostheses implants, he concluded that as long as the manufacture and metallurgical condition of the device conformed to international standards (e.g., BS 7252, ISO 5832 or ASTM F138), corrosion only made a minor contribution to most fatigue failures. However, Leclerc did note that the role of corrosion increases the longer the prosthesis is implanted in the patient. A later review by Zitter [23] in 1991 came to similar conclusions as Leclerc. In contrast, Morita *et al.* [53] reported that the *in-vivo* (rabbits) fatigue strength of 316 stainless steel and a CoCrNiFe alloy were considerably less than their values in air and they proposed that this was due to the corrosive action of body fluids on the materials.

In his review of clinical fatigue-related failures, Bechtol [54] claimed that the root cause of the problem was the failure of the bone-cement support interface which eventually led to a widening of the separation between the metal prosthesis and cement and finally to deformity of the metal stem. This was recently supported by von Knock *et al.* [55] who found no evidence of corrosion on 11 CoCr alloy femoral components retrieved after 2–15 years of service and speculated that the major component of micromotion between implant and bone occurs between the bone cement and the bone.

Hughes *et al.* [56] reported that the corrosion fatigue resistance of titanium has been shown to be almost independent of pH over the range of 2–7, whereas the fatigue strength of stainless steel declines rapidly below pH 4. This is consistent with the findings of Yu *et al.* [57] that pitting corrosion facilitates the initiation of corrosion fatigue in stainless steels. These authors also reported that the corrosion fatigue resistance of Ti6Al4V can be enhanced by nitrogen implantation and heat treatments to produce fine prior-β grain sizes.

The importance of material selection and design was again emphasized by Piehler *et al.* [58] who tested hip nail plates and found that large plates had better corrosion fatigue resistance than small ones and that Ti6Al4V outperformed 316L stainless steel.

3.3.2.5   *Fretting corrosion and mechanical wear*

If the passive oxide film is mechanically worn away, the underlying metal will immediately undergo active corrosion in an attempt to reform it. Since mechanical wearing does not involve the development of the aggressive chemical conditions associated with crevice corrosion (Section 3.2.2), as long as the process causing the wear does not occur frequently, only minimal corrosion is required to successfully complete the repassivation process. That is to say, the occasional scratch does not significantly cause long-term metal loss. However, with frequent wearing or fretting, the amount of metal loss in the periods of active corrosion increases accordingly. In the extreme case of near-continuous wearing, the passive film may never reform, resulting in rapid corrosion.

There are two common causes of wear. The first is the rapid flow of a solution across the surface of the metal and this leads to a phenomenon termed "erosion corrosion". However, in the case of medical applications, high solution flow rates are only likely to be encountered in a small number of applications such as at valves and pumps where the problem can often be solved by choosing a material that is highly resistant to erosion corrosion, such as titanium. The second common cause of wear is the rubbing of two solid surfaces, which leads to fretting corrosion. In fact, fretting corrosion represents the single most important form of attack on load-bearing surgical implants. This is because all the successful metallic implant materials are based on passive metals, and hence, any process that wears away the protective oxide film is of major concern [59].

However, in biomedical situations, such as the ball joint of a hip implant, it is likely that a thin film of solution will exist between the two rubbing surfaces. This has led to some debate on whether the corrosion that is observed is really due to fretting or if it is actually a form of crevice corrosion [60] (Section 3.2.2). Regardless of the true mechanism, corrosion at joints can be a serious problem as it not only results in metal loss but also increases the dimensions of the joint, causing fixation problems. Naturally, mechanical wear at joints can also lead to loss of the surrounding cement or bone, which, apart from being a serious problem in itself, increases the amount of movement of the implant, thereby increasing the likelihood of corrosion fatigue [54]. Naturally, mechanical wear at joints can also lead to loss of the surrounding cement or bone, but this is beyond the scope of this chapter.

All three major classes of prosthesis implant materials, namely, Ti alloys, CoCr alloys and stainless steels, suffer from fretting corrosion [61]. The situation is made worse by the fact that the corrosion products collect locally as particles. For example, black titanium oxide debris is often found, which causes further abrasion of the implant. The cause of the shearing micro-movements that eventually lead to the fretting corrosion appears to be the large differences between the elastic moduli of the solid metallic implants and the surrounding bone or PMMA cement [61]. The poor fretting resistance of the Ti6Al4V alloy represents its most serious drawback with regard to its use as an implant material, and thus there has been considerable effort dedicated to finding possible solutions [16, 62–64].

3.3.3 *Galvanic Corrosion (Bimetallic Corrosion)*

When two different metals are electrically coupled together, the anodic corrosion reaction of the base metal can be supported by cathodic reactions occurring on the more noble one. Effectively, the system forms a battery which leads to an increased corrosion rate on the base anode metal, while the more noble cathode metal is protected from corrosion. Galvanic corrosion, also known as bimetallic corrosion, not only occurs between two different metals but also can occur internally between different phases of a multiphase alloy, a phenomenon common in dental amalgams [65], or between particles of metallic impurities and the parent metal.

Unfortunately, the thermodynamically derived standard emf series for metals is insufficient to determine which one of any given two metals will be the more noble as the presence of passive films and complexing ions influence the relative corrosion potentials of different metals. Instead, it is necessary to use a galvanic series that has been experimentally determined in the medium of interest. Although there is insufficient data available to construct a full galvanic series for metals in body fluids, it is likely that the extensive galvanic series that has been produced for seawater can be used as a reasonable substitute [66].

Factors that influence the extent to which the galvanic coupling between two metals accelerates the respective corrosion rate of the anode include the following [67]:

(i) **Difference in the individual uncoupled corrosion potentials of the two metals:** This can be envisaged as the magnitude of the open-circuit voltage across the battery.

(ii) **Ratio between the exposed surface areas of the coupled metals:** This is also seen in the case of crevice corrosion where the large cathode area outside the crevice accelerates the corrosion of the small anode within (Section 3.2.2).

(iii) **Nature of the kinetics of the cathodic reactions on the coupled metals:** As the rates of the cathodic reaction can vary by up to 10 orders of magnitude [8], very small impurities or minor alloying additions of an efficient cathode can dominate the corrosion process.

(iv) **Conductivity of the surrounding medium:** A higher conductivity allows the two metals to interact over longer distances.

(v) **Polarizability of the two metals in the couple:** When the two metals are electrically coupled together, they must adopt a common potential, which entails shifting both of the metals from their individual uncoupled potentials to the new potential of the couple. The polarizability of a metal is a measure of how much current has to flow in order to shift its corrosion potential.

In the case of most biomedical devices, the last of these factors, polarizability, requires further consideration. From Figure 3.6, it can be seen that the actively corroding metals require large currents to shift their potentials, whereas within the passive regime, the currents are very small and virtually independent of potential. This means that for a metal in the passive state, i.e., for most practical biomedical devices, the galvanic couple is not expected to cause any significant change in the corrosion rate so long as the metal remains within the passive regime. Unfortunately, such a happy state of affairs is rarely found in practice, since although shifting a passive metal to a more positive potential may not increase its general corrosion rate, reference to Section 3.2 reveals that such a shift increases the likelihood of localized corrosion occurring. It is this increased threat of localized corrosion that is the major concern when considering the influence of galvanic corrosion on biomedical devices.

Furthermore, it is worth remembering that the conditions required to initiate localized corrosion are more aggressive than those required for its continued propagation. Therefore, if localized corrosion is initiated due to an accidental short-term galvanic coupling event, then breaking that galvanic couple will not stop the localized corrosion from continued propagation.

Rostoker *et al.* [68] found that 316L stainless steel suffered pitting corrosion in 1% NaCl solution at 37°C when it was coupled to either Ti6Al4V, CoCrMo alloy or graphite. No pitting corrosion was found when any two of the other three materials were coupled together.

In the event that titanium and any cobalt–chromium alloys are coupled together, it is likely that the passive titanium would become the cathode and thus accelerated corrosion of the CoCr alloy may be anticipated. However, titanium is a poor cathode, that is, the kinetics of the oxygen and water reduction reactions are slow on its surface, and because its passive current is virtually independent of potential, it is easily polarized. This means that the extent of accelerated corrosion caused to any metal from coupling to titanium should be small. This view has been confirmed in a literature review by Mears [69] and also for titanium–cobalt alloy combinations by the *in-vitro* experiments of Lucas *et al.* [30] and by clinical use, as reported by Jackson-Burrows *et al.* [70].

Galvanic corrosion in the oral cavity has caused particular concern as the high potential differences that can develop, say, for example, between a gold crown and an amalgam core, not only cause accelerated corrosion but also have been linked to a number of serious oral conditions, including leukoplakia and oral cancer [65].

3.3.4 *Selective Leaching*

Selective leaching, also referred to as "parting" and "dealloying", is the removal by corrosion of one element from a solid alloy. It differs from internal galvanic coupling in that it can occur within a single-phase alloy. Often, the dimensions of the alloy are not reduced. However, there is usually a drastic loss of strength. In terms of medical applications, selective leaching is of concern if it releases toxic elements in the body, e.g., mercury from dental alloys and chromium or nickel from stainless steel implants.

3.3.5 *Intergranular Attack*

Industrially, the most important form of this corrosion involves alloys that rely on the formation of a chromium oxide layer to maintain their passivity, such as stainless steels. Most of these alloys contain some carbon, which helps provide strength. However, during various forms of heat treatment, most notably under conditions encountered in welding, chromium can react with carbon to form chromium carbide. This leads to grain boundary areas that are depleted of free chromium, and hence the passive film is significantly weaker in these areas rendering them susceptible to corrosion. In practice, chromium depletion can be avoided by ensuring proper post-weld treatment or choosing one of the specially formulated low carbon alloys ($< 0.03\%$) denoted by the suffix L, e.g., 316L stainless steel, that are now available. Hence, although the intergranular attack was a problem with stainless steel implants prior to the 1960s [36], it should not be encountered in modern biomedical applications.

Dental amalgams are multiphase alloys. As such, these are susceptible to intergranular corrosion between the different phases. In terms of the mechanism, this can be considered a form of localized galvanic corrosion. In conventional amalgams, it is the phases that contain silver that are noble and cause accelerated corrosion of the non-silver phases, with the most vulnerable being the γ_2 phase (Sn_7Hg), which releases mercury when it corrodes [71]. The high copper amalgams contain no γ_2 phase and are more resistant to corrosion than silver-tin amalgams [72]. The most corrosion-prone phase in high-copper amalgams is the η' phase (Cu_6Sn_5), which does not lead to the release of mercury [73]. However, it has recently been shown that corrosion of dental amalgams only makes a minor contribution toward the total amount of mercury within the average human body, the vast majority $(> 90\%)$ enters via the food chain [74].

3.3.6 *Influence of Cold-Working*

Cold-working, without subsequent annealing, can have two effects on the corrosion of metals and alloys. The first is that cold-working not only increases the density of dislocations, which has the advantage of increasing the material's strength, but also causes the worked areas to be slightly more susceptible to corrosion than unworked areas. The second effect is that phase changes in the crystal structure may occur. For example, cold-working of the austenitic 304L stainless steels can result in the development of some areas of the hard martensite phase, which renders the material more susceptible to stress corrosion cracking. However, this occurs to a much smaller extent in 316L stainless steel used in biomedical applications.

Nevertheless, cold-working followed by short-term tempering has been reported to improve the static and fatigue strength of high nitrogen stainless steels without any detrimental effects on the corrosion behavior in NaCl solutions [75].

3.4 Environments Encountered in Biomedical Applications

3.4.1 *Surgical Implants*

The compositions of body fluids are complicated. However, from the perspective of corrosion, the most important characteristics are the chloride, dissolved oxygen and pH levels. A 0.9%, NaCl solution is considered to be isotonic with blood, and under normal conditions, most body fluids have a pH of 7.4 and a temperature of 37°C. In these respects, body fluids appear to be slightly less aggressive than seawater and this is reflected in the fact that for stainless steels, a pitting resistance number (PREN) of greater than 26 is recommended for surgical implants compared to the value of 40 usually required for stagnant seawater [23]. However, the dissolved oxygen levels in blood are lower than in saline solutions exposed to air atmospheres by a factor of about two for arterial blood and a factor of about six for venous blood. Conversely, bicarbonate levels are about 200 times higher in blood than in seawater [53].

The many other components in body fluids, e.g., phosphates, cholesterols, phospholipids, etc., are usually considered to either play no role in the corrosion process or exist at inconsequential levels. As a result, most *in-vitro* experiments have been conducted in either 0.9% NaCl or standard isotonic solutions, such as Ringer's or Hank's solution, in which the presence of bicarbonate and calcium chloride tends to be the main difference compared to the NaCl solution. A review by Solar [76] in 1979 concluded that inorganic solutions based on diluted NaCl were indeed satisfactory substitutes for human body fluids when studying the behavior of passive metals. However, usually, no attempt is made in the *in-vitro* experiments to lower the dissolved oxygen content of the isotonic solution to that of venous blood and this has been proposed as an explanation for some of the differences observed in the *in-vivo* and *in-vitro* corrosion behavior of implant materials [53, 56]. Furthermore, the minor components in blood have occasionally been blamed for accelerated *in-vivo* corrosion. For example, it has been postulated that sulfur present in amino acids may enhance crevice corrosion of stainless steels [19].

Figure 3.9 shows the typical environmental conditions expected within a range of different body fluids superimposed on the Pourbaix diagram for chromium in the presence of chloride ions. From this diagram, it can be predicted that stainless steels are likely to suffer corrosion in many of the environments found within the body. However, fortunately, passivation of stainless steel is likely to occur in the body fluids most likely to be encountered by an implant, e.g., blood typically has a redox potential in the vicinity of 0V and pH 7.4. Titanium can be expected to be in a passive state for virtually all the physiological solutions shown in Figure 3.9.

Finally, the surgical operation plus the presence of the implant itself may cause the surrounding tissue to undergo severe pathological changes that result in the development of a more corrosive environment [77]. Laing reported that the pH around a newly inserted surgical implant can drop to as low as 4.0, due to the build-up of hematomas, a condition that could last several weeks [1, 78].

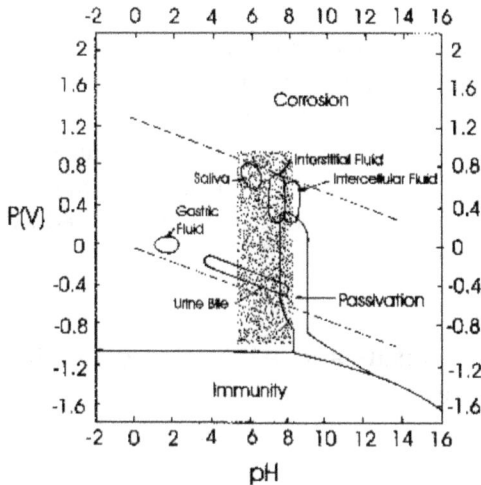

Figure 3.9. Representative environmental conditions for various body fluids superimposed on the Pourbaix diagram for chromium in solutions containing chloride. The shaded zone represents the conditions for physiological solutions, as suggested by Schenk [82].

Hydrogen peroxide may also be generated during the initial stages of the inflammatory response of the surrounding body tissue after the insertion of an implant [11,79]. The extent to which these pathological changes occur depends on the biological activity of any corrosion products emanating from the implant and also on its size and shape. The influences of size and shape mean that the extent of the pathological changes will vary across the surface of the implant, which could lead to the development of electrochemical cells [80]. Variations in the local pH on titanium alloys have even been observed during *in-vitro* experiments, which could also generate the potential gradients required to drive localized corrosion [81].

3.4.2 *Dental Applications*

The environment within the oral cavity is not well defined. Although there are a number of recipes for artificial saliva, the most popular being that of Fusayama (NaCl, $0.400\,\mathrm{g\,m^{-3}}$; KCl, $0.400\,\mathrm{g\,dm^{-3}}$; $CaCl_2.H2O$, $0.795\,\mathrm{g\,dm^{-3}}$; $NaH_2PO_4.H_2O$, $0.69\,\mathrm{g\,dm^{-3}}$; $Na_2S.9H_2O$, $0.005\,\mathrm{g\,dm^{-3}}$; pH5.5) [83], in reality, the make-up of human saliva varies considerably between individuals, especially in the sulfide content which can cause tarnishing of both silver- and gold-based amalgams. In any case, many foodstuffs are acidic with high chloride levels and are thus far more corrosive than salvia [84]. Moreover, oral hygiene has a strong effect on the corrosiveness of the oral environment. What rots the teeth is likely to corrode the amalgams and dental fixtures. Finally, many dental products and solutions contain fluoride, with some of the specialist varnishes used by dentists being over 2 wt% fluoride [85].

3.5   Common Metals and Alloys Used in Biomedical Applications

3.5.1   *Surgical Implants*

All the metals and alloys used for surgical implants rely on the development of a passive oxide film to reduce their corrosion rates to acceptable levels. The actual specifications of modern surgical implant alloys, including chemical compositions and heat treatments, are now covered by the international standard ISO 5832.

3.5.1.1   *Stainless steel*

Stainless steels are in fact a family of ferrous alloys that contain more than 12% chromium, and in the 1930s, these were the main implant materials [86]. With respect to surgical implants, usually, the more ductile austenitic stainless steels containing at least 8% nickel are generally used with the most important being grade 316L, which has a nominal composition of 17Cr, 8Ni, 2Mo, balance Fe, with an extremely low carbon content to prevent chromium depletion, hence their suffix 'L'. Occasionally, nitrogen is added at about the quarter-percent level to further improve the corrosion resistance of the alloy. The relative corrosion resistance of stainless steels can be estimated from their "pitting resistance number" (PREN):

$$\mathrm{PREN} = \%\mathrm{Cr} + 3.3 \times \%\mathrm{Mo} + 16 \times \%\mathrm{N}.$$

However, 316L stainless steel can corrode within the body, especially in regions where there is insufficient oxygen to maintain the passive film or where crevices are formed, e.g., under the heads of screws. In addition, stainless steel femoral components can fracture. Therefore, stainless steel is more suitable for temporary implant devices. Nevertheless, there are cases where 316L fracture plates have been removed from patients after more than 20 years of service, yet show no evidence of corrosion (see case histories in Section 3.8).

One final word of caution on stainless steels is that different grades should not be mixed as this can result in galvanic corrosion. Since it is not possible to visually distinguish one grade of stainless steel from another, careful quality control must be exercised. There have been examples of failures arising because just one of a group of screws holding a 316L fracture plate in position was fabricated from the lower 304L grade.

3.5.1.2 *Cobalt–Chrome alloys*

Of the cobalt–chrome alloys, the main ones used for surgical implants are based on either CoCrMo alloy, which has been used extensively in dentistry and more recently for artificial joints, or CoNiCrMo, which is used for making the stems of prostheses for heavily loaded joints. Cobalt–chrome alloys have very good resistance to most forms of corrosion, including crevice corrosion and stress corrosion cracking. However, corrosion fatigue can still cause failures.

A major concern with using these alloys is the potential release of chromium, a known carcinogen, into the body. This worry also applies to stainless steels since they too contain chromium, although at lower levels.

3.5.1.3 *Titanium and titanium alloys*

Titanium has an excellent strength-to-weight ratio, and it is this, allied to its excellent biocompatibility, which makes it such an attractive material for medical devices. During the 1950s and 1960s, it became the preferred choice of material [87]. Titanium has excellent corrosion resistance to most environments likely to be found *in vivo*, with the possible exception of anoxic regions where the protective passive oxide does not form. If this latter situation is a possibility, then the titanium should be alloyed with a small amount of palladium (Section 3.2.2.5.2). The ability of the passive oxide film to provide corrosion protection can be improved by anodizing, which results in a thicker film, or by simple "sealing". The latter can be achieved by simply heating in distilled water [17].

Titanium alloys have even better strength-to-weight ratios than pure titanium, such that the Ti6AL4V alloy has now become the most popular implant material. However, the titanium alloys do not have quite the same resistance to pitting corrosion as the parent metal and problems can be encountered if the local redox potential is high. Such a condition can result from a situation where hydrogen peroxide is produced during the initial stages of the inflammatory response after insertion of an implant. However, overall titanium alloys have better corrosion resistance than the cobalt–chrome alloys and stainless steels.

Despite their excellent corrosion resistance and biocompatibility, titanium and its alloys are not the perfect implant material as it has poor shear strength, making them unsuitable for screws, etc. Titanium also has a high coefficient of friction which means that wear particles may form if it rubs against bone or another implant surface. The latter case can also lead to fretting corrosion if the passive oxide film is worn away.

3.5.1.4 *Porous titanium*

Although titanium alloys have suitable corrosion characteristics for the construction of surgical implants, their elastic moduli are much higher than that of human bone. This means that stresses are not transferred to the surrounding bone effectively, and this can cause irregular bone growth. To overcome this problem, interest has focused on using porous implant materials, with lower elastic moduli that are closer to that of bone, instead of the traditional solid implants [88]. Porous materials not only encourage more regular bone growth but also allow the bone to grow into the implant itself, thereby improving retention. Unfortunately, the corrosion rate of porous titanium in simulated body fluids has been reported to be significantly higher than that of solid titanium [89, 90]. In part, the increased corrosion rate is due to the fact that a porous structure has a much larger surface area exposed to the surrounding environment than its solid counterparts. However, it also appears that crevice corrosion occurs within the porous matrix. Furthermore, techniques that improve the properties of the passive film on solid titanium (e.g., anodizing) are less effective on porous titanium [91].

3.5.1.5 *Nickel–Titanium alloy*

The NiTi alloy has interesting memory-shape properties [92] which have resulted in interest in its potential use in both surgical and dental applications [34]. Although the corrosion resistance of NiTi has not yet been fully assessed, it appears to be slightly more resistant than 316L stainless steel [93]. The most common form of corrosion on NiTi is pitting, which raises the concern of how much nickel (toxic and carcinogenic) may be released into the body. Initial studies suggest that the answer depends on the local environment, with tests in artificial saliva showing similar Ni release rates for NiTi and 316L stainless steel [94], while in physiological simulating fluids, the NiTi releases three times as much nickel [95].

3.5.1.6 *Magnesium alloy*

Magnesium alloys are starting to be used as degradable implants for musculoskeletal surgery. In this case, controlled corrosion is a desirable feature as magnesium ions encourage bone cell activation allowing bone regeneration as the metal corrodes as well as eliminating the need for secondary surgeries for implant retrieval [96]. Magnesium alloys also have a lower stress shielding ratio than titanium and stainless steels, minimizing bone resorption [97]. However, the challenge is to tailor the corrosion rates of the Mg alloy to match the bone regrowth rate, with the added concern that if excessive hydrogen is produced by the supporting cathodic reaction it could lead to the formation of bubbles, which could even result in mortality [98]. The situation is complicated by the observations of Witte *et al.* [99] that *in-vivo* corrosion rates are up to four orders of magnitude lower than *in-vitro* rates, meaning that the present standard *in-vitro* corrosion tests will need to be modified before they will be able to predict the *in-vivo* corrosion rates of magnesium alloys [100].

Presently, Mg–Al and Mg–RE [101] (RE = rare earth elements) are being used for biomedical purposes; however, there are concerns about possible detrimental implications of the aluminum and rare earth elements on the human body, so researchers have more recently turned to Mg–Zn alloys. Xu *et al.* [102] have recently reviewed the corrosion of magnesium alloys designed for biomedical applications.

3.5.1.7   *Additive manufactured printed alloys*

In the last decade, biomedical devices were being produced by 3D printing and the corrosion performance of additively manufactured alloys was reviewed by Sander *et al.* [103]. In most cases, the corrosion performance of 3D printed alloys is slightly worse than cast samples, often due to increased porosity enabling localized crevice corrosion to initiate or a less controlled microstructure resulting in undesirable internal galvanic coupling within the alloy. The exceptions are stainless steels, where the laser melting process involved in the 3D printing evaporates the sulfide inclusions or at least reduces their size, resulting in improved resistance to pitting corrosion, in a fashion similar to the previously mentioned vacuum melted 316LVM grade.

3.5.2   *Dental Materials*

3.5.2.1   *Amalgams*

Modern dental amalgams are prepared mainly from two types of alloys. Conventional silver tin amalgam is prepared from a silver–tin alloy containing small amounts of copper and zinc. High copper amalgams are prepared from either a mixture of silver–tin and silver–copper alloys (admixed alloys) or from a ternary silver–copper–tin alloy (single composition alloys). The high copper amalgams have been reported to possess superior clinical properties with higher resistance to corrosion [72]. However, the corrosion of both types of amalgam is of concern as it leads to the release of toxic mercury into the body.

Dental amalgams are multiphase alloys (as they require high strength), exposing them to localized galvanic or intergranular corrosion between the different phases. In conventional amalgams, it is the phases that contain silver that are noble and cause accelerated corrosion of the non-silver phases, with the most vulnerable being the γ_2 phase (Sn_7Hg), which releases mercury when it corrodes [71]. The high copper amalgams contain no γ_2 phase and are thus more resistant to corrosion than silver–tin amalgams. The most corrosion-prone phase in high-copper amalgams is the η' phase (Cu_6Sn_5). However, preferential corrosion of the η' phase does not release mercury [73].

The high percentage of gold and other precious metal amalgams appear to be highly corrosion-resistant in nearly all oral environments. The exception appears to be when high fluoride levels are introduced into the mouth during some dental cleaning procedures which can result in pitting corrosion in gold alloys and also in titanium [104, 105].

Furthermore, in some patients, both silver-and gold-based amalgams can suffer from tarnishing, in which a thin black layer (probably a sulfide) develops across the surface. Although tarnishing does not dramatically affect the performance of the amalgam, nor is it likely to increase mercury release rates, it is unsightly and is thus of concern. However, the solution to the problem is more likely to be eliminating the source of the sulfide, e.g., changing the patient's diet, than replacing the amalgam with a more corrosion-resistant material.

3.5.2.2 *Rare earth magnets*

There are a number of ternary alloys containing rare elements, such as the NdFeB family, which have remarkably strong magnetic properties. This makes them desirable for a number of specialized medical applications, for example, as dental keepers. Unfortunately, these rare earth magnets have very poor corrosion resistance, corroding rapidly in a humid atmosphere. One approach to prevent this has been to completely seal the magnet inside stainless steel cladding; however, the stainless steel must not reduce the effectiveness of the magnetization, which rules out the austenitic steels. Ferritic stainless steels with chromium levels as high as 55% have been used, which should be sufficiently corrosion-resistant to survive in the oral cavity; however, particular attention has to be paid to the stainless steel seal, which is normally achieved by laser welding.

3.6 Detection Methods

There are several methods of monitoring and measuring the corrosion rate of a metal in an electrolyte. Detailed explanations of each of the techniques are beyond the scope of the present work, so the interested reader is advised to consult one of a number of specialized corrosion texts [106, 107]. Technical standards for corrosion testing include ASTM G1 for metal loss calculation, ASTM G46 for analysis of localized corrosion and NACE TM-01 for corrosion testing.

The simplest method, which requires just the minimum of equipment with hardly any specialized instrumentation, is the weight-loss method. In this method, the specimen tested is weighed after being thoroughly dried before and after the corrosion test, and the difference in weight is calculated. This gives an indication of the extent of corrosion that the specimen has undergone. In addition, visual inspection of the test sample reveals the type of corrosion that has occurred, e.g., pitting or general corrosion. However, in practice, the formation of oxide films, which represent weight gains, impedes the accuracy of this simple technique. Nevertheless, this is still the only technique that lends itself well to *in-vivo* trails.

The second method, which is more sophisticated, is to construct a Tafel plot. This is obtained by polarizing the specimen over a range of potentials, typically 300 mV on either side of the corrosion potential, measuring the resulting current, plotting the log of the current against applied potential and extrapolating the linear regions back to the corrosion potential, yielding the corrosion current density. However, in practice, the linear regions, which also provide the Tafel slopes, are often ill defined such that extrapolation becomes difficult, leading to large errors because of the log scale. In addition, steady-state currents should be measured making the technique very time-consuming.

The third method is the linear polarization resistance (LPR) method in which the specimen is perturbed by the application of a small potential (10 mV) and the steady-state current is recorded after a few minutes. Alternatively, the potential may be applied in the form of a slow ramp with the current monitored continuously. In both cases, a charge transfer resistance (R_{ct}) can be calculated from the applied potential and the resulting current. Simple equations are then used to convert R_{ct} into a corrosion rate. However, this method neglects effects due to non-Faradaic processes, such as the resistance of the solution and the double-layer capacitance. Moreover, the equations used to convert R_{ct} to a corrosion rate require knowledge of the Tafel slopes, which as mentioned above, may be inaccurate or unavailable.

The fourth, and more modern, technique is electrochemical impedance spectroscopy (EIS), which is somewhat similar to the

LPR technique except that the perturbing potential is applied over a range of frequencies (0.01 Hz to 10 kHz). This takes into account all the non-Faradaic processes giving a more accurate value of Rct. However, although EIS is a great improvement over earlier techniques, the presence of oxide films and mass transport effects can make data interpretation difficult, and knowledge of the Tafel slopes is still required.

The fifth, and most modern technique is electrochemical noise, in which two identical specimens are coupled together via a device called a zero-resistance ammeter, and the small fluctuations in the current flowing between them and their corrosion potential are simultaneously recorded. The so-called "noise resistance" can be extracted from the standard deviations in the current and voltage fluctuations, and this is believed to be equivalent to the R_{ct} of the LPR method. The main advantage of the noise technique is that the specimen is not perturbed, so there is no danger of the experiment altering the corrosion rate. However, in practice, this requires more sophisticated equipment, and once again the Tafel slopes are required to calculate the corrosion rate. As a result, electrochemical noise has not yet obtained the status where it can surpass the EIS technique.

The final method is potentiodynamic polarization, in which a slow positive potential ramp (1 mV/s) is applied to a specimen until the measured current exceeds some predetermined value. Unlike the other techniques, this does not provide a corrosion rate. Instead, information is obtained on whether the specimen forms a passive oxide film in a given environment, and if it does, how much resistance this film can provide against localized corrosion, e.g., pitting. The more positive the potential at which the specified current limit is exceeded, the more corrosion-resistant the specimen is.

3.7 Corrosion Prevention

As mentioned at the beginning of this chapter, most of the traditional methods of controlling corrosion cannot be used for surgical implants as the environment within the human body is fixed. The only methods available are to fabricate the implants from a corrosion-resistant alloy or to use a coating that must be able to withstand any abrasion and wear to which the device may be subjected. Nevertheless, there are a number of things that can be done to reduce the risk of corrosion-related failures of surgical implants [108, 109].

3.7.1 *Coatings and Surface Treatment*

Paints and other forms of organic coatings have a very limited role (if any) in protecting implants since these are unable to withstand abrasion. Coatings that may be of use include titanium or titanium nitride films on Ni–Ti memory-shaped alloys [110] and very high chromium ferritic stainless steel claddings on rare earth magnets used as dental keepers. The poor fretting resistance of the Ti6Al4V alloy represents its most serious drawback with regard to its use as an implant material, and thus, there has been considerable effort dedicated to improving its surface properties. The techniques that have given the most encouraging results are anodizing [16] and generating titanium nitride coatings either by ion implantation [62], magnetron sputtering [111] or nitriding [63, 64].

3.7.2 *Quality Control*

Many of the corrosion-related failures of surgical implants can be traced to poor quality control. Problems usually stem from one of two points in the supply line. Firstly, the manufacturer has not followed the appropriate standards (e.g., BS 7252, ISO 5832 or ASTM F138) during fabrication, metallurgical conditioning or application of the surface finishing of the implant. Secondly, since it is impossible to tell the composition of a metallic alloy simply by visible inspection, it is vital that the type of alloy is clearly labeled on all components and different alloys are stored separately. This second problem has been particularly associated with screws, for example, type 304L stainless steel screws have been used by mistake instead of the more corrosion-resistant type 316L. The adoption of a quality assurance system, along the lines recommended in ISO 9000, would eliminate these failures.

3.7.3 *Reduce the Risk of Galvanic Corrosion*

Wherever possible, the coupling of different metals and alloys (including different grades of stainless steels) should be avoided. However, it is recognized that this may not always be possible, for example, titanium alloys do not process the necessary tensile strength to be used as screws or wires so a galvanic couple may be unavoidable if a titanium alloy implant needs to be screwed or wired into possible. If such a situation should occur, it should be remembered that of the common implant materials, stainless steels are the most vulnerable to galvanic corrosion and thus should only be used in a couple as a last result, i.e., for the case of securing a titanium alloy implant, it would be far better to use screws fabricated from a cobalt–chrome alloy than from any grade of stainless steel [68, 112, 113].

3.7.4 *Handling/Sterilization/Assembly*

Scratches or small cracks on a surface can act as initiation points for both fatigue and corrosion, so it is important to handle all implants with great care and to avoid their scratching by other surgical tools. It would be preferable to keep all implants in protective packaging until the time of use.

Chloride ions are aggressive toward most metallic alloys, particularly at elevated temperatures. So, sterilization in saline solutions should be avoided. Although the sterilization procedure may only take a short period of time, it is still sufficient for small pits to develop on the surface of the implants, which can then act as initiation points for further corrosion or fatigue.

Contamination of an implant's surface can also lead to corrosion. Such contamination can result from the transfer of metal from surgical tools to the implant. It is thus recommended that drill guides be used to prevent contact between the drill and plates [105]. When assembling implants, care must be taken not to introduce additional crevices and the importance of stable fixation cannot be overstressed in reducing the risk of mechanical fatigue, corrosion fatigue and fretting. Suggestions of how to improve the fixation include plasma spraying a titanium coating with a specific surface roughness on the surface of the Ti6Al4V [114]; engineering the shape, topography and composition of the implant to provide either in-growth of tissue or enhanced on-growth of mineralized bone [115]; or depositing strongly adhered hydroxyapatite coatings which should fuse with the growing bone [116].

3.7.5   *Education*

Both surgical teams and dentists need to be aware of the basic causes of corrosion and fatigue, particularly the importance of avoiding bimetallic couples, careful handling of implants and providing stable fixation.

3.8   Case Histories

Case study A: A housewife, born in 1941, who had a history of tuberculosis of the left hip, had a fusion of her hip done in 1947, with limb length corrective surgery subsequently done at the level of mid-shaft with a femoral plate and screws. The implant was an 8-cm four-hole bone plate, with four 4-mm diameter screws, 28 mm in length. The plate and screws were not removed until 1997 (50 years later) when the patient complained of thigh and knee pain with an associated swelling on the right side. Histology of the tissue surrounding the implant site showed features consistent with foreign body reaction. The fibrous tissue was observed to have deposits of a black foreign material. No malignancy was seen in the tissue specimens. In removing the plate, the proximal quarter with the two proximal screws had to be broken off to ease the removal of the implants. Figure 3.10 shows that one end of the plate was badly corroded, especially under the screw heads, while the screws and the other end of the plate were less affected. The X-ray image on the right-hand side of Figure 3.10 reveals that the less corroded end of the plate was protected by an overgrown layer of bone; the remains of a drill bit accidentally left in the patient at the time of the original operation can also be seen. Analysis revealed that the plate was constructed from a ferritic stainless steel containing only 12% Cr while the screws were austenitic 304 stainless steel. A level of only 12% Cr is insufficient to prevent pitting corrosion on the plate body fluids and the situation was aggravated by the galvanic coupling to the 304 stainless steel screws leading to severe crevice corrosion beneath the screw heads.

Case study B [117]: Fatigue/fatigue corrosion can be noted on type 316L straight bone plate. Figure 3.11 shows X-rays of a plate that was used to treat pseudarthrosis in the proximal femur. It can

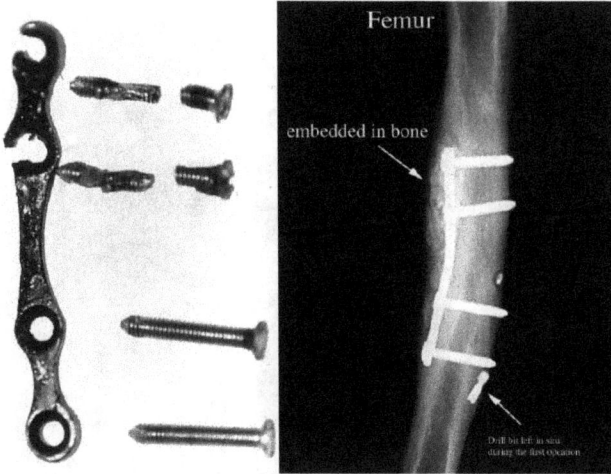

Figure 3.10. (Left) Sherman plate and screws removed from a patient after nearly 50 years of service. The 12%Cr plate is badly corroded, while the 304 stainless steel screws are in reasonable condition. (Right) X-ray showing that one end of the Sherman plate was covered by bone growth, which protected it from the corrosive environment.

be seen that because of an absence of bone in the area between screw hole numbers 5 and 6, no screws had been inserted at these locations. In Figure 3.11(a), a wide gap across the bone fracture is visible, which indicates instability. However, healing did not progress, so the plate was removed and replaced with an angled blade plate so that compression was exerted on the pseudarthrosis promoting bone healing. Investigation of the removed plate at high magnification revealed fatigue cracks on the top surface of a small section at the fifth screw hole, indicated by a box in Figure 3.11(a). Since hole number 5 was located at the transition between the bone and the defect, it was likely to have been exposed to high stress concentrations. However, no damage was seen at the other empty screw hole, number 6, which was located directly over the bone defect, where the elastic deformation could occur more uniformly. Slight fretting corrosion was also found at most of the screw/plate interfaces, being particularly noticeable in hole number 7. This hole was the closest to the fracture and had a relatively short screw, so it was the one likely to undergo the most motion, leading to the observed corrosion fatigue.

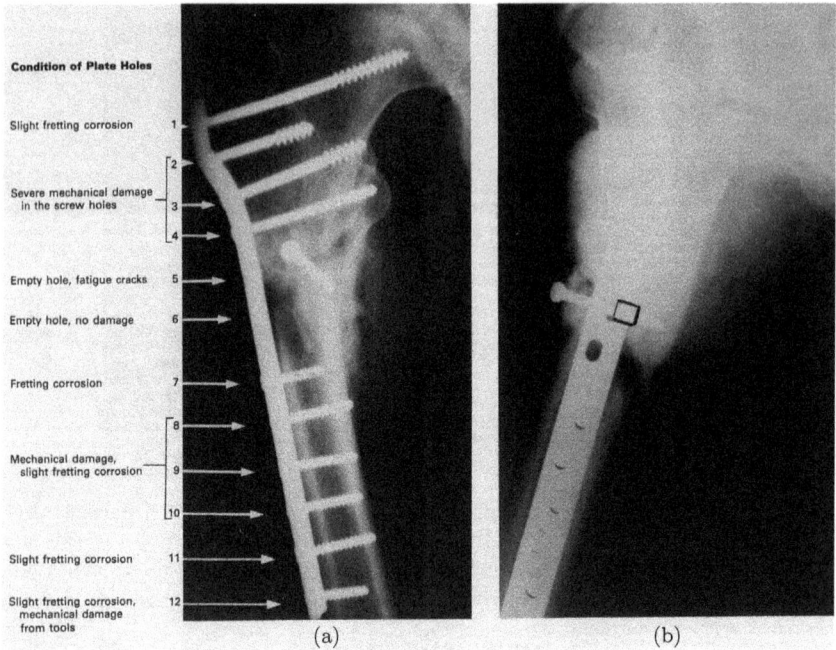

Figure 3.11. Crack initiation on type 316L stainless steel compression plate: (a) anterior–posterior X-ray; (b) lateral view, with a box indicating the location of fatigue crack initiation (Reproduced with permission from Ref. [109]).

Case study C [109]: Fretting and fretting corrosion can be noted between the screw head and the plate, both components being fabricated from type 316L stainless steel. Figure 3.12(a) shows that only grinding and polishing occurred over most of the contact area. However, at higher magnification of Figure 3.12(b), fine corrosion pits are visible. Evidence of intense mechanical material transfer from fretting in the form of a material tongue can be seen in the upper right corner of Figures 3.12(c) and 3.12(d). Figure 3.12(d) also shows a corrosion pit in front of the material tongue surrounded by a burnished surface texture, which may have broken open at some point. This is consistent with observations from other implants in which material layers are smeared over each other during wear and attacked by pitting corrosion [100]. Later, future wear causes these pits to be covered by a new burnished material film, which can then be broken open again. The products of this corrosion and wear process are transported in the surrounding tissue.

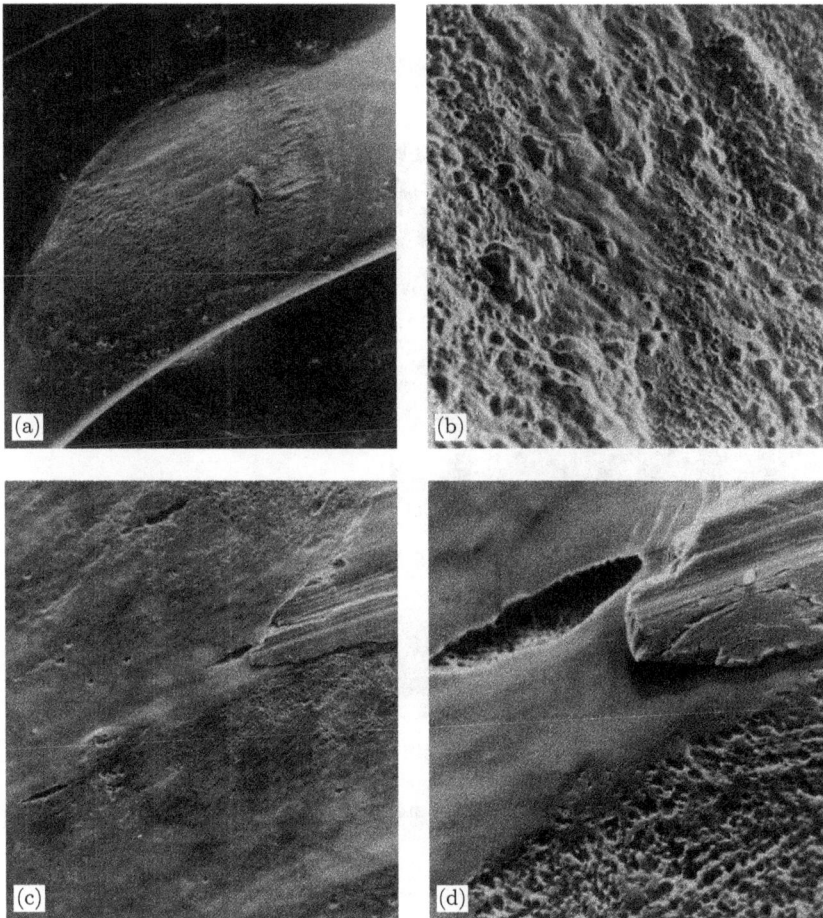

Figure 3.12. Fretting and fretting corrosion between screw head and plate, both components being fabricated from type 316L stainless steel. Magnifications: (a) 8x; (b) 190x; (c) 190x; (d) 345x (Reproduced with permission from Ref. [109]).

Case study D [109]: Broken stem of femoral head component of total hip prosthesis made from cast cobalt-base alloy can be seen in Figure 3.13. Radiotranslucency was visible around the collar of the femoral head prosthesis on an X-ray taken 5 months after implantation into a 65-year-old man. One month later, failure of the bond cement at the distal end of the stem occurred, and a small notch on the lateral edge of the prosthesis was visible, at this point the stem broke two weeks later. Figure 3.13(a) shows an X-ray of the broken

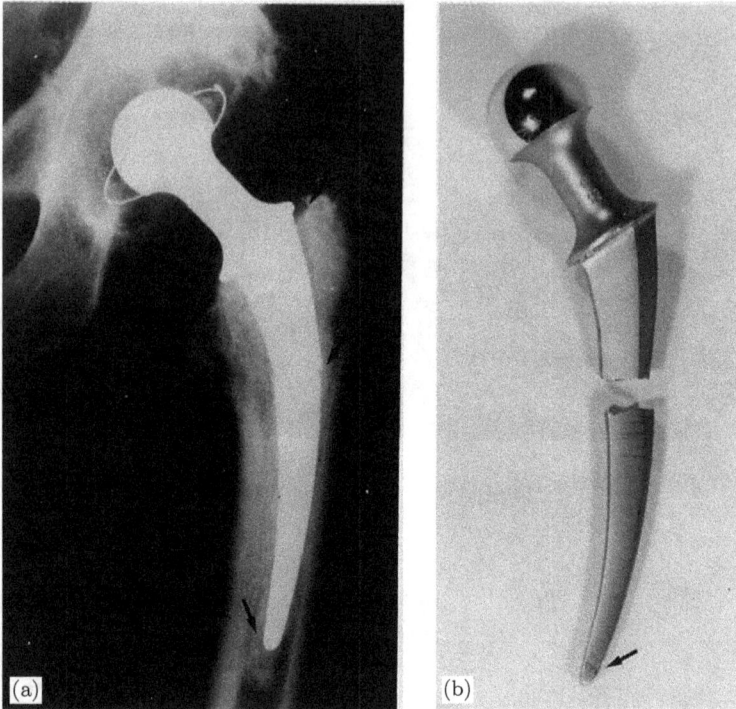

Figure 3.13. Broken CoCrMo alloy hip prosthesis: (a) X-ray of total hip prosthesis, with arrows showing areas of loosening; (b) fractured stem, with arrow showing area of heavy wear at base of stem (Reproduced with permission from Ref. [109]).

prosthesis from which the loosening of the implant can be observed as a gap between the lateral stem edge and the bone cement. The resultant movement under weight-bearing led to fatigue and eventual fracture. Figure 3.13(b) shows the broken prosthesis component, extensive rubbing against bone cement, due to the loosening, caused the heavy wear seen at the base of the stem (as marked by the arrow).

Case study E [105]: After a patient had complained of pain and disability in a repaired shoulder fracture, the screws were removed and analyzed (Figure 3.14). One was formed from CoCrMo, while the others were all stainless steel. The galvanic corrosion, along with the electrical currents generated by the electrochemical cell, was responsible for the patient's pain.

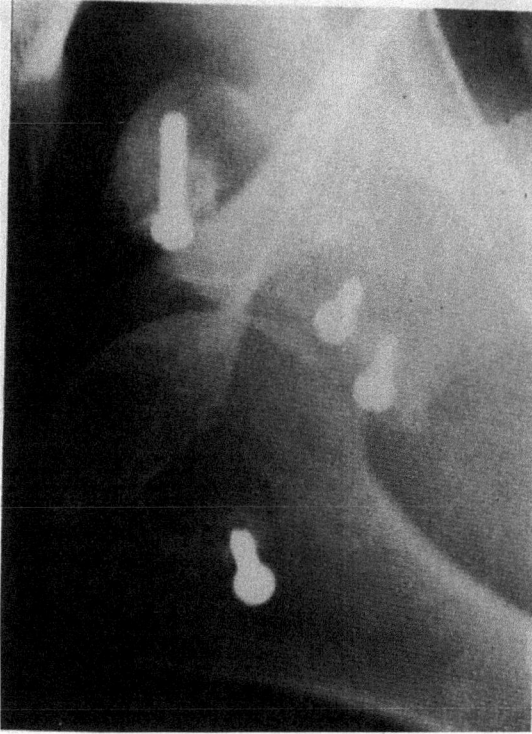

Figure 3.14. X-ray of a repaired shoulder. Examination of the screws revealed one to be CoCrMo and the others to be stainless steel. The resulting galvanic corrosion was the source of the patient's pain (Reproduced with permission from Ref. [105]).

Case study F: The male patient had previously fractured both his right ulna and radius at the mid-shift region in a road traffic accident. This was around 1960 when both fractures were closed with bone plates and screws. He was 13 years old then. In 1998, he again fractured his right radius and ulna in another road traffic accident. Both fractures were at the distal screws of the plate fixation (Figure 3.15). The old plates were removed, after being *in situ* for about 38 years, and the fracture was closed with two new plate implants. No inflammation or black material in the surrounding soft tissue was noted. The implants were 4-cm three-hole bone plates, each with three 3-mm diameter screws, 14-mm in length. Both plates and their respective screws were removed intact with remarkably little corrosion with just

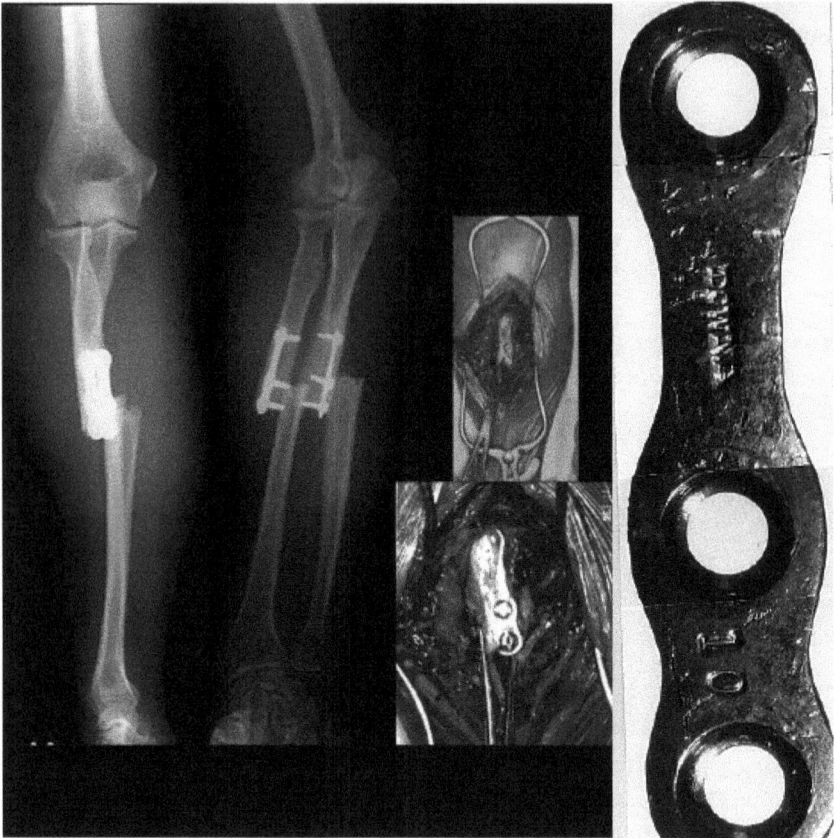

Figure 3.15. (Left) X-ray showing a 304 stainless steel Sherman plate that had to be removed after 38 years as the patient had a second road accident. (Right) Close-up of the Sherman plate on which the manufacturer's name (DOWN.A) can still be clearly seen.

a few scratches which were obtained during retrieval and the manufacturer's name "DOWN.A" was still clearly visible (Figure 3.15).

The surgeon who removed the plate and screws was sufficiently impressed to enquire why not all implants were made of such highly corrosion-resistant alloys. Surprisingly analysis of the plate and screws revealed that both were 304 stainless steel, a material that is now considered unsuitable for surgical implants due to its poor track record, particularly with respect to suffering pitting corrosion. It was proposed that the low dissolved oxygen levels found in human-body fluids make the long-term *in-vivo* environment much more benign than would be anticipated from *in-vitro* experiments. Furthermore, the Sherman plate was sufficiently small so that the surrounding tissue was not aggravated sufficiently to lead to the development of an environment aggressive enough to cause the pitting of 304 stainless steel.

3.9   Summary and Conclusions

Corrosion was a serious problem with early implant materials. However, knowledge of corrosion and mechanical properties of biomaterials has allowed the development of a number of extremely successful alloys, e.g., Ti6Al4V, 316LVM and the ASTM F1058 CoCrNiMo alloy, and it is certain that improved versions of these alloys will be developed in the future. As a result, as long as the chosen materials match the requirements of national and international standards, such as ISO 5832, the likelihood of a surgical implant suffering a corrosion-related failure is very small. Most modern failures tend to be due to poor quality control, leading to either the wrong choice of material or the use of mismatched materials, which results in galvanic corrosion.

Modern alloys have also reduced the extent to which potentially hazardous metallic ions leach out of biomedical devices. Nevertheless, the concern that extended exposure to even very low levels of corrosion products could result in medical complications remains in part due to a lack of knowledge as to what are safe levels for transition metal ions in the body. Thus, there is still a continuing need to further reduce passive corrosion rates.

References

[1]   M. F. LeClerc, Surgical implants, in *Corrosion*, Vol. 1, 3rd Edition, eds. L. L. Shrier, R. A. Jarman, and G. T. Burstein, (Butterworth Heinemann, Oxford, 1994) Chp. 2.13.

[2]   P. S. P. Thong, F. Watt, D. Ponraj, S. K. Leong, Y. He, and T. K. Y. Lee, Iron and cell death in Parkinson's disease: A nuclear microscopic study into iron-rich granules in the parkinsonian substantia nigra of primate models, *Nucl. Instrum. Methods Phys. Res., Sect. B*, 1999, 158:349–355.

[3] I. M. C. Lundstrom, Allergy and corrosion of dental materials in patients with oral lichen planus, *Int. J. Oral Surg.*, 1982, 12:1–9.

[4] J. Banoczy, B. Roed-Petersen, J. J. Pindborg, and J. Inovay, Clinical and histologic studies on electrogalvanically induced oral white lesions, *Oral Surg., Oral Med., Oral Pathol.*, 1979, 48:319–323.

[5] M. Pourbaix, *Atlas of electrochemical equilibria in aqueous solutions*, 2nd Edition (National Association of Corrosion Engineers, Houston, 1974).

[6] D. J. Blackwood, R. Peat, and A. M. Pritchard, In-situ imaging of corrosion processes, *Mater. Sci. Forum*, 1995, 192–193:693–709.

[7] L. L. Hench, Bioactive glasses and glass-ceramics, *Mater. Sci. Forum*, 1999, 293:37–63.

[8] Southampton Electrochemistry Group, *Instrumental Methods in Electrochemistry*, eds. R. Greef, R. Peat, L. M. Peter, D. Pletcher, and J. Robinson, (Ellis Horwood, Chichester, 1985) pp. 33–35, 233–242.

[9] G. T. Burstein, Passivity and localised corrosion, in *Corrosion*, Vol. 1, 3rd Edition, eds. L. L. Shrier, R. A. Jarman, and G. T. Burstein, (Butterworth Heinemann, Oxford, 1994) Chp. 1.5.

[10] L. Young, Anodic Oxide Films, (Academic Press, London, 1961).

[11] P. Tengvall and I. Lundstrom, Physico-chemical considerations of titanium as a biomaterial, *Clin. Mater.*, 1992, 9:115–134.

[12] N. B. Pilling and R. E. Bedworth, Oxidation of metals at high temperatures, *J. Inst. Met.*, 1923, 29:529–583.

[13] D. E. Williams and G. A. Wright, Nucleation and growth of anodic oxide films on bismuth. I. Cyclic voltammetry, *Electrochim. Acta*, 1976, 21:1009–1019.

[14] A. H. Tuthill and R. E. Avery, Specifying stainless steel surface treatments, *Adv. Mater. Process.*, 1992, 12:34–38.

[15] G. S. Frankel, Pitting corrosion of metals: A review of the critical factors, *J. Electrochem. Soc.*, 1998, 145:2186–2198.

[16] J. A. Disegi, Anodizing treatments for titanium implants, in *Proc. 16th South. Biomedical Eng. Conf.*, eds. J. D. Bumgardner and A. D. Pucknett (Institute of Electrical and Electronics Engineers, New York, 1997) pp. 129–132.

[17] D. J. Blackwood, L. M. Peter, and D. E. Williams, Stability and open circuit breakdown of passive films on titanium, *Electrochim. Acta*, 1988, 33:1143–1149.

[18] D. A. Jones, *Principles and Prevention of Corrosion*, 2nd Edition, (Prentice Hall, New Jersey 1996), pp. 187–188, 525–526.

[19] M. Traisnel, D. Le Maguer, H. F. Hildebrand, and A. Iost, Corrosion of surgical implants, *Clin. Mater.*, 1990, 5:309–318.

[20] K. Endo, Y. Abiko, M. Suzuki, H. Ohno, and T. Kaku, Corrosion resistance and biocompatibility of high-nitrogen stainless steels, *Zairyo to Kankyo*, 1998, 47:570–576.

[21] J. Stewart and D. E. Williams, The initiation of pitting corrosion on austenitic stainless steel: On the role and importance of sulfide inclusions, *Corros. Sci.*, 1992, 33:457–474.

[22] M. G. S. Ferreira, T. M. Silva, and A. Catarino, Electrochemical and laser Raman spectroscopy studies of stainless steel in 0.15M sodium chloride solution, *J. Electrochem. Soc.*, 1992, 145:3146–3151.

[23] H. Zitter, Case histories on surgical implants and their causes, *Werkst. Korros.*, 1991, 42:455–466.

[24] H. J. Mueller and E. H. Greener, Polarization studies on surgical materials in Ringer's solution, *J. Biomed. Mater. Res.*, 1970, 4: 29–41.

[25] B. C. Syrett and S. S. Wing, Pitting resistance of new and conventional orthopaedic implant materials, *Corrosion*, 1978, 34:138–145.

[26] B. C. Syrett and E. E. Davis, Crevice corrosion of implant alloys: A comparison of the in-vitro and in-vivo studies, *ASTM STP*, 1979, 684:229–244.

[27] F. R. Morral, Metallurgy of cobalt alloys: 1968 review, *JOM*, 1968, 20:52–59.

[28] J. Cohen and J. Wulff, Clinical failure caused by corrosion of a vitallium plate, *J. Bone Joint Surg.*, 1972, 54A:617–628.

[29] C. O. Clerc, M. R. Jedwab, D. W. Mayer, P. J. Thompson, and J. S. Stinson, Assessment of wrought ASTM F1058 cobalt alloy properties for permanent surgical implants, *J. Biomed. Mater. Res.*, 1997, 38:229–234.

[30] L. C. Lucus, R. A. Buchanan, J. E. Lemons, and C. D. Griffin, Susceptibility of surgical cobalt-base alloy to pitting corrosion, *J. Biomed. Mater. Res.*, 1982, 16:799–810.

[31] J. Cohen, Corrosion testing of orthopedic implants, *J. Bone Joint Surg.*, 1962, 44A:307–316.

[32] M. Chew, Electrodeposition of calcium phosphate on titanium and its alloys, BSc (Hons) thesis, (National University of Singapore, 2002) pp. 17–18.

[33] G. Rondelli, B. Vicentini, and A. Cigada, The corrosion behaviour of nickel titanium shape memory alloys, *Corro. Sci.*, 1990, 30:805–812.

[34] D. Mantovani, Shape memory alloys: Properties and biomedical applications, *JOM*, 2000, 52:36–44.

[35] K. H. W. Seah and X. Chen, A comparison between the corrosion characteristics of 316 stainless steel, solid titanium and porous titanium, *Corros. Sci.*, 1993, 34:1841–1851.

[36] J. T. Scales, G. D. Winter, and H. T. Shirley, Corrosion of orthopedic implants, *J. Bone Joint Surg.*, 1959, 41B:810–820.

[37] J. A. Disegi and L. D. Zardiackas, Microstructural features of implant quality 316L stainless steel, in *Advances in the Production and Use of Steel with Improved Internal Cleanliness*, ed. J. K. Mahaney, *ASTM STP*, 1999, 1361:49–56.

[38] J. Galante and W. Rostoker, Corrosion: Related failures in metallic implants and experimental study, *Clin. Orthop. Relat. Res.*, 1972, 86:237–244.

[39] K. H. W. Seah, R. Thampuran, and S. H. Teoh, The influence of pore morphology on corrosion, *Corros. Sci.*, 1998, 40:547–556.

[40] B. S. Becker and J. D. Bolton, Production of porous sintered Co-Cr-Mo alloys for possible surgical implant applications. Part 2: Corrosion behaviour, *Powder Metal*, 1995, 38:305–313.

[41] R. N. Parkins, Mechanisms of stress corrosion cracking, in *Corrosion*, Vol. 1, 3rd Edition, eds. L. L. Shrier, R. A. Jarman, and G. T. Burstein (Butterworth Heinemann, Oxford, 1994) Chp. 8.1.

[42] R. H. Jones and B. Craig, Environmentally induced cracking: Stress-corrosion cracking, in *Metals Handbook — Vol 13: Corrosion*, 9th Edition, eds. L. J. Korb, D. L. Olson, and J. R. Davis (ASM, Ohio, 1987) pp. 145–163.

[43] S. Tsujikawa, Y. Ishihara, and T. Shinohara, Failure analysis of stress corrosion cracking of type 304 steel tubes for hot-water use in Kusatsu town, Gunma Prefecture, *Zairyo to Kankyo*, 1993, 42: 20–26.

[44] K. Tamaki, S. Tsujikawa, and Y. Hisamatsu. T. Shinohara, and C. Liang, Development of a new test method for chloride stress corrosion cracking of stainless steels in dilute sodium chloride solutions, in NACE 9-*Advances in Localised Corrosion: Proc 2nd Inter. Conf. Localized Corrosion*, Orlando 1987, eds. H. Isaacs, U. Bertocci J. Kruger, and Z. Szklarska-Smialowska (National Association of Corrosion Engineers, Houston, 1990) pp. 207–214.

[45] T. Haruna and T. Shibata, Initiation and growth of stress corrosion cracks in type 316L stainless steel during slow strain rate testing,*Corrosion*, 1994, 50:758–791.

[46] S. Tsujikawa, T. Shinohara, and Y. Hisamatsu, The role of crevices in comparison to pits in initiating stress corrosion cracks of type 310S steel in different concentrations of magnesium chloride solutions at 80°C, in *Corrosion Cracking: Proc. Corros. Cracking Program Relat. Pap. 1985*, ed. V. S. Goel (ASM, Ohio, 1986) pp. 35–42.

[47] J. R. Cahoon and H. W. Paxton, Metallurgical analysis of failed orthopaedic implants, *J. Biomed. Mater. Res.*, 1968, 2:1–22.

[48] J. P. Sheehan, C. R. Morris, and K. F. Packer, Study of stress corrosion cracking susceptibility of type 316L stainless steel in vitro, in *Corrosion and Degradation of Implant Materials, 2nd Symposium*, eds. A. C. Fraker and C. D. Griffin (ATSM STP, West Conshohocken, PA, USA, 1985) Vol. 859, pp. 57–72.

[49] B. J. Edwards, M. R. Louthan, and R. D. Sission, Hydrogen embrittlement of Zimaloy: A cobalt-chromium-molybdenum orthopedic implant alloy, in *Corrosion and Degradation of Implant Materials, 2nd Symposium*, eds. A. C. Fraker and C. D. Griffin (ATSM STP, West Conshohocken, PA, USA, 1985) Vol. 859, pp. 11–29.

[50] K. J. Bundy and V. H. Desai, Studies of stress corrosion cracking susceptibility of type 316 stainless steel in-vitro, in *Corrosion and Degradation of Implant Materials, 2nd Symposium*, eds. A. C. Fraker and C. D. Griffin (ATSM STP, West Conshohocken, PA, USA, 1985) Vol. 859, pp. 73–90.

[51] R. C. Newman and R. P. M. Procter, Sress corrosion racking: 1965–1990, *Br. Corros. J.*, 1990, 25:259–269.

[52] M. F. Leclerc, A review of the factors influencing the mechanical failure of the femoral component used in total hip replacement, in *Proc. Eng, Ortho. Surg. Rehab.*, (Bioengineering Unit, Princess Margaret Rose Hospital, Edinburgh, 1982) pp. 36–48.

[53] M. Morita, T. Sasada, H, Hayashi, and Y. Tsukamoto, The corrosion fatigue properties of surgical implants in a living body, *J. Biomed. Mater. Res.*, 1988, 22:529–540.

[54] C. O. Bechtol, Failure of femoral implant components in total hip replacement operations, *Orthop. Rev.*, 1975, 4:23–29.

[55] M. von Knoch, A. Bluhm, M. Morlock, and G. von Förster, Surface roughness changes of non-polished femoral components of artifical hip joints during 2 to 15 years in service, *J. Arthroplasty*, 2003, 18:471–477.

[56] A. N. Hughes, B. A. Jordan, and S. Orman, The corrosion fatigue properties of surgical implant materials: Third progress report — May 1973, *Eng. Med.*, 1978, 7:135–141.

[57] J. Yu, Z. J. Zhao, and L. X. Li, Corrosion fatigue resistances of surgical implant stainless steels and titanium alloy, *Corros. Sci.*, 1993, 35:587–597.

[58] H. R. Piehler, M. A. Portnoff, L. E. Sloter, E. J. Vegdahl, J. L. Gilbert, and M. J. Weber, Corrosion-fatigue performance of hip nails: The influence of materials selection and design, in *Corrosion and Degradation of Implant Materials, 2nd Symposium*, eds. A. C. Fraker and C. D. Griffin (ATSM STP, West Conshohocken, PA, USA, 1985) Vol. 859, pp. 93–104.

[59] B. C. Syrett and S. S. Wing, An electrochemical investigation of fretting corrosion of surgical implant materials, *Corrosion,* 1978, 34:379–386.

[60] M. G. Fontana, *Corrosion Engineering,* 3rd Edition (McGraw-Hill, Singapore, 1987) p. 109.

[61] J. Rieu, L. M. Rabbe and P. Combrade, Fretting wear corrosion of surgical implant alloys: Effects of ion implantation and ion nitriding on the fretting behavior of metals/PMMA contacts, in *Proc. 8th Inter. Conf. Surf. Modification Tech.,* Nice, 1994, eds. T. S. Sudarshan and M. Jeandin (Institute of Materials, London, 1995) pp. 43–52.

[62] R. A. Buchanan, E. D. Rigney, and J. M. Williams, Ion implantation of surgical Ti-6Al-4V for improved resistance to wear-accelerated corrosion, *J. Biomed. Mater. Res.,* 1987, 21:355–366.

[63] A. Shenhar, I. Gotman, S. Radin, P. Ducheyne, and E. Y. Gutmanas, Titanium nitride coatings on surgical titanium alloys produced by powder immersion reaction assisted coating method: Residual stresses and fretting behaviour, *Surf. Coat. Technol.,* 2000, 126: 210–218.

[64] D. Starosvetsky, A. Shenhar, and I. Gotman, Corrosion behaviour of PIRAC nitrided Ti-6Al-4V surgical alloy, *J. Mater. Sci.: Mater. Med.,* 2001, 12:145–150.

[65] J. A. von Fraunhofer, Corrosion in the oral cavity, in *Corrosion,* Vol. 1, 3rd Edition, eds. L. L. Shrier, R. A. Jarman, and G. T. Burstein, (Butterworth Heinemann, Oxford, 1994) Chp. 2.14.

[66] H. P. Hack and D. Taylor, Evaluation of galvanic corrosion, in *Metals Handbook — Vol 13: Corrosion,* 9th Edition, eds. L. J. Korb, D. L. Olson, and J. R. Davis, (ASM, Ohio, 1987) pp. 234–241.

[67] M. J. Pryor and D. J. Astley, Bimetallic corrosion, in *Corrosion,* Vol. 1, 3rd Edition, eds. L. L. Shrier, R. A. Jarman, and G. T. Burstein (Butterworth Heinemann, Oxford, 1994) Chp. 1.7.

[68] W. Rostoker, C. W. Pretzel, and J. O. Galante, Couple corrosion among alloys for skeletal prostheses, *J. Biomed. Mater. Res.,* 1974, 8:407–419.

[69] D. C. Mears, The use of dissimilar metals in surgery, *J. Biomed. Mater. Res. (Symp.),* 1975, 6:133–148.

[70] H. Jackson-Burrows, J. N. Wilson, and J. T. Scales, Excision of tumors of humerus and femur with restoration of internal prostheses, *J. Bone Joint Surg.,* 1975, 57B:148–59.

[71] J. A. von Fraunhofer and P. J. Staheli, Corrosion of dental amalgam, *Nature,* 1972, 240:304–306.

[72] N. K. Sarkar and C. S. Eyer, The microstructural basis of creepin dental amalgam, *J. Oral Rehab.,* 1987, 14:27–33.

[73] B. M. Eley, The future of dental amalgam: A review of the literature. Part 1: Dental amalgam structure and corrosion, *Brit. Dent. J.*, 1997, 182:247–249.

[74] T. Newton, Dental fillings, *Chem. Br.*, 2002, 38(10):24–27.

[75] P. Mueller, and C. Rodig, Dispersion hardening behavior of cold-formed X2CrNiMoN18.12 steel for surgical implants, *Neue Huette*, 1989, 34:378–381.

[76] R. J. Solar, Corrosion resistance of titanium surgical implant alloys: A review, in *Corros. Degradation Implant Mater.*, eds. B. C. Syrett and A. Acharya, *ASTM STP*, 1979, 684:259–273.

[77] B. Jacobson and J. B. Webster, Surgery, in *Medicine and clinical engineering*, eds. B. Jacobson and J. B. Webster, (Prentice-Hall, New Jersey, 1977) Chp. 10.

[78] P. G. Liang, Compatibility of biomaterials, *Orthop. Clinc. Nor. Am.*, 1973, 4:249–273.

[79] P. Thomsen and L. E. Ericson in *The Bone-Biomaterial Interface*, ed. J. E. Davis (University of Toronto Press, Toronto, 1991) pp. 153–164.

[80] N. D. Greene, Corrosion of surgical alloys: A few basic ideas, in *Corrosion and Degradation of Implant Materials, 2nd Symposium*, eds. A. C. Fraker and C. D. Griffin (ATSM STP, West Conshohocken, PA, USA, 1985) Vol. 859, pp. 5–10.

[81] S. Ciolac, E. Vasilescu, P. Drob, M. V. Popa, and M. Anghel, Long-term in vitro study of titanium and some titanium alloys used in surgical implants, *Rev. Chim. (Bucharest)*, 2000, 51:36–41.

[82] R. Schenk in *Titanium in Medicine: Material Science, Surface Science, Engineering, Biological Responses, and Medical Applications*, eds. D. M. Brunette, P. Tengvall, M. Textor, and P. Thomsen, (Springer, Berlin, 2001) pp. 145–170.

[83] T. Fusayama, T. Katayori, and S. Nomoto, Corrosion of gold and amalgam placed in contact with each other, *J. Dent. Res.*, 1963, 42:1183–1197.

[84] A. U. J. Yap, B. L. Ng, and D. J. Blackwood, Corrosion behaviour of high copper dental amalgams, *J. Oral Rehab.*, 2004, 31:595–599.

[85] S. Joyston-Bechal and E. A. M. Kidd, Update on the appropriate uses of fluoride, *Dental Update*, 1994, 21:366–371.

[86] A. C. Fraker, Corrosion of metallic implants and prosthetic devices, in *Metals Handbook — Vol 13: Corrosion*, 9th Edition, eds. L. J. Korb, D. L. Olson, and J. R. Davis (ASM, Ohio, 1987) pp. 1325–1335.

[87] G. H. Hille, Titanium for surgical implants, *J. Materials*, 1966, 1:373–383.

[88] M. Spector, M. J. Michno, W. H. Smarook, and G. T. Kwiatkowski, A high-modulus polymer for porous orthopedic implants: Biomechanical compatibility of porous implants, *J. Biomed. Mater. Res.*, 1978, 12:665–677.

[89] K. H. W. Seah, R. Thampuran, X. Chen, and S. H. Teoh, A comparison between the corrosion behaviour of sintered and unsintered porous titanium, *Corros. Sci.*, 1995, 37:1333–1340.

[90] D. J. Blackwood, A. W. C. Chua, K. W. H. Seah, R. Thampuran, and S. H. Teoh, Corrosion behaviour of porous titanium-graphite composites designed for surgical implants, *Corros. Sci.*, 2000, 42:481–503.

[91] D. J. Blackwood and S. K. M. Chooi, Stability of protective oxide films films formed on porous titanium, *Corros. Sci.*, 2002, 44:395–405.

[92] F. X. Gil, J. M. Manero, and J. A. Planell, Relevant aspects in the clinical applications of NiTi shape memory alloys, *J. Mater. Sci.: Mater. Med.*, 1996, 7:403–406.

[93] J. Ryhänen, E. Niemi, W. Serlo, E. Niemelä, P. Sandvik, H. Pernu, and T. Salo, Biocompatibility of nickel-titanium shape memory metal and its corrosion behavior in human cell cultures, *J Biomed Mater Res.*, 1997, 35:451–457.

[94] R. D. Barrett, S. E. Bishara, and J. K. Quinn, Biodegradation of orthodontic appliances. Part 1. Biodegradation of nickel and chromium in vitro, *Am. J. Orthod. Dentofacial. Orthop.*, 1993, 103:8–14.

[95] G. Rondelli, Corrosion resistance tests on NiTi shape memory alloy, *Biomaterials*, 1996, 17:2003–2008.

[96] F. Witte, V. Kaese, H. Haferkamp, E. Switzer, A. Meyer-Lindenberg, C. J. Wirth, and H. Windhagen, In vivo corrosion of four magnesium alloys and the associated bone response, *Biomaterials*, 2005, 26:3557–3563.

[97] O. Kurdi, Rusnaldy, A. Suprihanto, Muchammad, H. Rachma, A. R. Leoni, and I. Yulianti, Determination of stress shielding due to magnesium internal bone fixation, *AIP Conf. Proc.*, 2020, 2262:030018.

[98] D. Noviana, D. Paramitha, M. F. Ulum, and H. Hermawan, The effect of hydrogen gas evolution of magnesium implant on the postimplantation mortality of rats, *J. Orthop. Transl.*, 2016, 5: 9–15.

[99] F. Witte, J. Fischer, J. Nellesen, H. A. Crostack, V. Kaese, A. Pisch, F. Beckmann, and H. Windhagen, In vitro and in vivo corrosion measurements of magnesium alloys, *Biomaterials*, 2005, 27:1013–1018.

[100] K. X. Kuah, S. Wijesinghe, and D. J. Blackwood, Toward understanding in vivo corrosion: Influence of interfacial hydrogen gas build-up on degradation of magnesium alloy implants, *J. Biomed. Mater. Res. A*, 2023, 111:60–70.

[101] X. Gu, Y. Zheng, Y. Cheng, S. Zhong, and T. Xi, In vitro corrosion and biocompatibility of binary magnesium alloys, *Biomaterials*, 2009, 30:484–498.

[102] L. Xu , X. Liu, K. Sun, R. Fu, and G. Wang, Corrosion behavior in magnesium-based alloys for biomedical applications, *Materials*, 2022, 15:2613.

[103] G. Sander, J. Tan, P. Balan, O. Gharbi, D. R. Feenstra, L. Singer, S. Thomas, R. G. Kelly, J. R. Scully, and N. Birbilis, Corrosion of additively manufactured alloys: A review, *Corrosion*, 2018, 74:1318–1350.

[104] L. Reclaru and J. M. Meyer, Effects of fluorides on titanium and other dental alloys in dentistry, *Biomaterials,* 1998, 19:85–92.

[105] E. Lenz, Der einfluss von fluoriden auf das korrosionsverhalten von titan, *Dtsch. Zahnärztl. Z.*, 1997, 52:351–354.

[106] R. G. Kelly, J. R. Scully, D. W. Shoesmith, and R. G. Buchheit, *Electrochemical Techniques in Corrosion Science and Engineering* (Marcel Dekker, New York, 2002).

[107] K. R. Trethewey and J. Chambe rlain, *Corrosion for science and engineering*, 2nd edition, (Longman Harlow, Essex, 1995).

[108] U. Kamachi Mudali, T. M. Sridhar, N. Eliaz, and B. Raj, Failure of stainless steel implants: Causes and remedies, *Corrosion Reviews*, 2003, 21:231–267.

[109] D. Sharan, The problem of corrosion in orthopaedic implant materials, *Orthop. Update (India)*, 1999, 9:1–5.

[110] D. Starosvetsky and I. Gotman, Corrosion behavior of titaniumnitride coated Ni-Ti shape memory surgical alloy, *Biomaterials,* 2001, 22:1853–1859.

[111] R. Hubler, Hardness and corrosion protection enhancement behavior of surgical implant surfaces treated with ceramic thin films, *Surf. Coat. Technol.,* 1999, 116–119:1111–1115.

[112] C. D. Griffin, R. A. Buchanan, and J. E. lemons, In vivo electrochemical corrosion study of coupled surgical implant materials, *J. Biomed. Mater. Res.*, 1983, 17:489–500.

[113] J. B. Park and R. S. Lakes, Metallic implant materials, in *Biomaterials: An Introduction* (Plenum Press, New York 1992) pp. 75–115.

[114] B. Normand, F. Renaud, C. Coddet, and F. Tourenne, The effect of spraying conditions on the corrosion resistance of titanium

coatings for surgical implants, in *Proc. 9th Natl. Thermal Spraying Conf.*, ed. C. S. Berndt (ASM, Materials Park, Ohio, 1996) pp. 73–78.

[115] J. E. Lemons, Surface modifications of surgical implants, *Surf. Coat. Technol.*, 1998, 103–104:135–137.

[116] K. Hayashi, T. Mashima, and K., Uenoyama, The effect of hydroxyapatite coating by bony ingrowth into grooved titanium implants, *Biomaterials*, 1999, 20:111–119.

[117] E. M. Ortrun, Failures of metallic orthopaedic implants, in *Metals Handbook — Vol 11: Failure Analysis and Prevention*, 9th Edition, eds. R. J Shipley and W. T. Becker, (ASM, Ohio, 1986) pp. 670–694.

Chapter 4

Surface Modification of Metallic Biomaterials

Takao Hanawa

Institute of Biomaterials and Bioengineering,
Tokyo Medical and Dental University,
2-3-10 Kanda-Surugadai, Chiyoda-ku, Tokyo 101–0062, Japan
hanawa.met@tmd.ac.jp

When a metallic material is implanted into a human body, an immediate reaction occurs between its surface and the living tissues. In other words, the immediate reaction at this initial stage straightaway determines and defines a metallic material's tissue compatibility. Since conventional metallic biomaterials are usually covered with metal oxides, surface oxide films on metallic materials play an important role not only against corrosion but also in tissue compatibility. The surface properties of a metallic material may be controlled using surface modification techniques. To develop and apply the appropriate surface modification technique, knowledge of the material's surface composition is absolutely necessary. This is because surface modification is a process that improves surface property by changing the composition and structure while leaving the mechanical properties of the material intact. Since surface properties are critically important in biomaterials, issues closely related to this aspect of metallic biomaterials are discussed here: surface compositions of metallic biomaterials; how surface compositions change due to interaction with human tissues; how to control surface compositions and morphologies using surface modification techniques.

4.1 Surface of Metals

The definition of "surface" varies in situations. In this section, only the general concept is explained.

Atoms in metallic materials located at the surface are considered partly reactive to the environment because atomic configuration terminates at the surface. The surface represents a property different from that inside the material. Due to high surface energy, a single molecular layer forms easily on a solid surface where gas molecules are adsorbed at 1 Pa in 10^{-4} seconds. For example, in the presence of oxygen atoms, oxygen and metal atoms chemically bond together to form an oxide layer. This phenomenon occurs even at the surface of gold, which is the most noble metal. Unlike ceramics and polymers, enrichment of component elements occurs easily on metal surfaces. This means that the surface composition of a metal is different from its inside composition in the order of nanometers. Therefore, the variant surface composition of a metallic material contributes significantly to defining the overall properties of the material.

A metal surface is usually covered with a surface oxide film. The surface oxide layer, on the other hand, is always covered with surface hydroxyl groups that are adsorbed by water (Figure 4.1). Of particular interest in this chapter is the surface oxide film.

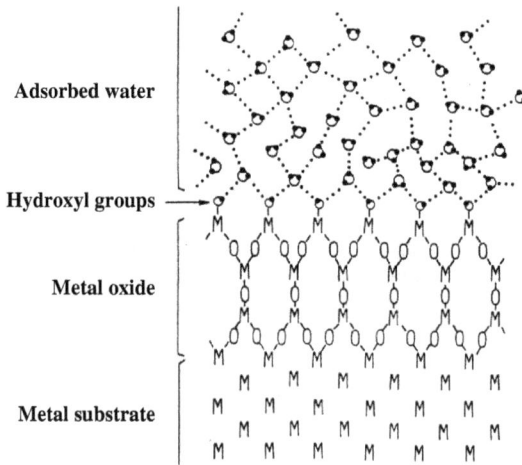

Figure 4.1. Schematic model of the structure of surface layer consisting of oxide layer, hydroxyl group layer and adsorbed water layer on metals and alloys.

4.2 Surface Oxide Film

Except in reduction environments, the corrosion process always causes a reaction film to form on metallic materials. Passive film is one such reaction film and is particularly significant for corrosion protection. When solubility is extremely low and pores are absent, the adhesion of film, which is formed in an aqueous solution, to the substrate will be strong. The film then becomes a corrosion-resistant or passive film. Passive film is about 1–5 nm thick and transparent. Due to the tremendously fast rate at which it is formed, passive film readily becomes amorphous. For example, film on a titanium metal substrate was generated in 30 seconds. This was estimated from the time transient of current of titanium at 1 V vs. SCE after exposing the metal surface, as shown in Figure 4.2. Since amorphous films hardly contain grain boundary and structural defects, they are corrosion-resistant. However, corrosion resistance decreases with crystallization. Fortunately, passive films contain water molecules that promote and maintain amorphousness.

Metallic materials, such as stainless steels, cobalt–chromium alloys, commercially pure titanium, and titanium alloys, used for biomedical devices are covered by their characteristic passive films.

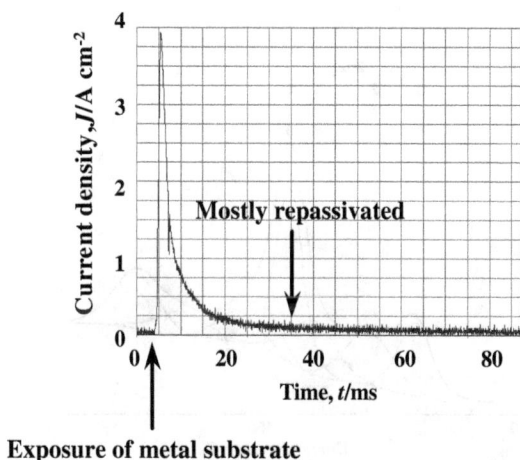

Figure 4.2. Time transient of anodic current of titanium in Hanks' solution under 1 V charge vs. a saturated calomel electrode (SCE); anodic current is generated with the dissolution and repassivation of titanium.

These films self-repair when they are disrupted by some causes (as given in Figure 4.2). Noble metals and alloys such as dental alloys are also covered with an oxide layer. While the oxide layer protects against corrosion, it is not chemically strong like the passive film.

4.2.1 *Titanium*

When titanium was polished in deionized water and analyzed using X-ray photoelectron spectroscopy (XPS), the Ti 2p spectrum obtained from the titanium gave four doublets according to valence: Ti^0, Ti^{2+}, Ti^{3+}, and Ti^{4+}. Published data [1] were used to determine the binding energy of each valence. Figure 4.3 shows an example of the decomposition of the Ti 2p spectrum.

A distinct Ti^0 peak at the metallic state was observed, which accounted for a very thin surface oxide film at less than a few nanometers. Besides, Ti^{4+} (TiO_2), Ti^{3+} (Ti_2O_3), and Ti^{2+} (TiO) were detected. Though Ti^{2+} oxide existed in the surface oxide film, Ti^{2+} formation is always thermodynamically less favorable than Ti^{3+} formation at the surface. The surface film on titanium consisted mainly of amorphous or low-crystalline and non-stoichiometric TiO_2, and the film stood firm against chloride ions.

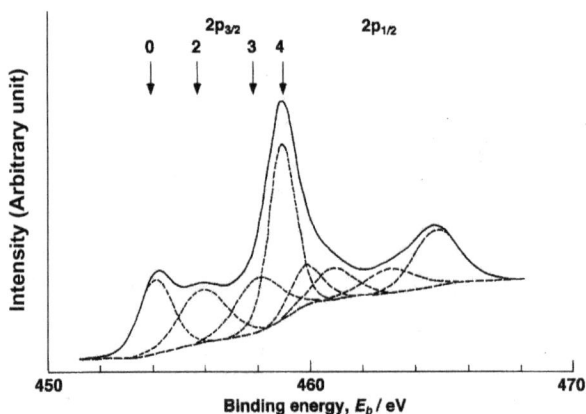

Figure 4.3. Decomposition of Ti 2p XPS spectrum obtained from titanium abraded and immersed for 300 seconds in water into eight peaks (2p$_{3/2}$ and 2p$_{1/2}$ electron peaks in four valences); numbers with arrows are valence numbers.

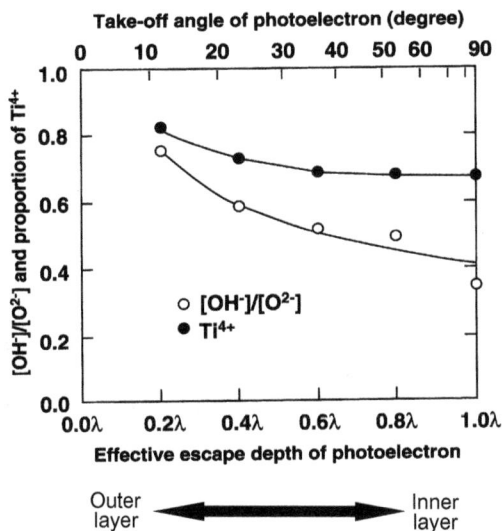

Figure 4.4. The proportional ratio of OH^- concentration to that of O^{2-} (i.e., $[OH^-]/[O^{2-}]$), and the proportion of cationic fraction of Ti^{4+} among titanium species in surface oxide film of titanium polished in water plotted against the average effective escape depth of photoelectrons for angle-resolved XPS measurements [2]. Lambda (λ) is the average escape depth of O 1s and Ti $2p_{3/2}$ photoelectrons, and the effective escape depth is obtained by (escape depth x sine[take-off-angle]). The values at small take-off angles of photoelectron (or effective escape depths of photoelectron) represent outer region information and those larger ones represent inner region information.

Since a considerable portion of oxidized titanium stayed as Ti^{2+} and Ti^{3+} in the surface film, the oxidation process might proceed to the end just at the uppermost part of the surface film. As shown in Figure 4.4, the proportion of Ti^{4+} among titanium cations (Ti^{2+}, Ti^{3+} and Ti^{4+}) in the film decreased with an increase in the photoelectron take-off angle [2], indicating that more Ti^{4+} existed near the outer layer in the film. From the take-off angle dependence of $[OH^-]/[O^{2-}]$ in Figure 4.4, it can be deduced that the oxygen atoms in the hydroxyl group were mainly located in the outer part of the surface film. This means that dehydration proceeded inside the surface film and only partly for Ti^{4+} oxide.

The thickness of the film was about 2 nm just after polishing and about 5 nm one week after polishing (as shown in Figure 4.5). Note also that the thickness of the surface oxide film increased according

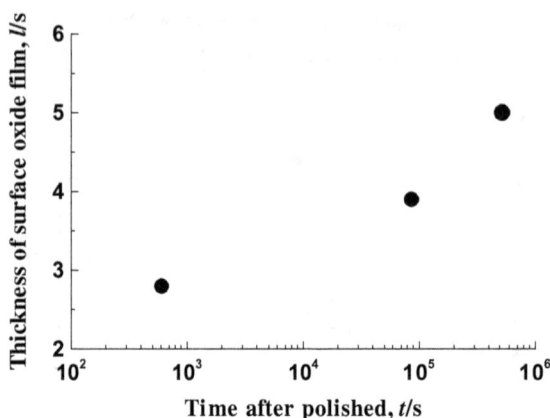

Figure 4.5. Thickness of the surface oxide film on titanium as a function of time after polishing.

to the logarithmic rule which is common in the initial growth of oxide films of metallic materials.

4.2.2 Titanium Alloys

The film on the Ti–6Al–4V alloy was almost the same as that on titanium, containing a small amount of aluminum oxide [3, 4]. In other words, the surface oxide film on Ti–6Al–4V was a TiO_2 containing small amounts of Al_2O_3, hydroxyl groups, and bound water. Vanadium contained in the alloy was not detected in the oxide film after the alloy was polished.

The Ti–56Ni shape memory alloy was covered by TiO_2-based oxide, with minimal amounts of nickel in both the oxide and metallic states [3, 4]. The film on Ti–56Ni was a TiO_2 containing small amounts of metallic nickel, NiO, hydroxyl groups, and bound water.

In the Ti–Zr alloy, the surface oxide film consisted of titanium and zirconium oxides [5]. The relative concentration ratio of titanium to zirconium in the film was almost the same as that in the alloy (Figure 4.6). In the surface oxide film, titanium and zirconium were uniformly distributed along the depth. The thickness of the film increased with an increase in the zirconium content. The chemical state of zirconium was more stable than that of titanium in the film.

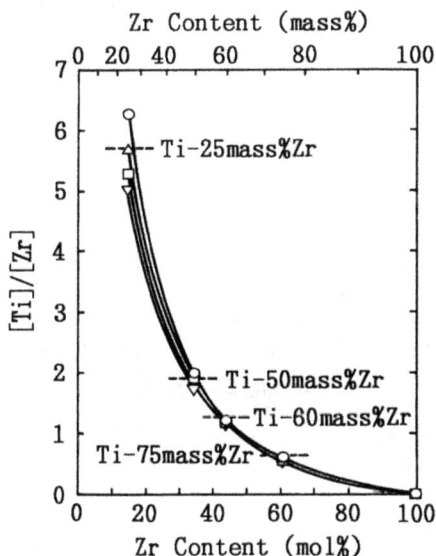

Figure 4.6. Change in ratio of the concentration of titanium to that of zirconium, [Ti]/[Zr], as the zirconium content increases [5]; dashed lines indicate the [Ti]/[Zr] values from nominal compositions of specimens.

4.2.3 *Stainless Steel*

Compositions of surface oxide films on stainless steels are well understood in the field of engineering. In an austenitic stainless steel, the surface oxide film consists of iron, chromium, and a small amount of molybdenum, but it does not contain nickel while in the air and in chloride solutions [6, 7].

On the other hand, the surface oxide film on 316L steel polished mechanically in deionized water consists of oxide species of iron, chromium, nickel, molybdenum, and manganese, and its thickness is about 3.6 nm [8]. The surface film contains a large amount of OH^- — the oxide which is hydrated or oxyhydroxidized (Figure 4.7). The surface oxide film is also enriched with iron, while the alloy substrate just under the film is enriched with nickel, molybdenum, and manganese.

4.2.4 *Co–Cr–Mo Alloy*

The surface oxide film of a Co–Cr–Mo alloy is characterized as containing oxides of cobalt and chromium without molybdenum [9].

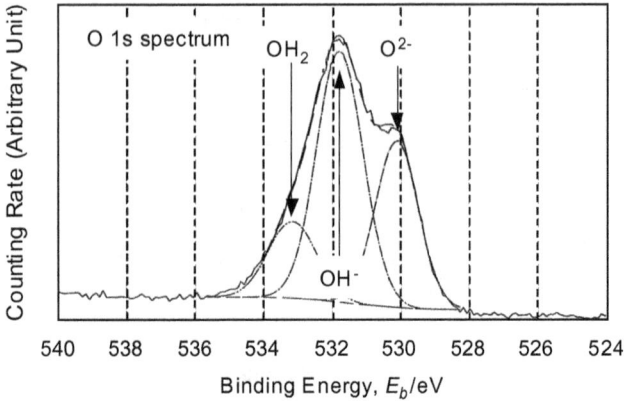

Figure 4.7. Typical O 1s spectrum obtained from 316L austenitic stainless steel and its deconvolution into O^{2-}, OH^-, and H_2O components.

On the other hand, the surface oxide film on another Co–Cr–Mo alloy polished mechanically in deionized water consists of oxide species of cobalt, chromium, and molybdenum, and its thickness is about 2.5 nm [10]. This surface film contains a large amount of OH^- — the oxide which is hydrated or oxyhydroxidized. There are also more traces of chromium and molybdenum distributed at the inner layer of the film.

4.2.5 *Noble Metal Alloys*

Au–Cu–Ag alloys and Ag–Pd–Cu–Au alloys for dental restoration are covered by copper oxide and/or silver oxide [11]. An Ag–In alloy is covered by zinc oxide and indium oxide, and an Ag–Sn–Zn alloy is covered by tin oxide and zinc oxide. Dental amalgams (Ag–Sn–Cu–Hg alloys) are covered by tin oxide [12]. While these oxides serve as a protective film against corrosion, they are not as chemically strong as the passive film.

4.3 Reconstruction of Surface Oxide Film

The composition of the surface oxide film varies according to environmental changes, though the film is macroscopically stable. Passive surfaces co-exist in close contact with electrolytes, undergoing a

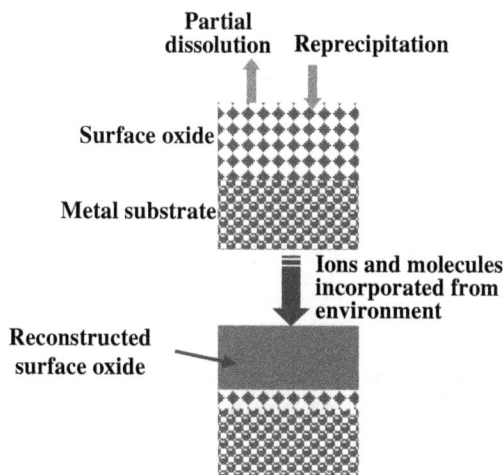

Figure 4.8. Schematic reconstruction model of surface oxide film on metallic biomaterials.

continuous process of partial dissolution and re-precipitation from the microscopic viewpoint. In this sense, surface composition is always changing according to the environment (Figure 4.8).

Due to abrasion with bone and other materials, the surface oxide film may be scratched and destroyed during insertion and implantation into living tissues. Fretting corrosion also leads to film destruction. Fortunately, the surface oxide is immediately regenerated in a biological environment where biofluid surrounds the metallic material. However, the composition and properties of the oxide film regenerated in a biological environment may be different from those in water.

4.3.1 *Titanium*

When titanium which has been surgically implanted into the human jaw is characterized using Auger electron spectroscopy (AES), its surface oxide film reveals constituents of calcium, phosphorus, and sulfur [13, 14]. By immersing titanium and its alloys in Hanks' solution (Figure 4.9) and other solutions [3–5, 15], preferential adsorption of phosphate ions occurs, leading to the formation of calcium phosphate on their surfaces [16].

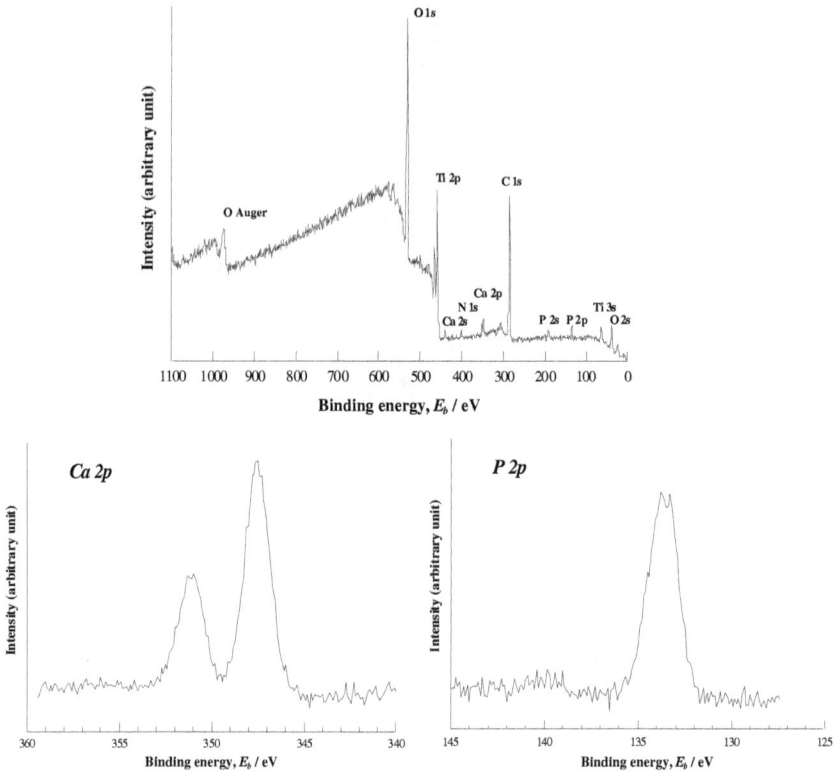

Figure 4.9. XPS spectra of survey: Ca 2p and P 2p regions obtained from titanium immersed in Hanks' solution for one day. Peak binding energies of Ca 2p and P 2p regions reveal that calcium and phosphorus exist as calcium phosphate.

Hanks' solution, whose pH is 7.4, is an artificial biofluid. Its inorganic composition is similar to extracellular fluid. Hydrated phosphate ions are adsorbed by a hydrated titanium oxide surface during the release of protons [15]. Calcium ions are then adsorbed by phosphate ions, which are adsorbed on the titanium surface, thus leading to calcium phosphate being formed eventually. On the same note, when titanium is immersed in Hanks' solution containing albumin, a non-uniform and porous albumin-containing apatite[a] is formed [17]. The above phenomena are characteristic of titanium and its alloys [4].

---

[a]Apatite is a general term referring to similar crystals, and the predominant apatite is hydroxyapatite. Here, apatite refers to hydroxyapatite.

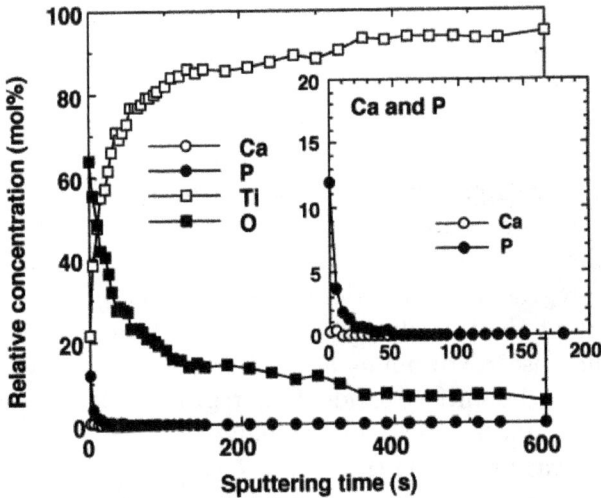

Figure 4.10. AES depth profiles of relative concentrations of elements at the surface of titanium abraded and immersed for 300 seconds in Hanks' solution [2].

The surface oxide film regenerated in Hanks' solution contains phosphate ions in the outermost layer. Phosphate ions are preferentially taken up during the regeneration of surface oxide film on titanium. The resultant film comprises titanium oxide and titanium oxyhydroxide, and the latter contains titanium phosphate. Following regeneration, calcium and phosphate ions are adsorbed to the film, thus forming calcium phosphate or calcium titanium phosphate on the outermost surface, as shown in Figure 4.10 [2].

Calcium phosphate precipitates faster on a surface film regenerated in a biological system than in water because seeds of calcium phosphate already exist on the regenerated film. Extrapolating from here, it can be assumed that bone formation is faster on titanium implanted in hard tissue simply because the surface oxide film is titanium oxide. On this basis, surface modification was attempted on titanium using this repassivation reaction [18].

4.3.2 *Titanium Alloys*

Calcium phosphate is also formed on Ti–6Al–4V and Ti–56Ni alloys after immersion in Hanks' solution, but the [Ca]/[P] ratios are smaller than that in titanium [3, 4]. On the other hand, only phosphate without calcium is formed on Ti–Zr alloys that contain over 50 mass%Zr [5].

Ti–6Al–4V, Ti–56Ni, and Ti–xZr (x = 0, 25, 50, 60, 75, 100 in mass%) alloys were abraded and kept for 300 seconds in water and Hanks' solution [19]. The regenerated surface oxide film in Hanks' solution was characterized using XPS. As summarized in Tables 4.1–4.3, phosphate ions are preferentially taken up in the surface oxide film during regeneration. Besides calcium and phosphate, other ionic constituents of Hanks' solution were absent from the surface oxide film. In the case of titanium and Ti–6Al–4V, calcium phosphate was found in the surface oxide film regenerated in Hanks' solution. However, for Ti–56Ni, Ti–Zr, and zirconium, phosphate without calcium was formed on the surfaces instead. These results are in good agreement with those of titanium alloys immersed in Hanks' solution.

Table 4.1. XPS results for relative concentrations of elements in surface oxide film on Ti–6Al–4V (Ti–10.2at%Al–3.6at%V) regenerated in water and in Hanks' solution during 300-second immersion [33].

Abraded in	Relative concentration (at %)					
	Ti	Al	V	O	Ca	P
Water	24.5 (0.9)*	3.8 (1.1)	0.0 (0.0)	71.8 (0.1)	0.0 (0.0)	0.0 (0.0)
Hanks	21.4 (0.1)	3.2 (0.2)	0.0 (0.0)	73.2 (0.3)	0.1 (0.0)	2.2 (0.0)

Note: *Standard deviations.

Table 4.2. XPS results for relative concentrations of elements in surface oxide film on Ti–56Ni (Ti–50at%Ni) regenerated in water and in Hanks' solution during 300-second immersion [33].

Abraded in	Relative concentration (at %)				
	Ti	Ni	O	Ca	P
Water	23.4 (0.1)*	7.2 (0.7)	69.4 (0.6)	0.0 (0.0)	0.0 (0.0)
Hanks	24.0 (0.4)	5.6 (0.7)	69.0 (0.6)	0.0 (0.0)**	1.4 (0.2)

Notes: *Standard deviations.
**Trace amount.

Table 4.3. XPS results for relative concentrations of elements in surface oxide film on titanium, zirconium, and Ti–Zr alloys regenerated in water (top values) and in Hanks' solution (bottom values) during 300-second immersion [33].

	Relative concentration (at %)				
	Ti	**Zr**	**O**	**Ca**	**P**
Ti	29.6	0.0	70.4	0.0	0.0
	28.6	0.0	70.6	0.2	0.7
Ti–mass25Zr	29.4	4.7	65.9	0.0	0.0
(18.7at%Zr)	24.1	4.0	70.2	0.0	1.7
Ti–mass50Zr	23.7	12.0	64.3	0.0	0.0
(40.8at%Zr)	18.2	9.1	70.7	0.0	1.9
Ti–mass60Zr	18.6	15.5	65.9	0.0	0.0
(50at%Zr)	16.1	11.8	70.5	0.0	1.7
Ti–mass75Zr	12.7	20.9	66.4	0.0	0.0
(67.4at%Zr)	10.0	15.5	72.4	0.0	2.1
Zr	0.0	32.1	67.9	0.0	0.0
	0.0	20.6	77.5	0.0	1.9

4.3.3 *Stainless Steel*

In pins and wires made from 316L austenitic stainless steel, calcium and phosphorus are present in the surface oxide [20]. The corrosion product of 316L steel implanted in the femur, as part of an artificial hip joint, consists of chromium combined with sulfur, and/or iron combined with phosphorus (where the latter contains calcium and chlorine) [21].

Five surface oxide specimens of stainless steel were prepared according to the following methods [8]:

- polishing in deionized water;
- autoclaving;
- immersion in Hanks' solution;
- immersion in cell culture medium;
- incubation with cultured cells.

Next, XPS was performed to find out the following:

- composition of surface oxide film;
- composition of the substrate;
- thickness of surface oxide film.

For 316L steel polished in deionized water, the surface oxide film consisted of iron and chromium oxides which contained small amounts of nickel, molybdenum, and manganese oxides. The surface oxide also contained a large amount of OH$^-$.

For specimens immersed in Hanks' solution and in cell culture medium, as well as incubated with culture cells, calcium phosphate was formed. Sulfate was adsorbed by the surface oxide film and reduced to sulfite in the cell culture medium and with the cultured cells. The results of this study suggest that nickel and manganese are depleted in the oxide film. The surface oxide changes into iron and chromium oxides, where a small amount of molybdenum oxide will be present in the human body.

4.3.4 Co–Cr–Mo Alloy

In the Co–Cr–Mo alloy, cobalt was dissolved during immersion in the Hanks' solution and in the cell culture medium, as well as during incubation in a cell culture [10]. After dissolution, the surface oxide consisted of chromium oxide (Cr^{3+}), which contained molybdenum oxide (Mo^{4+}, Mo^{5+}, and Mo^{6+}). Results from angle-resolved XPS revealed that chromium and molybdenum were more widely distributed in the inner layer than in the outer layer of the oxide film.

In body fluids, cobalt is completely dissolved. The surface oxide changes into chromium oxide containing a small amount of molybdenum oxide. Calcium phosphate is also formed on the top surface. The above process is shown using a schematic illustration in Figure 4.11.

4.4 Adsorption of Proteins

When a metallic material is implanted into a human body and in contact with its living tissues, proteins are immediately adsorbed by the material (as shown in Figure 4.12).

Protein adsorption influences material corrosion, and subsequently, cell adhesion. Likewise, protein denaturalization and fragmentation (which occur due to adsorption) may affect the function of the host body. To characterize proteins adsorbed to metals and metal oxides, various techniques can be used [22], especially that of

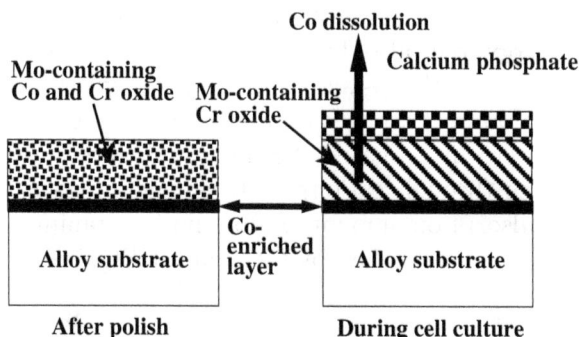

Figure 4.11. Schematic illustration of reconstruction of surface oxide film on a Co–Cr–Mo alloy after polishing and during cell culture [10].

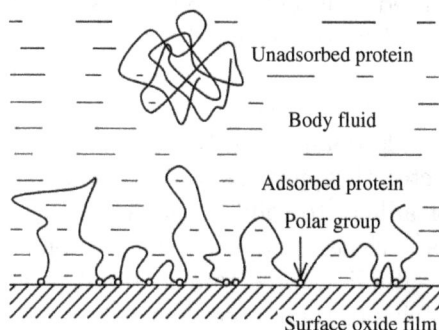

Figure 4.12. Possible model of protein adsorption by metals.

ellipsometry [23]. To predict protein adsorption, the wettability test is used where a liquid droplet is applied to the material [24].

The adsorption behavior of albumin to a metal surface varies according to the metallic element as follows [25]:

- **Titanium, aluminum, molybdenum, cobalt, nickel, and tantalum:** Adsorption amount of albumin is small both at the initial and later stages.
- **Vanadium:** Small adsorption amount is noted at the initial stage, but the amount increases at the later stage.
- **Silver, gold, and copper:** Large adsorption amount is noted at the initial stage, and the amount increases further at the later stage.

These results reveal that protein adsorption is governed not only by surface energy but also by a metal's electrostatic force. The adsorption of fibronectin, α-lacto albumin, α-amylase and albumin, bovine serum albumin, and glycosaminoglycan by titanium or titanium dioxide were investigated. Serum proteins were adsorbed by titanium surface through cations such as calcium ions in a $CaCl_2$ solution. The adsorption amount of albumin by titanium dioxide, on the other hand, was controlled by Ca^{2+} and HPO_4^{2-}.

4.5 Adhesion of Cells

Affinity for cells is one important property for biomaterials because they are always used adjacent to living tissues. Qualitatively, cell adhesion is evaluated by observing the cells adhering to the surface under a microscope. However, to develop new biomaterials with superior biocompatibility, it is absolutely necessary to evaluate a material's affinity for cells quantitatively. This is because cell adhesion is a significant factor that governs a material's tissue compatibility. Since cells do not adhere to solid surfaces directly, but through cell adhesion proteins such as fibronectin and vitronectin (as shown in Figure 4.13), the adhesion force to a material is determined by the adsorption of proteins to the material surface and the activity of the cell itself.

The adhesion of osteoblasts and fibroblasts to titanium, titanium alloys and a Co–Cr alloy was investigated from the viewpoint of hard tissue compatibility [26], while the adhesion of epithelial cells to titanium was investigated from the viewpoint of a dental implant [27]. In these studies, the effects of surface roughness, pores, grooves, and surface treatment on cell adhesion were investigated: a stretch of cells, for example, resided in the grooves [26]. In the case of osteoblasts and osteoblastic cells, osteoid tissue formation was also investigated [28].

One method to quantitatively evaluate a material's affinity for cells is to measure the detachment force of an adherent cell on the material. A new system was developed to measure directly the shear force required to detach a cell from a material [29]. Using a microcantilever, the detachment force was measured in the cell culture medium by applying a lateral load to the cell which adhered to the material. The schematic illustration of the system is shown in

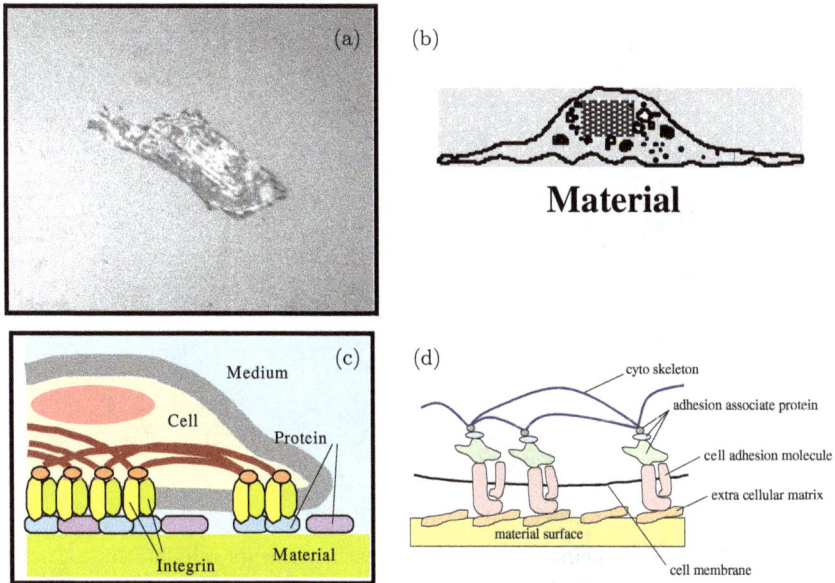

Figure 4.13. (a) Interference reflection microscopic image of human fibroblast cells IMR-90 adhered to a glass surface; (b) schematic image of cell adhesion to a material; (c, d) schematic models of cell adhesion mechanism to a material.

Figure 4.14. Adhesive properties of L929 to sputter-deposited metal films depend on the types of metal to which they adhere (as shown in Figure 4.14). Among titanium, chromium, aluminum, gold, silver, and palladium, cells on chromium and titanium had the highest cell adhesive shear strength and cell detachment surface energy — almost close to those of glass materials [30].

4.6 Surface Modification

Surface modification is a process that changes a material's surface composition, structure and morphology, leaving the bulk of mechanical properties intact. With surface modification, chemical and mechanical durability, as well as tissue compatibility of the surface layer could be improved. Surface property is particularly significant for biomaterials, and thus, surface modification techniques are particularly useful to biomaterials. Dry processes (using ion beams) and hydro-processes (which are performed in aqueous solutions) are

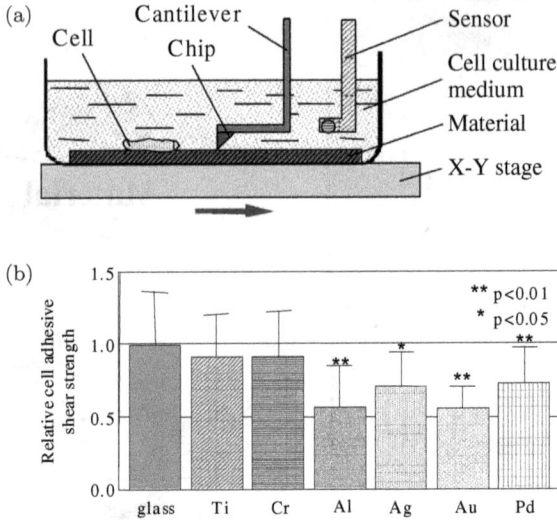

Figure 4.14. (a) Principle of shear force measurement for cell detachment from a material using a newly developed instrument, and force–displacement curves obtained with the instrument [29]; (b) relative cell adhesive shear strength of L929 to thin metal films normalized by cell adhesive shear strength of L929 to glass [30].

predominant surface modification techniques. Apatite coating on titanium with plasma spray, titanium nitride coating with sputter deposition, and titanium oxide growth with morphological control by electrolysis are already available for commercial use (as shown in Figure 4.15).

4.6.1 *Purpose*

In biomaterials, the chief purpose of surface modification is to improve corrosion resistance, wear resistance, antibacterial properties, and tissue compatibility. Shown in Figure 4.16 are schematic illustrations of an artificial hip joint, bone plate, and screws.

When the sliding interface between the head and socket is worn, wear debris will be generated. Fretting fatigue and crevice corrosion may occur at the fixation site of the plate with screws. Metallic elements are released as ions and wear debris due to corrosion and wear, causing metallosis of the surrounding tissue and loosening at the fixation site. Although commercial metallic biomaterials are

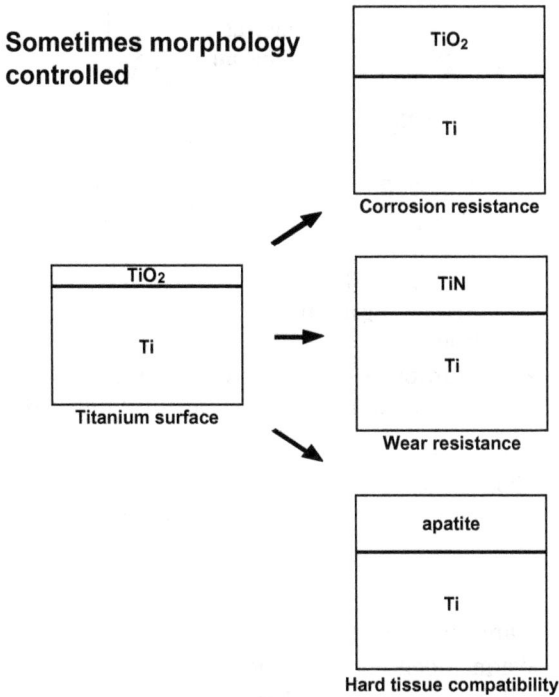

Sometimes morphology controlled

TiO₂ / Ti — Corrosion resistance

TiO₂ / Ti — Titanium surface

TiN / Ti — Wear resistance

apatite / Ti — Hard tissue compatibility

Figure 4.15. Commercially used surface modification techniques of titanium (when it is used as biomaterial).

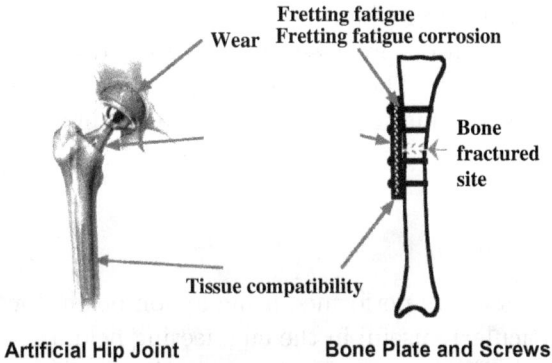

Figure 4.16. Schematic illustrations of the artificial hip joint, bone plate and screws, and problems sometimes occurring in clinical use.

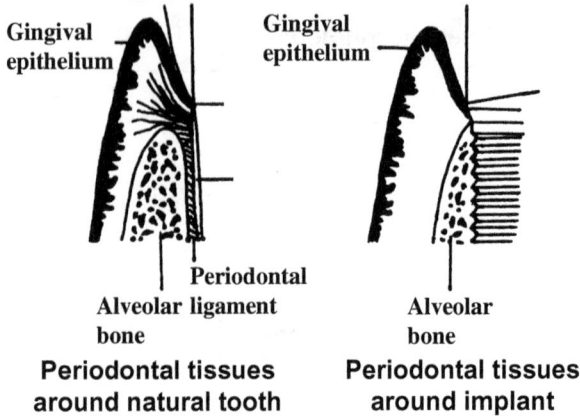

Figure 4.17. Schematic illustrations of periodontal tissues around natural tooth and dental implant material. Bacteria may invade from the pocket between gingival epithelium and dental implant. Dental implant must fix with alveolar bone.

corrosion-resistant, trace metal ions may be released because of characteristic corrosion mechanism in the human body. In bone implant materials, rapid bone conductivity is required. In cardiovascular devices, blood compatibility or antithrombogenecity is required. In dental implants, soft tissue compatibility is required to prevent bacteria invasion from the crevice, which is between the dental implant and gingival epithelium (Figure 4.17).

Surface modification processes are categorized into dry processes and hydro-processes. The surface modification techniques being investigated are summarized in Table 4.4 according to their objectives.

4.6.2 Dry Process

Most dry processes are performed using an ion beam. Ion beam technology is particularly useful in the engineering field, especially in silicon technology. Ion beam technology permits the formation of thin films at atomic and molecular levels, as well as low-temperature syntheses utilizing ionic effects. The process is thermal unequilibrium, thus making it possible to synthesize unnatural substances.

Table 4.4. Surface modification techniques for metallic biomaterials.

Purpose	Techniques	
Improve corrosion resistance	Immersion	
	Anodic polarization or electrolysis	
	Noble metal ion implantation	
Improve wear resistance	TiN layer deposition	
	Nitrogen ion implantation	
Improve hard tissue compatibility	Apatite layer formation	Immersion
		Electrochemical deposition
		Plasma spray
		Ion plating
		RF magnetron sputtering
		Pulse laser deposition
	Non-apatite layer formation	Immersion in alkaline solution and heating
		Immersion in H_2O_2
		Calcium ion implantation
		Calcium ion mixing
		Hydrothermal treatment
		Biomolecule unmobilization
Improve blood compatibility	Polymer unmobilization	
	Biomolecule unmobilization	

Ion beam technology has contributed significantly to the modification of biomaterial surfaces. It can be classified according to the effects on solid surfaces: film formation, sputtering, and ion implantation. When an ion impacts a material surface, attaching, sputtering, and implantation effects occur according to the ion's energy (Figure 4.18).

By utilizing these effects, thin film formation, graded-composition layer, and unequilibrium layer are obtained. Figure 4.18 also presents surface modification techniques as a function of ion energy and thickness of the resultant surface-modified layer. This figure serves only as a guide and need not be true for advanced techniques. Figure 4.19 shows the key principles of predominant dry processes, plasma spray, and ion implantation.

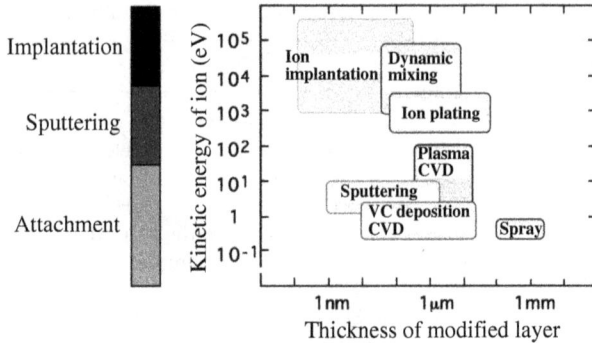

Figure 4.18. Effects of ion irradiation on a solid surface due to ion energy (hence the ion beam technique as a function of kinetic ion energy) and the resultant thickness of the modified layer.

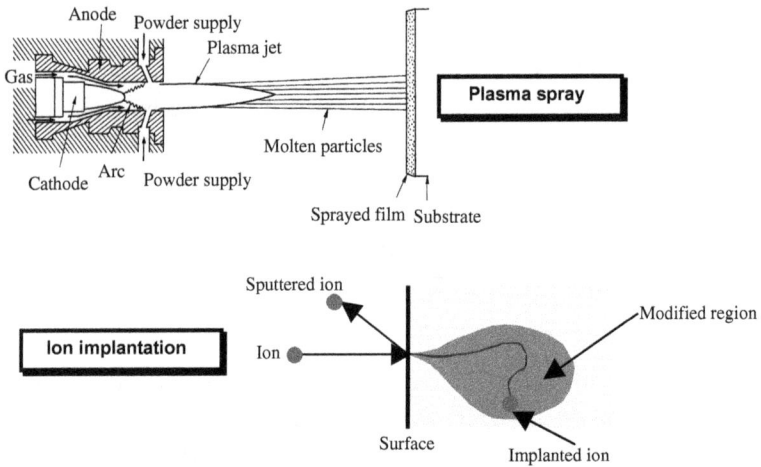

Figure 4.19. Principles of plasma spray and ion implantation.

4.6.3 *Hydro-Process*

Hydro-process is performed in aqueous solutions. This process does not require large facilities and cost as immersion or electrolysis in aqueous solutions is a basic process. The resultant modified layer changes according to changes in the following parameters:

- composition and pH of aqueous solution;
- potential gain due to electrolysis;
- current density of electrolysis.

4.7 Apatite Film Formation

4.7.1 *Apatite Formation with Dry Process*

The chief purpose for surface modification of titanium is to improve its hard-tissue compatibility. This is done by forming a calcium phosphate film on the titanium surface. Currently, plasma spraying of apatite on metallic materials is widely used to form the apatite layer — the nucleus for active bone formation and conductivity. In the case of plasma-sprayed apatite, however, the apatite–titanium interface or apatite itself may fracture under relatively low stress because of low interface bonding strength and low toughness of the sprayed layer itself [31]. To overcome this weakness, dynamic ion mixing is applied to form an apatite with high interface bonding strength. Calcium ions are implanted during the mixing process to induce strong bonding between the apatite film and the titanium substrate, with implanted calcium ions serving as a binder (as shown in Figure 4.20). Sputter deposition of apatite is now done by using RF magnetron sputtering and laser-pulse deposition.

The solubility of ceramics increases as its crystallinity decreases. The crystallinity of a thin film formed with an ion beam is low and the solubility is high. The crystallinity of coated apatite is an important factor because crystallinity governs solubility in the human body. Low-crystalline film on titanium dissolves rapidly when the titanium is implanted into a human body. This is because the pH of body fluid can reach as low as 5. Thus, heat treatment of apatite film is

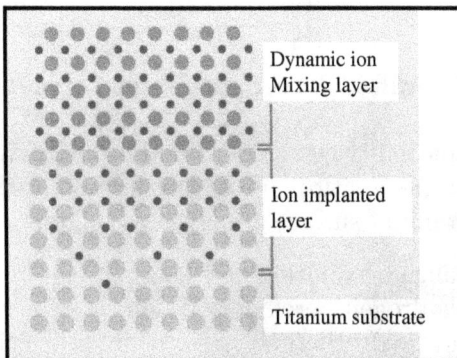

Figure 4.20. Surface-modified layer produced by ion mixing techniques with calcium ion implantation and sputter deposition of hydroxyapatite.

necessary to increase its crystallinity and reduce its solubility [31]. Therefore, based on the discussion thus far in this section, the following issues must be carefully considered when the ion beam technique is to be used to form the apatite layer:

- composition of apatite layer;
- coating efficiency;
- bonding strength of apatite to the substrate;
- crystallinity of apatite.

4.7.2 *Apatite Formation with Hydro-Process*

Titanium has a unique property that enables calcium phosphate to form on its surface in simulated biofluids [3–5, 15]. When both the composition and pH of a solution are selected properly, apatite can be formed on titanium in the solution. The apatite formed by this technique contains a large amount of carbonate. Control of morphology, volume, and composition in the precipitate is difficult. Moreover, the apatite film is mechanically weak.

Electrochemical treatment [32, 33] is used commonly to form an apatite layer on titanium. Through an electrochemical process, carbonate-containing apatite with desirable morphology such as plate, needle, and particle could be precipitated on titanium substrate. Figure 4.21 shows an example of morphology control using electrolysis techniques [32]. This process could also be used to coat substrates of complex designs. When titanium with apatite fabricated by this process is implanted into rat femur, apatite-formed titanium shows larger bonding strength than untreated titanium.

4.8 Surface-Modified Layer for Bone Formation

Hard-tissue compatibility can be improved by modifying the titanium surface instead of the apatite film. In this section, various techniques to modify the titanium surface are given as follows:

- immersion in alkaline solution and heating;
- immersion in hydrogen peroxide solution;
- immersion and hydrothermal treatment in calcium-containing solution;
- calcium ion implantation.

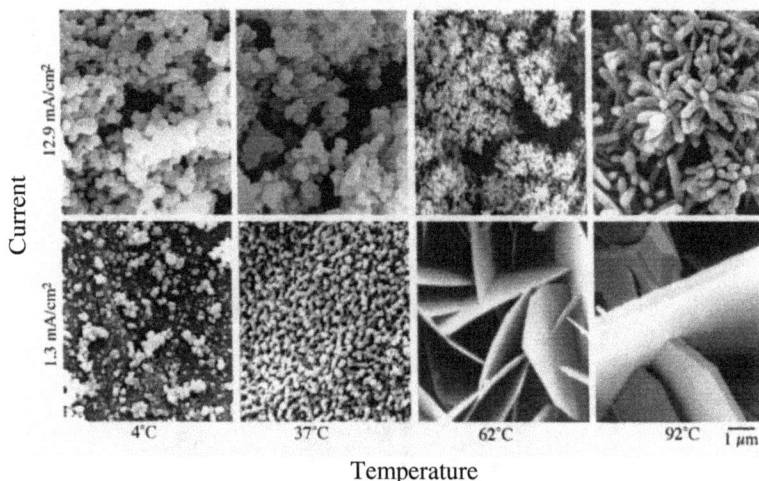

Figure 4.21. Hydroxyapatite precipitates with various morphologies according to different current and temperature readings in electrolysis [32].

4.8.1 *Immersion in Alkaline Solution and Heating*

When titanium is immersed in NaOH or KOH alkaline solution, a hydrated titanium oxide gel containing alkaline ions (gel-like titanium oxide containing hydroxyl groups) with 1 μm thickness is formed on the titanium substrate, as shown in Figure 4.22 [34]. Upon heating, the gel layer condenses and the gel bonds to the substrate strongly.

When titanium, with the gel, is immersed in a simulated biofluid, alkaline ions are released from the layer to the solution. Simultaneously, hydronium ions are soaked up by the layer, eventually forming titania hydrogel. This increases the magnitude of supersaturation of hydroxyapatite in the solution near the surface. The gel induces apatite nucleation, and the apatite layer is rapidly formed. This process is expected to accelerate bone formation on titanium in hard tissue.

4.8.2 *Immersion in Hydrogen Peroxide Solution*

When a material is implanted into a human body, macrophages will attach themselves to the material. The macrophages generate active oxygen species, which then react with the material. When

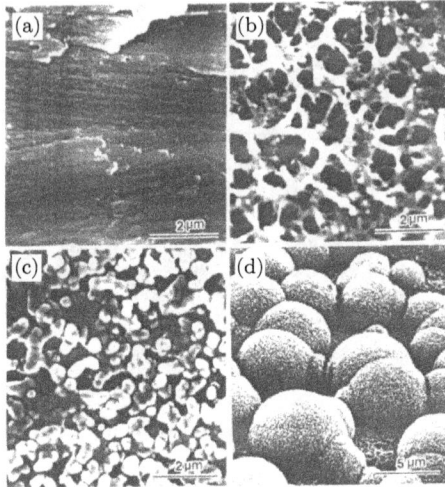

Figure 4.22. (a) Titanium surface before treatment; (b) after alkaline treatment; (c) after heat treatment; (d) after immersion in a simulated body fluid in alkaline and heat treatments [34].

titanium was incubated with macrophages, titanium dissolution was significantly accelerated in the presence of macrophages [35]. Hydrogen peroxide is an active oxygen species, and the reaction between titanium and hydrogen peroxide was investigated [36]. As shown in Figure 4.23, this reaction was applied to induce the formation of a titanium oxide gel on titanium [37].

Immersion of titanium in $TaCl_2$-containing H_2O_2 accelerates apatite formation in a simulated body fluid. The pull-out test of specimens from rat tibia reveals increased bonding strength of titanium to the bone.

4.8.3 *Immersion and Hydrothermal Treatment in Calcium-Containing Solution*

A titanium oxide layer, which contains calcium hydroxide, is formed whenever titanium is immersed in any of the following calcium-containing solutions [38]:

- calcium nitrate (pH 3.9);
- calcium chloride (pH 7.4);
- calcium hydroxide (pH 12.6).

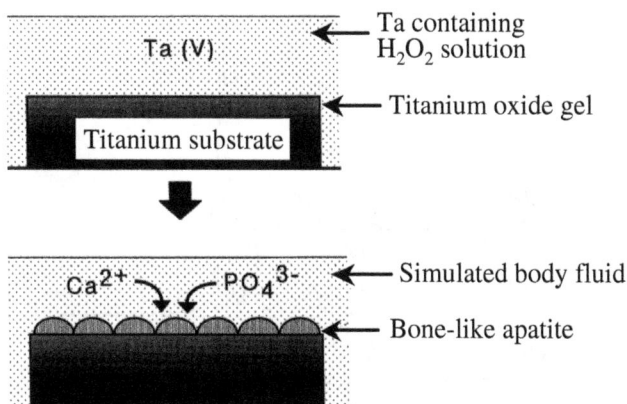

Figure 4.23. Schematic illustration of treating titanium with tantalum-containing hydrogen peroxide [37].

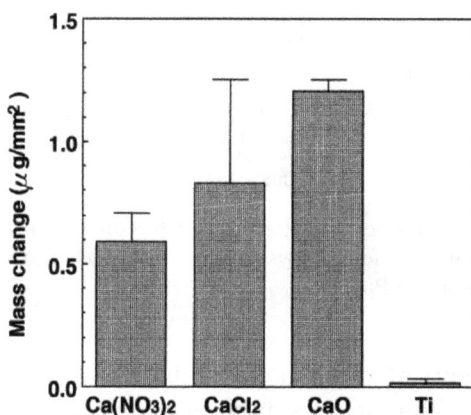

Figure 4.24. Mass changes of titanium specimens with and without modification in calcium nitrate, calcium chloride, and calcium oxide solutions before and after immersion in Hanks' solution [38].

The oxide layer catalyzes the precipitation of calcium phosphate on titanium when immersed in Hanks' solution. As shown in Figures 4.24 and 4.25, the catalytic function was confirmed by mass changes, X-ray diffractometry, and XPS. It was also observed that the most effective means to precipitate apatite was immersion in alkaline solutions.

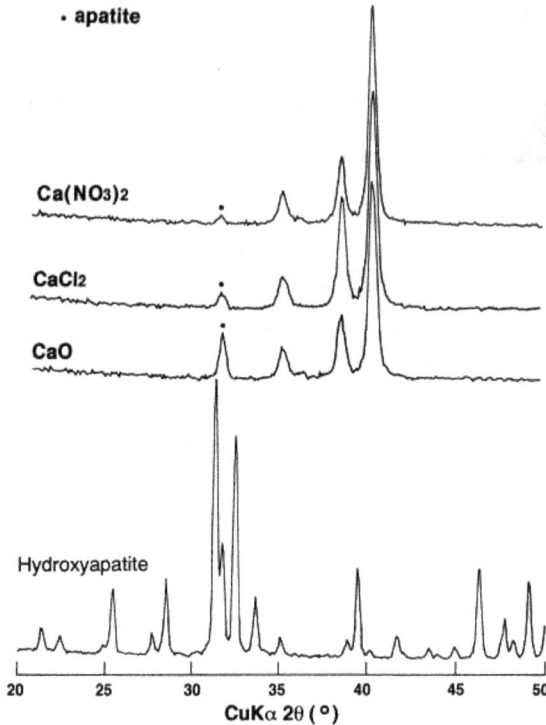

Figure 4.25. X-ray diffraction patterns of surface-modified titanium immersed in Hanks' solution at 37°C for 30 days and heated at 600°C for 30 minutes under a reduced pressure of 100 Pa [38].

While in identical calcium-containing solutions, hydrothermal modification of titanium was performed using an autoclave [39]. Apatite precipitation in Hanks' solution was the largest on titanium modified in calcium hydroxide solution. On the other hand, apatite precipitation was prevented on titanium modified in calcium chloride solution. It was also noted that surface modification of titanium in calcium hydroxide was more effective with an increase in temperature or pressure.

4.8.4   Calcium Ion Implantation

Calcium ion implantation is another surface modification technique used to improve the hard-tissue compatibility of titanium. When

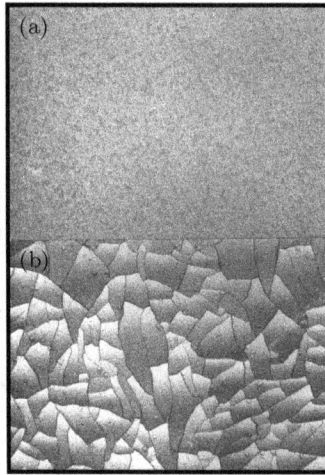

Figure 4.26. Scanning electron micrographs of (a) titanium and (b) calcium-ion-implanted titanium [40].

calcium ions are implanted into titanium, calcium phosphate precipitation in an electrolyte is speeded up [40] (as shown in Figure 4.26). MC3T3–E1 cells on titanium were activated to form osteoid tissue and tissue formation was accelerated when calcium ions were implanted [41].

In Figure 4.27, both unimplanted titanium and calcium-ion-implanted titanium were incubated with MC3T3–E1 cells. Calcium phosphate formed only on calcium-ion-implanted titanium, but not on unimplanted titanium. Moreover, new osteoid tissue was formed earlier on calcium-ion-implanted titanium than on unimplanted titanium as early as two days after implantation into rat tibia [42]. This superiority of calcium-ion-implanted titanium is due to the modified surface by calcium ion implantation.

In Figure 4.28, the depth distribution of substances on calcium-ion-implanted titanium is illustrated schematically. The modified surface of calcium-ion-implanted titanium comprised titanium oxide, which contained calcium in the chemical state of calcium titanate [43]. Compared to the unimplanted titanium surface, the calcium-ion-implanted titanium surface was more positively charged due to the dissociation of hydroxyl radicals [44], as schematically illustrated in Figure 4.29. As a result, the number of charging sites was bigger.

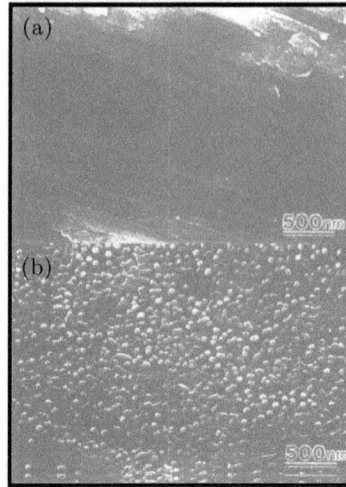

Figure 4.27. Surfaces of (a) titanium and (b) calcium-ion-implanted titanium after scraping off osteogenic cells with which these specimens are incubated for 14 days [41].

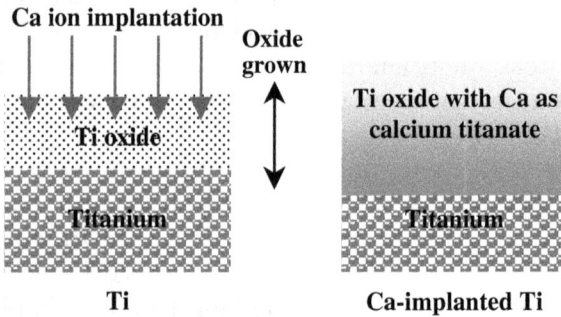

Figure 4.28. Change in the surface layer of titanium with calcium ion implantation.

More phosphate ions in the body fluid adsorb onto the calcium-ion-implanted titanium surface because of electric charge attraction. The more phosphate ions adsorbed, the more calcium ions attracted, and the more calcium phosphate is precipitated. Simultaneously, calcium ions are released from the surface of calcium-ion-implanted titanium [45, 46], leading to the supersaturation of calcium ions in body fluid near the surface and resulting in accelerated calcium phosphate precipitation.

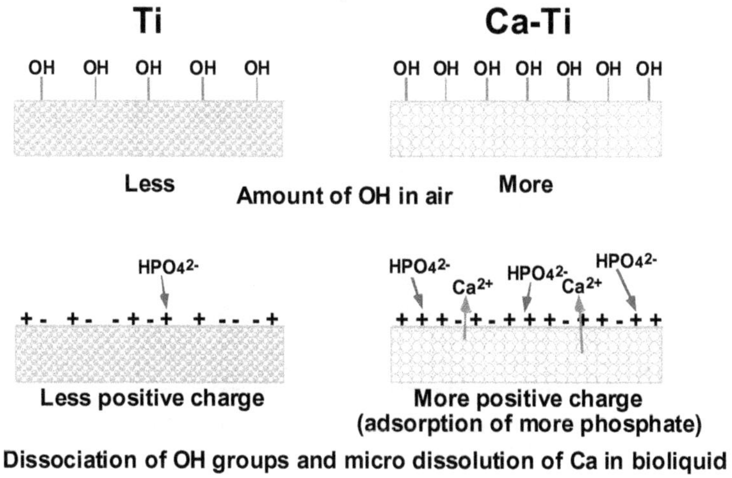

Figure 4.29. Acceleration mechanism of calcium phosphate precipitation on titanium with calcium ion implantation.

To obtain a surface composition that is the same as a modified layer (where the latter is modified by calcium ion implantation), advanced techniques such as $CaTiO_3$ sputter deposition with argon ion or titanium ion mixing can be used.

4.9 Titanium Oxide Layer Formation

The easiest way to increase the corrosion resistance of titanium is either by anodic oxidation in an acidic solution or by high-temperature oxidation in the air (see Figure 4.15). Sputter deposition of a thin TiO_2 film is also effective in improving corrosion resistance. By iridium ion implantation into Ti–6Al–4V, the electro-chemical properties of the alloy approached those of iridium, eventually improving corrosion resistance. Improving corrosion resistance, however, does not always ensure bone conductivity.

Electrolysis in aqueous solution is effective for forming porous or irregular-shaped titanium oxide layer on titanium substrate (as shown in Figure 4.30). This technique is already applied to control the surface morphology of dental implants. Nowadays, titanium oxide film is used as coloring to categorize devices.

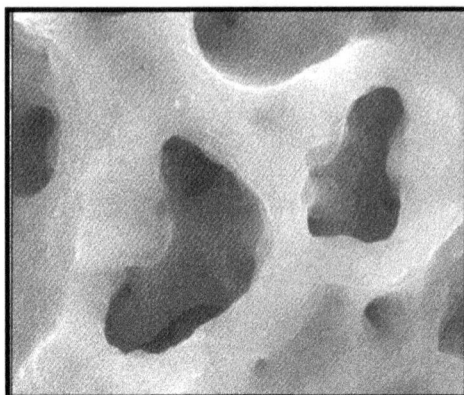

Figure 4.30. Porous titanium oxide surface [from Brånemark System®
TiUnite™ Catalogue, Nobel Biocare].

4.10 Titanium Nitride Layer Formation

Nitrogen ions are implanted onto titanium to improve wear resistance
and hard-tissue compatibility, and into Ti–6Al–4V to improve corrosion resistance. A thin nitride film formed on titanium with high
wear resistance is already used commercially in bone plates, dental
implants, and artificial hip joints (see Figure 4.15). Thin films of TiN
show gold color — the film is used to categorize devices.

4.11 Modification with Biomolecules and Polymers

In the design of bone-substituting and blood-contacting materials for
both medical implants and bioaffinity sensors, it is a major challenge
to generate surfaces and interfaces that are able to withstand protein
adsorption.

To accelerate bone formation surrounding implant materials,
the materials are modified with biomolecules. Several phosphonic
acids were synthesized and grafted onto titanium. Proliferation,
differentiation, and protein production of rats' osteoblastic cells
on the titanium were then investigated [47]. Type I collagen production increased with modification by ethane–1,1,2–triphosphonic
acid and methylenediphosphonic acid. To improve hard tissue
response, bone morphogenetic protein–4 (BMP–4) was immobilized

on Ti–6Al–4V alloy through lysozyme [48]. To improve tissue compatibility, attempts were made for silane chemistry to couple proteins to the oxidized metal surfaces of Co–Cr–Mo, Ti–6Al–4V, Ti, and Ni–Ti [49].

Platelet adhesion, adsorption of proteins, peptides and antibodies, and DNA can likewise be controlled by modifications. A class of copolymers based on poly(L–lysine)–g–poly(ethylene glycol), PLL–g–PEG, was found to spontaneously adsorb from aqueous solutions onto TiO_2, $Si_{0.4}Ti_{0.6}O_2$, and Nb_2O_5 to develop blood-contacting materials and biosensors [50]. Poly(ethylene glycol)–poly(DL–lactic acid) (PEG–PLA) copolymeric micelles were attached to functionalized TiO_2 and Au. The micelle layer enhanced the protein resistance of the surfaces by up to 70%.

Silicon and titanium oxide surfaces (SiO_2/Si and TiO_2/Ti) were covalently modified with bioactive molecules (e.g., peptides) in a simple three-step procedure to control cellular and biomolecular functions on the surfaces. Bioactive surfaces were synthesized by first immobilizing N–(2–aminoethyl)–3–aminopropyl–trimethoxysilane (EDS) to polished quartz disks, polished silicon wafers, or sputter-deposited titanium films. Subsequently, a maleimide-activated surface, amenable to tethering molecules, with a free thiol (e.g., cysteine) was created by coupling sulfosuccinimidyl 4–(N–maleimidomethyl) cyclohexane–1–carboxylate (sulfro–SMCC) to the terminal amine on EDS. Peptides with terminal cysteine residues were immobilized on maleimide-activated oxides [51].

The surface of stainless steel was first modified by the silane coupling agent (SCA), (3–mercaptopropyl)trimethoxysilane. The silanized stainless steel surface (SCA–SS surface) was subsequently activated by argon plasma and then subjected to UV-induced graft polymerization of poly(ethylene glycol)methacrylate (PEGMA). The PEGMA graft-polymerized stainless steel couple (PEGMA–g–SCA–SS) with a high graft concentration, and thus a high PEG content, was found to be very effective in preventing bovine serum albumin and γ-globulin adsorption [52].

Metal oxide surfaces (Ta_2O_5, Al_2O_3, Nb_2O_5, ZrO_2, SiO_2) were coated by self-assembled monolayers (SAMs) of dodecyl phosphate ($DDPO_4$) and 12–hydroxy dodecyl phosphate ($OH–DDPO_4$). The coating was done by a novel surface modification protocol based on the adsorption of alkyl phosphate ammonium salts from aqueous

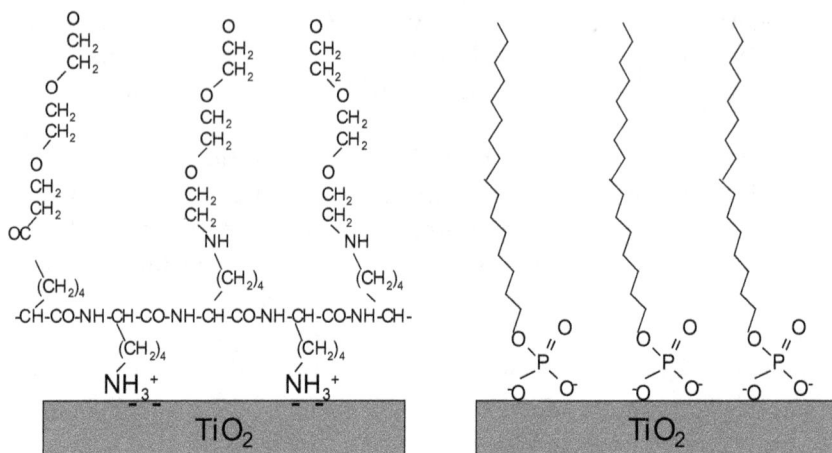

Figure 4.31. Examples of polymer immobilization model on titanium [53].

solution for application to biochemical analyses and biosensors [53]. To apply a surface plasmon resonance (SPR) to biosensors, a sandwich immunoassay was performed on a thin gold film set in an SPR cell. The molecular motion of self-assembled monolayers on gold was examined using SPR under an electric field. Two examples of polymer modification of TiO_2 are shown in Figure 4.31.

4.12   Morphological Modification

The morphology of an implant surface influences the bonding strength of the bone-implant interface. In other words, the surface structure of an implant has a significant influence on both its anchorage and strength of adhesion to the tissue. A smooth implant surface with a small contact area with the tissue will show lower adhesion strength than a rough surface. The ingrowth of bone into surface cavities has a favorable influence on adhesion strength. Cell growth is unaffected by grooves or pores on the implant surface. Figure 4.32 shows how cell growth was expanded alongside the grooves on titanium which was vaporized on a silicon substrate.

Surface structuring or morphological control was performed to increase the anchoring or bonding of bone to implants. For structured surfaces, various types were formed by casting, surface roughening,

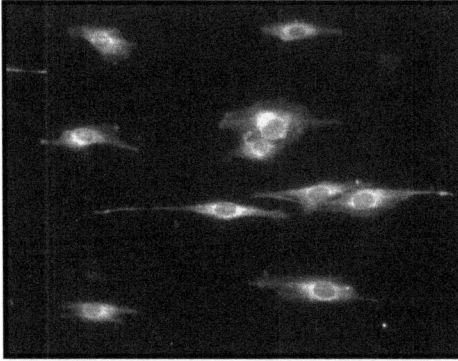

Figure 4.32. Fluorescent microscopic image of human endothelial cell type HGTFN expanding along to fill grooves present in gold, which is deposited on a silicon substrate. Grooves are not apparent in this picture, but transverse directional grooves exist on gold.

or through lacunae holes and porous coating produced by sintering or plasma spraying. With corresponding wax models, a roughened surface can be produced by investment casting, while a special open-cell, porous, sponge structure can be produced by precision casting.

In terms of morphological control, various morphologies of the implant surface were designed: beads, grooves, cancellous structure, fiber mesh, and porous coating. Rough pores were prepared using metallic beads with casting. The pore size was 0.4–1.5 mm, and the pore fraction was up to 70%. Micro-porous porosities of 0.1–0.4 mm with porosity values of 35–50% were produced using one of these methods: sintering of metal beads or diffusion welding of metal fibers. A smaller pore size of 0.02–0.2 mm was obtained through plasma spraying of titanium powder. To evaluate the effect of porous surface structures on fatigue strength, a surface layer consisting of beads or wires which corresponded to a porous coating was used. All pores were interconnected and superficially linked to the outer demarcation of the coating. Typical surface patterns are shown in Figure 4.33.

Many studies were conducted to examine the effect of pores (see Figure 4.30) on the ingrowth of tissues or cells to titanium. The host bone came into contact with a surface relief of the plasma-sprayed coating, which was then characterized using an open microstructure with variable height at any part of a surface Animal tests confirmed the advantage of a rough surface Several studies have been conducted

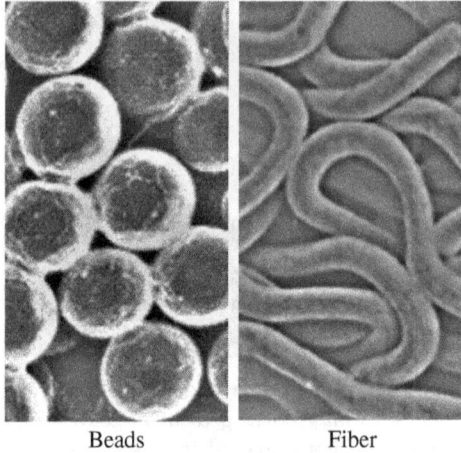

Beads   Fiber

Figure 4.33. Beads and fibers of titanium.

on bone ingrowth into porous systems with different pore sizes. The diameter of interconnecting pores seems to dictate the quality of tissue growing into porosity space. When pore sizes were down to 50 μm, there was effective bone ingrowth into porous coatings. However, for the regeneration of mineralized bone, the interconnections of porosity must be larger than 100 μm. When the pore size was larger than 1 mm, fibrous tissues were sometimes formed. Based on these readings, the optimal pore size for mineralized bone ingrowth was concluded at 100–400 μm [54].

Titanium fiber mesh (see Figure 4.30) was used as a scaffold for tissue engineering with cultured osteogenic cells [47, 55]. After titanium fiber mesh was seeded with osteogenic cells, bone formation was generated more effectively in a shorter culture time.

4.13 Surface Analysis

Surface analysis and surface modification are inseparably related to each other. Following surface modification, surface analysis techniques will be used to characterize composition, crystallinity, and other critical surface properties of modified surfaces.

A surface analysis technique consists of two components. The first component is the probe that irradiates a material surface. The second component refers to the signal used for analysis. Summarized

Table 4.5. Examples of surface analysis instruments: original probe and detected signal.

	Probe		
Signal	**(a) X-ray or Light**	**(b) Electron**	**(c) Ion**
1. Photo electron	X-ray Photoelectron Spectroscopy (XPS)		
2. Auger electron		Auger Electron Spectroscopy (AES)	
3. Secondary electron		Scanning Electron Spectroscopy (SEM)	
4. Ion	Laser Microprobe Mass Spectrometry (LAMMA)		Secondary Ion Mass Spectroscopy (SIMS)
5. X-ray or light	X-ray Diffractometry (XRD)	Energy Dispersive Spectroscopy (EDS) Electron Probe Microanalysis (EPMA)	Particle-Induced X-ray Emission (PIXE)
6. Backscattering ion		Scanning Electron Spectroscopy (SEM)	Rutherford Backscattering Spectrometry (RBS)

in Table 4.5 are the probe-signal permutations of various surface analytical instruments.

XPS, AES, SIMS, and RBS are surface-sensitive techniques used to characterize thin films and layers at the nanometer level. On the other hand, SEM, EDS, and EPMA are conventional tools that analyze specimens' morphologies and compositions.

4.14 Future of Surface Engineering of Metallic Biomaterials

Metallic materials are widely used in medicine not only for orthopedic implants but also as cardiovascular devices and for other purposes. Biomaterials are always used in close contact with living tissues.

Therefore, interactions between material surfaces and living tissues must be well understood. This knowledge is essential to developing new novel materials.

In particular, metal surface–biomolecule reactions and/or metal surface–cell reactions are important. A good knowledge of these reactions can help to add biofunctions to metallic materials that already have excellent mechanical properties. Finally, through surface modification techniques such as multi-layer coating and patterning of multi-functional layers, it is possible to arrive at an optimal range of biofunctions in a biomaterial.

References

[1]   K. Asami, S. C. Chen, H. Habazaki, and K. Hashimoto, The surface characterization of titanium and titanium–nickel alloys in sulfuric acid, *Corros. Sci.*, 1993, 35:43–49.

[2]   T. Hanawa, K. Asami, and K. Asaoka, Repassivation of titanium and surface oxide film regenerated in simulated bioliquid, *J. Biomed. Mater. Res.*, 1998, 40:530–538.

[3]   T. Hanawa and M. Ota, Calcium phosphate naturally formed on titanium in electrolyte solution, *Biomaterials*, 1991, 12:767–774.

[4]   T. Hanawa, Titanium and its oxide film: A substrate for formation of apatite, in *The Bone-biomaterial Interface*, ed. J. E. Davies, (University of Toronto Press, Toronto, 1991) pp. 49–61.

[5]   T. Hanawa, O. Okuno, and H. Hamanaka, Compositional change in surface of Ti–Zr alloys in artificial bioliquid, *J. Jpn. Inst. Met.*, 1992, 56:1168–1173.

[6]   P. Bruesch, K. Muller, A. Atrens, and H. Neff, Corrosion of stainless steels in chloride solution — An XPS investigation of passive films, *Appl. Phys.*, 1985, 38:1–18.

[7]   S. Jin and A. Atrens, ESCA-studies of the structure and composition of the passive film formed on stainless steels by various immersion times in 0.1 M NaCl solution, *Appl. Phys.*, 1987, A42:149–165.

[8]   T. Hanawa, S. Hiromoto, A. Yamamoto, D. Kuroda, and K. Asami, XPS characterization of the surface oxide film of 316L stainless samples that were located in quasi-biological environments, *Mater. Trans.*, 2002, 43:3088–3092.

[9]   D. C. Smith, R. M. Pilliar, J. B. Metson, and N. S. McIntyre, Preparative procedures and surface spectroscopic studies, *J. Biomed. Mater. Res.*, 1991, 25:1069–1084.

[10]   T. Hanawa, S. Hiromoto, and K. Asami, Characterization of the surface oxide film of a Co–Cr–Mo alloy after being located in quasibiological environments using XPS, *Appl. Surf. Sci.*, 2001, 183: 68–75.

[11]   K. Endo, Y. Araki, and H. Ohno, *In vitro* and *in vivo* corrosion of dental Ag–Pd–Cu alloys, *Trans. Int. Cong. Dent. Mater.*, 1989, 226–227.

[12]   T. Hanawa, H. Takahashi, M. Ota, R. F. Pinizzotto, J. L. Ferracane, and T. Okabe, Surface characterization of amalgams using X-ray photoelectron spectroscopy, *J. Dent. Res.*, 1987, 66:1470–1478.

[13]   J. E. Sundgren, P. Bodo, and I. Lundstrom, Auger electron spectroscopic studies of the interface between human tissue and implants of titanium and stainless steel, *J. Colloid Interface Sci.*, 1986, 110: 9–20.

[14]   M. Espostito, J. Lausmaa, J. M. Hirsch, and P. Thomsen, Surface analysis of failed oral titanium implants, *J. Biomed. Mater. Res. Appl. Biomater.*, 1999, 48:559–568.

[15]   T. Hanawa and M. Ota, Characterization of surface film formed on titanium in electrolyte, *Appl. Surf. Sci.*, 1992, 55:269–276.

[16]   K. E. Healy and P. Ducheyne, The mechanisms of passive dissolution of titanium in a model physiological environment, *J. Biomed. Mater. Res.*, 1992, 26:319–338.

[17]   A. P. Serro, A. C. Fernandes, B. Saramago, J. Lima, and M. A. Barbosa, Apatite desorption on titanium surfaces — The role of albumin adsorption, *Biomaterials*, 1997, 18:963–968.

[18]   T. Hanawa, S. Hiromoto, K. Asami, H. Ukai, and K. Murakami, Surface modification of titanium utilizing a repassivation reaction in aqueous solutions, *Mater. Trans.*, 2002, 43:3005–3009.

[19]   T. Hanawa, S. Hiromoto, K. Asami, O. Okuno, and K. Asaoka, Surface oxide films on titanium alloys regenerated in Hanks' solution, *Mater. Trans.*, 2002, 43:3000–3004.

[20]   J. E. Sundgren, P. Bodo, I. Lundstrom, A. Berggren, and S. Hellem, Auger electron spectroscopic studies of stainless steel implants, *J. Biomed. Mater. Res.*, 1985, 19:663–671.

[21]   J. Walczak, F. Shahgaldi, and F. Heatley, *In vivo* corrosion of 316L stainless steel hip implants: Morphology and elemental compositions of corrosion products, *Biomaterials*, 1998, 19:229–237.

[22]   B. Ivarsson and I. Lundström, Physical characterization of protein adsorption on metal and metal oxide surfaces, *CRC Critic. Rev. Biocompatibility*, 1986, 2:1–96.

[23]   H. Elwing, Protein adsorption and ellipsometry in biomaterial research, *Biomaterials*, 1998, 19:397–406.

[24] R. D. Bagnall and P. A. Arundel, A method for the prediction of protein adsorption on implant surfaces, *J. Biomed. Mater. Res.*, 1983, 17:459–466.

[25] R. L. Williams and D. F. Williams, Albumin adsorption on metal surfaces, *Biomaterials*, 1988, 9:206–212.

[26] M. Ahmad, D. Grawronski, J. Blum, J. Goldberg, and G. Gronowicz, Differential response of human osteoblast-like cells to commercially pure (CP) titanium grades 1 and 4, *J. Biomed. Mater. Res.*, 1999, 46:121–131.

[27] L. Raisanen, M. Kononen, J. Juhanoja, P. Varpavaara, J. Hautaniemi, J. Kivilahti, and M. Hormia, Expression of cell adhesion complexes in epithelial cells seeded on biomaterial surfaces, *J. Biomed. Mater. Res.*, 2000, 49:79–87.

[28] J. E. Davies, B. Lowenberg, and A. Shiga, The bone-titanium interface *in vitro*, *J. Biomed. Mater. Res.*, 1990, 24:1289–1306.

[29] A. Yamamoto, S. Mishima, N. Maruyama, and M. Sumita, A new technique for direct measurement of the shear force necessary to detach a cell from a material, *Biomaterials*, 1998, 19:871–879.

[30] A. Yamamoto, S. Mishima, M. Sumita, and T. Hanawa, Measurement of cell adhesive shear strength and cell detachment surface energy of a single murine fibroblast adhering to thin metal films, *J. Jpn. Soc. Biomater.*, 2000, 18:87–94.

[31] J. L. Ong and L. C. Lucas, Post-deposition heat treatment for ion beam sputter deposited calcium phosphate coatings, *Biomaterials*, 1994, 15:337–341.

[32] S. Ban and S. Maruno, Morphology and microstructure of electro-chemically deposited calcium phosphates in a modified simulated body fluid, *Biomaterials*, 1998, 19:1245–1253.

[33] H. Ishizawa and M. Ogino, Formation and characterization of anodic titanium oxide films containing Ca and P, *J. Biomed. Mater. Res.*, 1995, 29:65–72.

[34] H. M. Kim, F. Miyaji, T. Kokubo, and T. Nakamura, Preparation of bioactive Ti and its alloys via simple chemical surface treatment, *J. Biomed. Mater. Res.*, 1996, 32:409–417.

[35] Y. Mu, T. Kobayashi, M. Sumita, A. Yamamoto, and T. Hanawa, Metal ion release from titanium with active oxygen species generated by rat macrophages *in vitro*, *J. Biomed. Mater. Res.*, 2000, 49: 238–243.

[36] P. Tengvall, I. Lundstrom, L. Sjoqvist, H. Elwing, and L. M. Bjursten, Titanium-hydrogen peroxide interaction: Model studies of the influence of the inflammatory response on titanium implants, *Biomaterials*, 1989, 10:166–175.

[37] C. Ohtsuki, H. Iida, S. Hayakawa, and A. Osaka, Bioactivity of titanium treated with hydrogen peroxide solutions containing metal chlorides, *J. Biomed. Mater. Res.*, 1997, 35:39–47.

[38] T. Hanawa, M. Kon, H. Ukai, K. Murakami, Y. Miyamoto, and K. Asaoka, Surface modification of titanium in calcium-ion-containing solutions, *J. Biomed. Mater. Res.*, 1997, 34:273–278.

[39] K. Hamada, M. Kon, T. Hanawa, K. Yokoyama, Y. Miyamoto, and K. Asaoka, Hydrothermal modification of titanium surface in calcium solutions, *Biomaterials*, 2002, 23:2265–2272.

[40] T. Hanawa, S. Kihara, and M. Murakami, Calcium phosphate precipitation on calcium-ion-implanted titanium in electrolyte, in Characterization and performance of calcium phosphate coatings for implants, eds. E. Horowitz and J. E. Parr, (American Society for Testing and Materials, Philadelphia) ASTM STP 1196, pp. 170–184.

[41] T. Hanawa, Y. Nodasaka, H. Ukai, K. Murakami, and K. Asaoka, Cell compatibility of calcium-ion-implanted titanium, *J. Jpn. Soc. Biomater.*, 1994, 12:209–216.

[42] T. Hanawa, Y. Kamiura, S. Yamamoto, T. Kohgo, A. Amemiya, H. Ukai, K. Murakami, and K. Asaoka, Early bone formation around calcium-ion-implanted titanium inserted into rat tibia, *J. Biomed. Mater. Res.*, 1997, 36:131–136.

[43] T. Hanawa, H. Ukai, and K. Murakami, X-ray photoelectron spectroscopy of calcium-ion-implanted titanium, *J. Electron Spectrosc.*, 1993, 63:347–354.

[44] T. Hanawa, M. Kon, H. Doi, H. Ukai, K. Murakami, H. Hamanaka, and K. Asaoka, Amount of hydroxyl radical on calcium-ion-implanted titanium and point of zero charge of constituent oxide of the surface-modified layer, *J. Mater. Sci. Mater. Med.*, 1998, 9:89–92.

[45] T. Hanawa, K. Asami, and K. Asaoka, Microdissolution of calcium ions from calcium-ion-implanted titanium, *Corros. Sci.*, 1996, 38:1579–1594.

[46] T. Hanawa, K. Asami, and K. Asaoka, AES studies on the dissolution of surface oxide from calcium-ion-implanted titanium in nitric acid and buffered solutions, *Corros. Sci.*, 1996, 38:2061–2067.

[47] C. Viornery, H. L. Guenther, B. O. Arronson, P. Pechy, P. Descouts, and M. Gratzel, Osteoblast culture on polished titanium disks modified with phosphonic acids, *J. Biomed. Mater. Res.*, 2002, 62:149–155.

[48] D. A. Puleo, R. A. Kissling, and M. S. Sheu, A technique to immobilize bioactive proteins, including bone morphogenetic protein–4 (BMP–4), on titanium alloy, *Biomaterials*, 2002, 23:2079–2087.

[49] A. Nanci, J. D. Wuest, L. Peru, P. Brunet, V. Sharma, S. Zalzal, and M. D. McKee, Chemical modification of titanium surfaces for

covalent attachment of biological molecules, *J. Biomed. Mater. Res.*, 1998, 40:324–335.

[50] N. P. Huang, R. Michel, J. Vörös, M. Textor, R. Hofer, A. Rossi, D. L. Dlbert, J. A. Hubbell, and N. D. Spencer, Poly(L–lysine)–g–poly(ethylene glycol) layers on metal oxide surfaces: Surface analytical characterization and resistance to serum and fibrinogen adsorption, *Langmuir*, 2001, 17:489–498.

[51] S. J. Xiao, M. Textor, N. D. Spencer, and H. Sigrist, Covalent attachment of cell-adhesive, (Arg–Gly–Asp)-containing peptides to titanium surfaces, *Langmuir*, 1998, 114:5507–5516.

[52] F. Zhang, E. T. Kang, K. G. Neoh, P. Wang, and K. L. Tan, Surface modification of stainless steel by grafting of poly(ethylene glycol) for reduction in protein adsorption, *Biomaterials*, 2001, 22:1541–1548.

[53] M. Textor, L. Ruiz, R. Hofer, A. Rossi, K. Feldman, G. Hähner, and N. D. Spencer, Structural chemistry of self-assembled monolayers of octadecylphosphoric acid on tantalum oxide surfaces, *Langmuir*, 2000, 16:3257–3271.

[54] R. D. Bloebaum, K. N. Bachus, N. G. Momberger, and A. A. Hoffman, Mineral apposition rates of human cancellous bone at the interface of porous-coated implants, *J. Biomed. Mater. Res.*, 1994, 28:537–544.

[55] J. W. M. Vehof, A. E. de Ruijter, P. H. M. Spauwen, and J. A. Jansen, Influence of rh BMP–2 on rat bone marrow stromal cells cultured on titanium fiber mesh, *Tissue Eng.*, 2001, 7:373–383.

Chapter 5

Biomaterials in Restorative Dentistry

Adrian U. Jin Yap[*,†,‡] **and Na Yu**[†,§]

*Department of Dentistry, Ng Teng Fong General Hospital and
Faculty of Dentistry, National University Health System, Singapore
†National Dental Research Institute Singapore,
National Dental Centre Singapore and Duke-NUS Medical School,
Singapore Health Services, Singapore
‡tmdsleepden@gmail.com
§nayu0909@gmail.com

Dentistry is a science and art concerned with the prevention, diagnosis, and treatment of diseases of the teeth and adjacent tissues, and the restoration of missing dental and maxillo-facial structures. Every dental restorative procedure requires the use of materials. This chapter introduces the restorative materials used in clinical dentistry. Dental biomaterials can be broadly classified into ceramics, polymers, and metals. Many restorative materials are fixed permanently into the patient's mouth or are removed only occasionally for cleaning. The materials have to withstand the effects of a hostile environment. Temperature variations, wide variations in acidity or alkalinity, and high stresses all affect the durability of restorative materials. Most restorative materials are managed entirely by clinicians and their assistants. Some are, however, associated with the work of dental technologists or the use of computer-aided design and manufacturing (CAD/CAM) at dental laboratory to produce customized dental restoration to reconstruct patient-specific tooth anatomy. Successful restorative dentistry is dependent on the correct selection of material for a given application and the ability to carry out customized manipulative procedures to arrive at the optimum properties of the material.

5.1 Introduction

Dentistry is a science and art concerned with the prevention, diagnosis, and treatment of diseases of the teeth and adjacent tissues, and the restoration of missing dental and maxillo-facial structures. Every dental restorative procedure requires the use of materials. As the former makes up the bulk of clinical work, a dentist spends much of his/her professional career handling materials. The success or failure of restorative treatment depends upon the "correct choice of material for a given application" and the "ability to carry out manipulative procedures to arrive at the optimum properties" of that material [1]. Restorative materials in dentistry can be broadly classified into ceramics, polymers, and metals (Figure 5.1). As many of these materials are fixed into the patient's mouth or are removed only occasionally, they have to withstand the effects of a very hostile environment. Normal mouth temperature varies between 32°C and 37°C. Intake of hot or cold drinks or food extends this temperature range from 0 to 70°C. The pH of oral fluids ranges from 4 to 8.5 and extends from pH 2 to 11 with the consumption of acidic juices and alkaline medications [2]. As the load on teeth and restorations can reach up to 170 N, most restorative materials must have high mechanical properties [3].

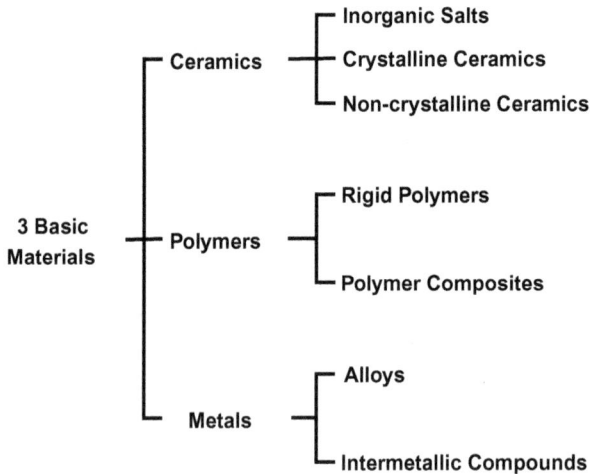

Figure 5.1. The three basic materials used in restorative dentistry.

Although many restorative materials are managed entirely by the dentist and his assistant, others are generally fabricated by dental technologists. A third group of materials links the dental surgery to the laboratory, e.g., impression material. This group of materials is beyond the scope of this chapter and will not be deliberated. This chapter serves to introduce the restorative materials used in clinical dentistry with special emphasis on materials science, engineering, and processing.

5.2 Ceramics

5.2.1 *Inorganic Salts (Dental Cements)*

Dental cements are typically formulated as powders and liquids. The powders are basic (proton acceptors) in nature while the liquids are acidic (proton donors). A viscous paste is formed when the powder and liquid are mixed. This subsequently hardens to a solid mass. The equation for the cement-forming reaction [1] can be simplified as follows:

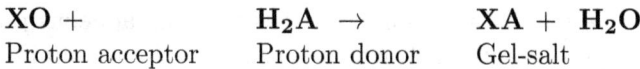

$$\text{XO} + \qquad \text{H}_2\text{A} \rightarrow \qquad \text{XA} + \text{H}_2\text{O}$$

Proton acceptor	Proton donor	Gel-salt

As only a part of the powder reacts with the liquids, the set cement is heterogeneous and composed of unreacted powder particles surrounded by a matrix of gel-salt (reaction product). Five main types of acid–base cements can be derived from two types of powders (Figure 5.2).

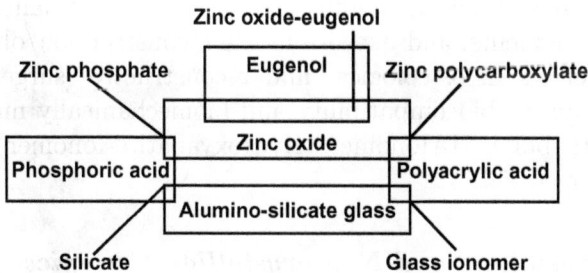

Figure 5.2. Five main types of dental cements.

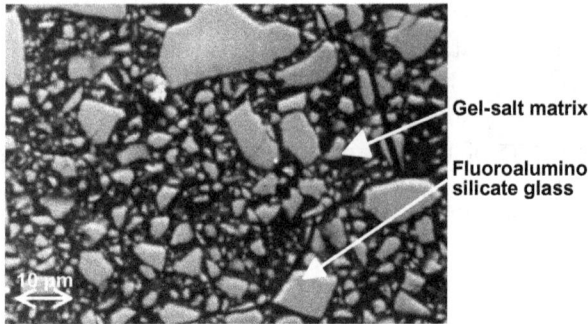

Figure 5.3.   SEM of a typical glass ionomer.

Clinical usage of these cements includes temporary and permanent restoration of teeth:

- cementing of inlays, crowns, bridges, and orthodontic brackets,
- lining of cavities, and
- filling of root canals,
- preserving tooth pulp tissues.

Among the various inorganic salts, the glass ionomer cements are worthy to be highlighted. They are derived from aqueous polymeric acid and a glass component, which is usually a fluoroalumino silicate (Figure 5.3). The glass is obtained by fusing silica, alumina, and calcium fluoride at high temperature, followed by fine-grinding the shocked-cooled molten mass. They have the dual advantages of chemical adhesion to teeth (hydroxyapatite) and sustained fluoride release. The lack of exotherm during setting, the absence of monomer as well as the improved release of incorporated therapeutic agents have led to the development of glass ionomer cements for biomedical applications. They have been successfully used to stabilize implanted devices and bony fragments, and likewise in the reconstruction/obliteration of bony defects in osteological and reconstructive surgery [4]. In order to improve biocompatibility and biomechanically match glass ionomers to bone, HAIonomer (Hydroxyapatite-Ionomer) cements were developed [5].

5.2.2   *Crystalline and Non-crystalline Ceramics*

Crystalline ceramics like silica and alumina are used to reinforce polymers and porcelain. Dental porcelain is essentially a non-crystalline

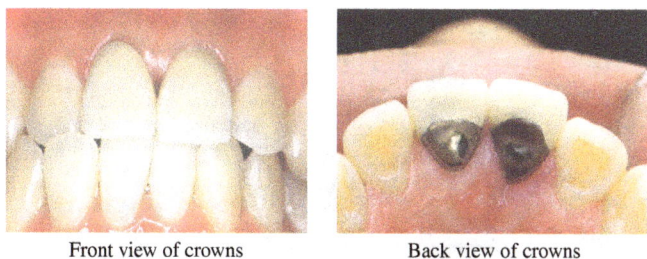

| Front view of crowns | Back view of crowns |

Figure 5.4. Porcelain-fused-to-metal (PFM) crowns.

ceramic (glass) prepared from high-purity feldspar. Ceramics are inherently brittle and must not be subjected to large tensile stresses. The latter can lead to catastrophic failures. One method of reducing the influence of the brittleness of ceramics is to fuse them to a material of higher toughness (e.g., metal), as with porcelain-fused-to-metal prostheses (Figure 5.4). Ceramics can also be reinforced with dispersions of alumina or a core of pure alumina.

Feldspathic porcelain was the traditional ceramic material used for veneers, inlays, and onlays. It is composed of a mixture of glass and crystalline phases. Aluminous porcelain containing aluminum oxide was introduced in the 1950s to improve strength and wear resistance. Glass-ceramics, encompassing leucite-reinforced and lithium disilicate porcelains, were developed in the 1960s–1970s. These materials provided increased strength and durability, extending their use as crowns in posterior load-bearing teeth. Zirconia-based ceramics, such as yttria-stabilized zirconia, became popular in the 2000s. They have excellent mechanical properties, including high strength as well as fracture resistance, and biocompatibility and are indicated for crowns, bridges, and implant prostheses.

The fabrication process of ceramic dental restorations comprises several essential steps [6]. First, impressions of the patient's prepared teeth are acquired physically with silicone materials or digitally with the use of intraoral scanners (Figures 5.5 and 5.6). Second, the impressions are employed to create physical and digital models. Third, the choice of ceramic materials is decided upon considering the restoration designs and mechanical as well as aesthetic requirements. Fourth, the restorations are manufactured through combinations of sintering, pressing, and computer-aided design and manufacturing (CAD/CAM) processes depending on the type of

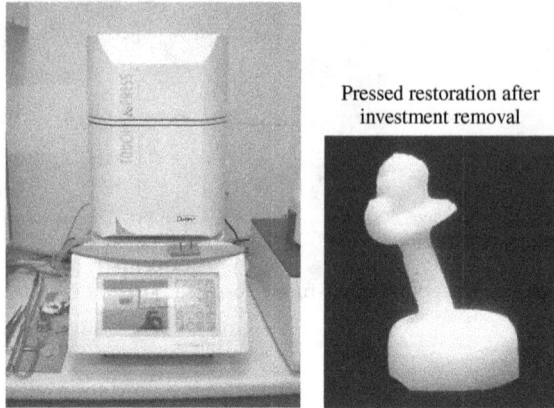

Pressed restoration after
investment removal

Figure 5.5. Injection and pressed ceramic systems involve the use of "loss-wax" technique.

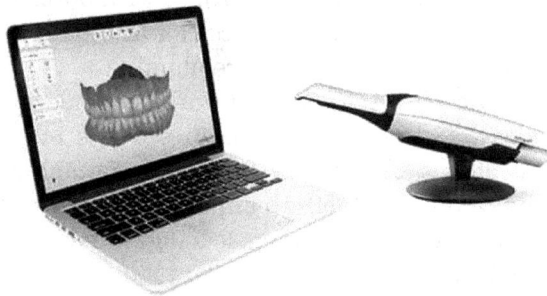

Figure 5.6. Intraoral scanner.

material and restoration. CAD/CAM processes involve the milling of ceramic blocks (Figures 5.7 and 5.8) and possibly 3D-ceramic printing. In the final stage, the manufactured restorations are adjusted to the desired forms, polished, and/or glazed to obtain a smooth finish before clinical fitting.

Advances in technology, especially CAD/CAM systems and digital impressions, have significantly enhanced the accuracy and efficiency of fabrication processes, resulting in improved quality and longevity of ceramic dental restorations. Using proprietary CAD software, dental professionals or technicians can import digital impression data, manipulate digital models, design, and customize restorations for individual patients. The software offers tools for the virtual shaping of restorations, contour/contact adjustments, and

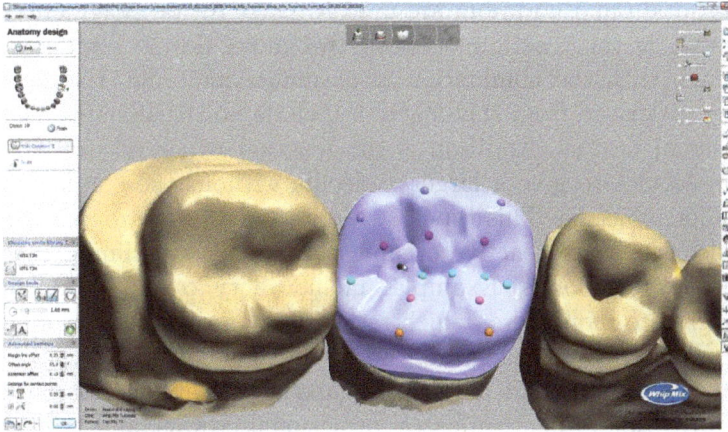

Figure 5.7. Computer-aided design software.

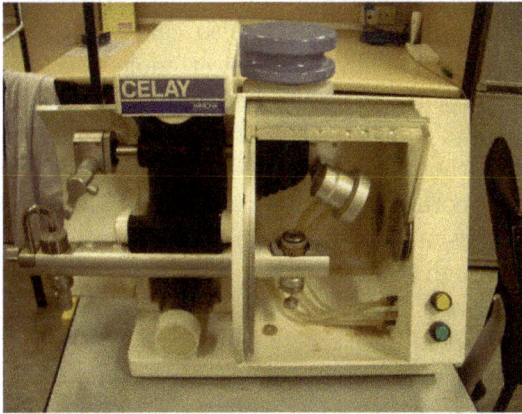

Figure 5.8. The Celay copy-milling system.

material selection. Once the design is finalized, the CAD software generates the instructions for the computer-controlled production.

5.3 Polymers

5.3.1 *Rigid Polymers*

Polymers are long-chain molecules derived from many repeating units called monomers. Two types of chemical polymerization reactions, condensation and addition, are used to make dental polymers. Condensation is the reaction between two molecules to form a larger molecule, with the elimination of a smaller molecule. Examples of polymers derived from this reaction include polycarbonates used for provisional crowns. Addition is the reaction which occurs between two molecules to give a larger molecule without the elimination of a smaller molecule. This type of reaction takes place for vinyl compounds, which are reactive organic compounds containing carbon–carbon double bonds. Examples include acrylic acids and methyl methacrylate monomers, which respectively form poly(acrylic acid) and poly(methyl methacrylate) or acrylic. The latter (acrylic) is the most widely used rigid polymeric material. Its applications include the fabrication of denture bases, provisional crowns, and bridges.

Acrylic materials can be heat- or self-cured. The composition of self-cured materials is similar to heat-cured materials except that activators, such as dimethyl-p-toluidine, are present in the liquid component. Self-cured acrylics are also called autopolymerizing or cold-curing materials. They have lower molecular weights, higher residual monomer contents, poorer rheological properties, poorer color stability, and greater porosity and are weaker than heat-cured acrylics. Although acrylic prostheses (e.g., dentures and dental splints) can theoretically be processed by a number of techniques including compression and injection molding, the most commonly used one is the dough technique. In this technique, a dough is formed from a mixture of the monomer (liquid) and polymer (powder). This is subsequently packed into a mold and polymerized under the appropriate conditions to give a solid prosthesis (Figures 5.9 and 5.10). For heat-cured acrylics, two alternative heating techniques are used: (a) heat at 72°C for at least 16 hours or (b) heat at 72°C for two hours followed by continued heating at 100°C for a further two hours [1]. The latter heating technique enables prosthesis to be produced in a shorter time but increases the likelihood of warpage. Microwave curing techniques have also been suggested. The free radical addition polymerization reactions in light-cured acrylic materials are initiated by visible light via tungsten halogen lamps with a light wavelength of 400–500 nm.

Polymer-based prostheses could be also produced with CAD/CAM. Employing the same procedures for ceramics, CAD/CAM technology can be used to mill high-quality acrylic temporary

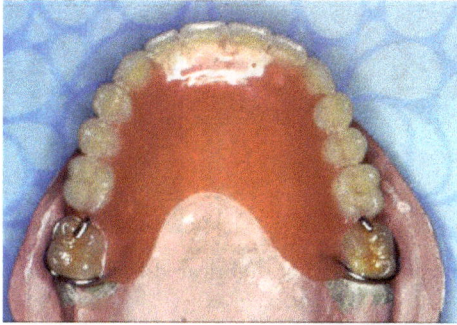

Figure 5.9. Acrylic dentures on cast.

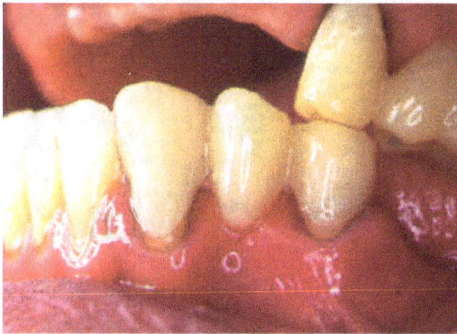

Figure 5.10. Acrylic provisional bridge in patient.

restorations. Additionally, high-performance polymers such as Polyetheretherketone (PEEK) are used together with computer numerical control (CNC) milling to produce frameworks for partial dentures and implant-supported prostheses [7]. Polyethylene is also emerging as a viable CAD/CAM material for partial denture fabrication (Figure 5.11). Its pliability imparts flexibility to the denture frameworks [8]. In 3D printing, polyurethane-based materials could serve as substrates for elastic denture bases and liners increasing patient comfort and adaptability.

5.3.2 *Polymer Composites*

Composites can be defined as three-dimensional combinations of at least two chemically different materials with a distinct interface.

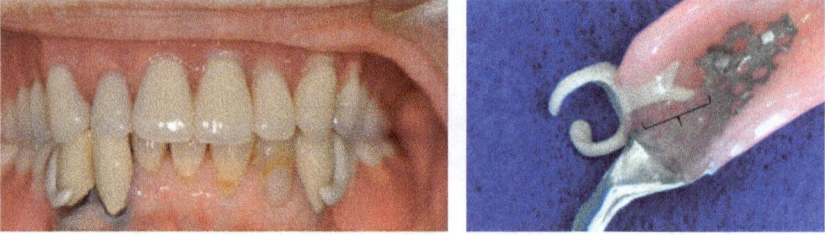

Figure 5.11. CAD/CAM fabricated PEEK denture clasps.

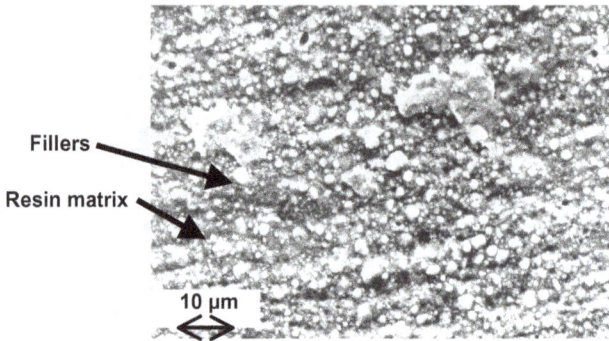

Figure 5.12. Microstructure of a dental composite.

Dental composites (Figure 5.12) essentially comprise a resin matrix (organic phase), a filler-matrix coupling agent (interface), filler particles (dispersed phase), and other minor additions including polymerization initiators, stabilizers, and coloring pigments. Fillers are used in dental composites to provide strengthening, increase stiffness, reduce dimensional change when heated or cooled, reduce setting contraction, impart radiopacity, enhance aesthetics, and improve handling. Most current composites are filled with radiopaque silicate particles based on oxides of barium, strontium, zinc, aluminum, or zirconium. The resin matrix usually contains dimethacrylate monomers of which Bisphenol A–glycidyl methacrylate (BisGMA) is most popular. The hardening of dental composites is the result of a chemical reaction between the resin monomers. A rigid and well-cross-linked polymer network that surrounds the inert fillers is produced. The degree of cure is influenced by many parameters, which include the following [9]:

- addition of polymerization promoters and inhibitors,
- chemical structure of the monomers,
- chemical or light energy imparted to activate the reactions,
- filler composition, and
- composite shade.

Due to the well-recognized anticariogenic effects of fluoride, fluoride-releasing and polyacid-modified composites (compomers) are developed. These composites contain either one or both essential components of glass ionomer cements. The components, however, do not react as part of the setting process — they undergo an acid–base reaction only after hydration. Three different approaches to the development of fluoride-releasing composites have been reported. These approaches involve the addition of water-soluble fluoride salts, matrix-bound fluoride, or fluoride-releasing fillers [10]. The first approach is not ideal because soluble fluoride salts are easily washed out, resulting in a porous structure. This can compromise the physio-mechanical properties of the composite. The second group of materials has been intensely investigated, and fluoride-releasing resin systems are currently used in some commercial composites. The fluoride-releasing filler system approach has been adopted by most commercially available fluoride-releasing composites. More recently, bioactive composites that release fluorides and other therapeutic ions such as calcium were developed to suppress biofilms/acid production, neutralize acids, and replace lost minerals.

Composite restorative techniques may be categorized into three groups:

- direct techniques which consist of only intraoral procedures and require only one appointment (Figure 5.13),
- semi-direct techniques which include both intraoral and extraoral procedures to produce luted restorations, and
- indirect techniques which require several appointments and the support of a dental laboratory.

In both semi-direct and indirect techniques, composites are subjected to photothermic treatment in special ovens. This procedure allows for optimal resin conversions, which results in increased hardness and wear resistance [11, 12]. Both techniques can also employ

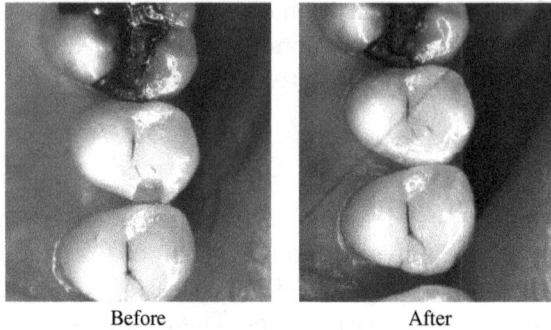

Before   After

Figure 5.13. Direct restorative technique for dental composites.

Table 5.1. Difference between ceramic and composite restorations.

Evaluation Parameters	Ceramics	Composites
Ease of clinical procedures	Satisfactory	Good
Ease of laboratory procedures	Satisfactory	Good
Intraoral repair	Poor	Excellent
Aesthetics	Excellent	Good
Surface polish	Good	Excellent
Wear resistance	Excellent	Good
Brittleness	Satisfactory	Good
Intraoral chemical stability	Excellent	Satisfactory

CAD/CAM milling of photothermic treated and cure composite blocks.

Fiber-reinforced composites have been introduced for the laboratory and chairside fabrication of bridges. Different types of reinforcing fibers are used, including glass, polyethylene, and carbon. The fibers may be arranged in various configurations. Unidirectional, long continuous, and parallel fibers are the most popular, followed by woven and braided fibers. Typically, the fibers are about 7–10 μm in width and span the length of the prosthesis or appliance.

Table 5.1 shows the differences between composite and ceramic restorations. Both are bonded to tooth via micromechanical retention, and both involve the acid-etching of tooth tissues followed by the application of resin primers and/or adhesives.

5.4   Metals

5.4.1   *Alloys*

Since the introduction of investment casting to dentistry in the early 1900s, alloys have been used for different types of prostheses, including crowns, bridges, dentures, and implants. An alloy is a mixture of two or more metallic elements. The constituents can be a metalloid or a non-metal, provided that the resultant mixture exhibits metallic properties. Dental alloys for fabrication of crowns/bridges can be broadly divided into precious metal casting alloys and alloys for porcelain-fused-to-metal restorations. Precious or high-gold-content alloys are used for inlays, full-cast crowns, and partial-veneer crowns (Figure 5.14) as they are soft and burnishable. Precious metal alloys contain mainly gold, palladium, platinum (which are classified as noble metals), and silver. They also contain limited amounts of non-precious alloying elements, like iron, tin, and indium.

Due to aesthetic requirements, most crowns and bridge works are of the porcelain-fused-to-metal (PFM) type. They constitute the majority of all cast restorations used clinically. Alloys intended for use in PFM restorations have several special requirements, such as the following:

- melting temperatures must be above that of porcelain application,
- close matching of thermal properties to those of porcelain,
- high modulus of elasticity, and
- good corrosion resistance.

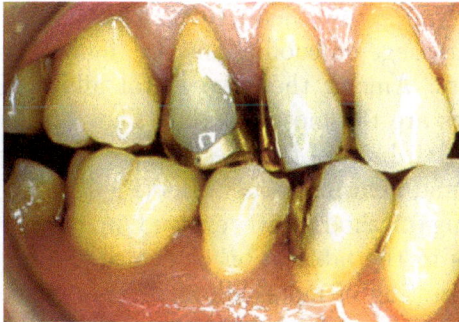

Figure 5.14.   Gold inlay and partial-veneer restorations.

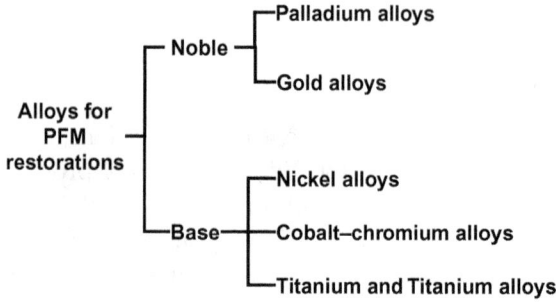

Figure 5.15.   Classification of porcelain-fused-to-metal alloys.

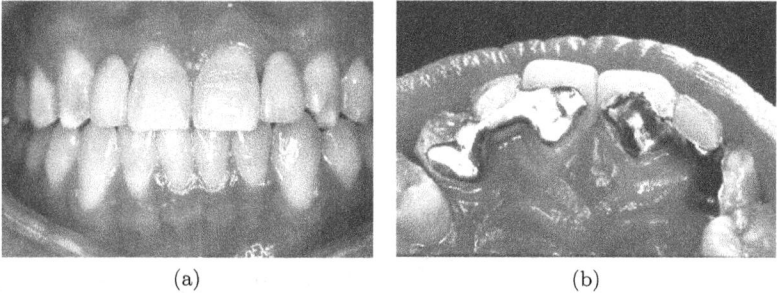

(a)   (b)

Figure 5.16.   (a) Co–Cr acid-etch bridges (front view). (b) Co–Cr acid-etch bridges (back view).

Two groups of alloys are used for PFM applications: noble metal alloys and base metal alloys (Figure 5.15).

Ni–Cr–Be alloys are not popular as nickel is allergenic and beryllium is toxic. The processing of these alloys in the laboratory may be hazardous. They are also difficult to cast because of their low density and high shrinkage on cooling and are difficult to finish because of their hardness. Among the base metal alloys, Co–Cr (cobalt–chromium) alloys are the most popular. They are used for the fabrication of acid-etch bridges (bridges bonded by composite resins to etched enamel) and denture frameworks (Figures 5.16 and 5.17).

Metal printing methods have evolved in recent years, offering new possibilities in the fabrication of dental prostheses. Compared to milling, 3D printing of metal alloys is more economical and efficient. Among the many 3D printing techniques, selective laser melting (SLM) is the most promising. SLM of CoCr [13] and titanium (Ti)

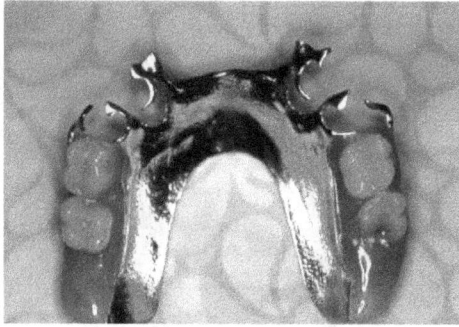

Figure 5.17. Co–Cr denture.

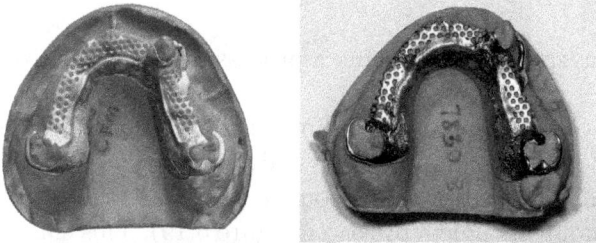

Figure 5.18. CAD/CAM denture framework.

alloys [14] has been extensively used in the construction of removable partial denture frameworks and implant-supported prostheses. The process begins with the generation of a patient-specific 3D model (Figure 5.18). A uniform layer of alloy powder is deposited on a build platform, serving as the foundational material. A high-power laser then meticulously traces the contours of the dental restoration, selectively melting and fusing the alloy particles layer by layer. This additive process yields intricately detailed restorations that are customized to individual patients. Post-processing steps encompass support structure removal and surface finishing/refinements.

Despite their high biocompatibility, Ti and Ti alloys are not commonly used for PFM restorations. This is due primarily to processing difficulties, including high casting temperature (2000°C), rapid oxidization, and reactions with investments [15]. Melting of titanium and titanium alloys has to be done in special furnaces with argon atmosphere. Pure titanium PFM restorations may be fabricated by

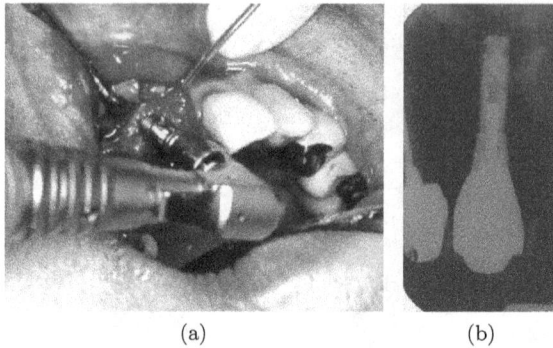

(a)   (b)

Figure 5.19. (a) Surgical placement of dental implant; (b) radiograph of an implant after restoration with a PFM crown (Courtesy of Dr. Keson BC Tan).

machining/spark erosion using a process developed by Nobelpharma AB.

The most common use of Ti and Ti alloys is for dental implants. In general, dental implants are classified as endosseous, subperiosteal, or transosteal. Root-form endosseous implants are the most commonly used implants in clinical practice (Figure 5.19). This class of implants is the only one for which good long-term clinical data are available. Success rates for implants in the lower jaw are approximately 96%, 94%, and 86% at 5, 10, and 15 years, respectively. For the upper jaw, success rates are 88%, 82%, and 78% at the same time intervals [16]. Clinicians' expertise and surgical techniques are two important factors that determine the clinical outcome. They are significantly more important than the specific implant itself. Due to the need to develop a stable interface prior to biomechanical loading, bioceramic coatings and surface roughening have been used to accelerate tissue apposition to implant surfaces. The general requirement for the use of dental implants is available bone to support the implant. Bone augmentation materials (i.e., bone grafts or bone graft substitutes) are used to replace bone deficits and defects.

Noble metals (Figure 5.20) are defined based on their resistance to oxidation and attack by acids. Three noble metals are widely used in dental alloys. They are gold, palladium, and platinum. High-gold alloys (80–90% Au) bond well to porcelain, but creep of alloy may occur during porcelain firing due to their comparatively low melting range. As their moduli are low, a minimum alloy thickness of 0.5 mm is required. Gold–palladium alloys have better creep properties than

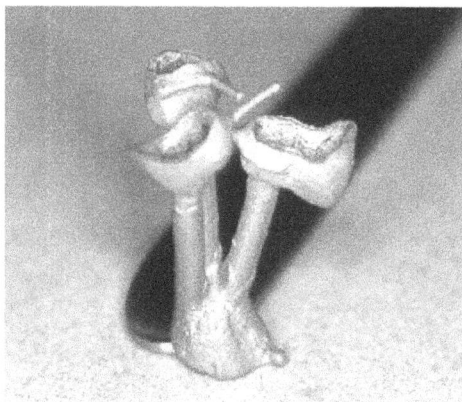

Figure 5.20. Noble metal crowns after casting and prior to addition of porcelain.

high-gold alloys and are more economical. Palladium–silver alloys have similar mechanical properties to high-gold alloys but have high shrinkage and are difficult to cast. They may also have problems with discoloration (greening) when used with certain porcelains. The observed bond between gold alloys and porcelain is believed to result from a combination of the following factors:

- mechanical bonding between fused porcelain and small irregularities on the metal surface,
- chemical bonding between surface film of oxide and porcelain if tin or indium is present,
- compressive bonding resulting from the contraction of porcelain.

While bonding between gold alloys and porcelain is multi-faceted, bonding between base metals is predominantly chemical in nature.

5.4.2 *Intermetallic Compounds*

Metals with chemical affinity for each other can form intermetallic compounds. The most well-known intermetallic compound in dentistry is probably dental amalgam. Amalgam was the material of choice for direct posterior restorations for more than 150 years. The reason for its popularity lies in its ease of manipulation, relatively low cost, and long clinical service. Recently, biological and environmental concerns have arisen due to the mercury it contains. It is, however, presently believed that amalgam presents an acceptable

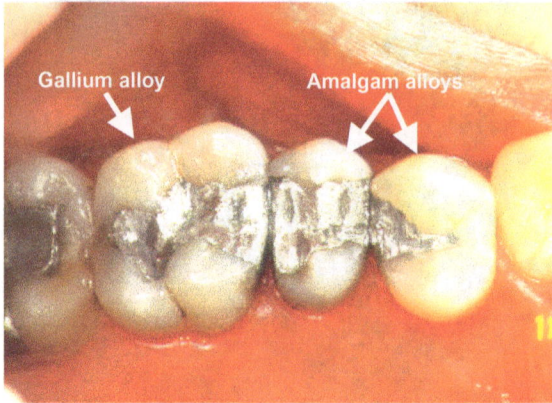

Figure 5.21. Amalgam and gallium alloy restorations (Courtesy of Dr. Jennifer CL Neo).

risk-to-benefit ratio when properly used. An exception to this position has been taken in several parts of Europe where concerns have been raised regarding their use in populations thought to be more susceptible to mercury exposure. The latter includes children as well as pregnant women.

Contemporary amalgams have high copper contents (Figure 5.21) and are classified into lathe-cut, spherical, and admixed types. Lathe-cut alloy particles are milled from a cast ingot and sifted to the appropriate particle size distribution. Spherical alloys are created by means of an atomizing process where a spray of tiny drops is allowed to solidify in an inert atmosphere. Admixed alloys are a mix of lathe-cut and spherical powders. The amalgamation reaction of traditional amalgam alloys can be represented as follows:

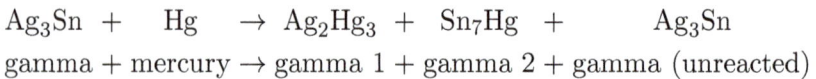

$$Ag_3Sn \; + \quad Hg \quad \rightarrow Ag_2Hg_3 \; + \; Sn_7Hg \; + \qquad Ag_3Sn$$

gamma + mercury → gamma 1 + gamma 2 + gamma (unreacted)

In high-copper blended compositions (where traditional and high-copper phases are mechanically blended together), the gamma 2 phase is removed via the following reaction:

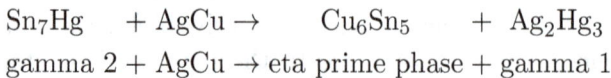

$$Sn_7Hg \quad + AgCu \rightarrow \quad Cu_6Sn_5 \quad + \; Ag_2Hg_3$$

gamma 2 + AgCu → eta prime phase + gamma 1

In single-composition systems (where components are melted together), the eta prime phase is also formed during the amalgamation reaction. The reaction is, however, thought to be $2Cu_3Sn + 3Sn \rightarrow Cu_6Sn_5$ as the source of copper is in the epsilon phase. Absence of the weak gamma 2 phase improves corrosion, strength, and creep properties as well as the marginal durability of amalgam restorations.

In an attempt to circumvent the problems with mercury, gallium alloys (Figure 5.21) were introduced. The melting temperature of gallium can be kept below room temperature with the addition of indium and tin. This liquid can be triturated with spherical silver–tin–copper alloy powder as with other amalgam alloys [15]. Palladium has been added to the alloy powder to improve corrosion properties. Clinical data pertaining to the long-term performance of gallium alloys are currently not available. Significant changes in luster and surface roughness have, however, been reported as early as four months after placement [17].

5.5   Conclusions

An overview of the restorative materials used in clinical dentistry has been presented. Dental biomaterials can be broadly classified into ceramics, polymers, and metals. The success of these restorations is dependent on the correct selection of materials for a given application and the ability to carry out manipulative procedures to arrive at the optimum properties of the material.

References

[1]   E. C. Combe, *Notes on Dental Materials* (Longman, Singapore, 1992).

[2]   J. F. McCabe, *Applied Dental Materials* (Blackwell Science Publications, Oxford, 2008).

[3]   H. W. Fields, W. R. Proffit, J. C. Case, and K. W. L. Vig, Variables affecting measurement of vertical occlusal forces, *J. Dent. Res.*, 1986, 65:135–138.

[4]   I. M. Brook and P. V. Hatton, Glass ionomers: Bioactive implant materials, *Biomaterials*, 1998, 19:565–571.

[5] A. U. J. Yap, Y. S. Pek, R. A. Kumar, P. Cheang, and K. A. Khor, Experimental studies on a new bioactive material: HAIonomer cements, *Biomaterials*, 2002, 23:955–962.

[6] G. Davidowitz and P. G. Kotick. The use of CAD/CAM in dentistry, *Dent. Clin. North Am.*, 2011, 55:559-70.

[7] I. Papathanasiou, P. Kamposiora, G. Papavasiliou, and M. Ferrari. The use of PEEK in digital prosthodontics: A narrative review, *BMC Oral Health*, 2020, 20:217.

[8] T. Ichikawa, K. Kurahashi, L. Liu, T. Matsuda, and Y. Ishida. Use of a polyetheretherketone clasp retainer for removable partial denture: A case report. *Dent J. (Basel)*, 2019, 7:4.

[9] J. L. Ferracane, Current trends in dental composite, *Crit. Rev. Oral. Biol. Med.*, 1995, 6:302–318.

[10] J. Arends, G. E. H. M. Dijkma, and A. G. Dijkman, Review of fluoride release and secondary caries reduction by fluoride-releasing composites, *Adv. Dent. Res.*, 1995, 9:367–376.

[11] A. J. de Gee, P. Pallav, A. Werner, and C. L. Davidson, Annealing as a mechanism of increasing wear resistance of composites, *Dent. Mat.*, 1990, 6:266–270.

[12] K. Shinkai, S. Susuki, K. F. Leinfelder, and Y. Katoh, How heat treatment and thermal cycling affect wear of composite inlays, *J. Am. Dent. Assoc.*, 1994, 125:1467–1472.

[13] V. A. P. Chia, Y. L. See Toh, H. C. Quek, Y. Pokharkar, A. U. Yap, and N. Yu. Comparative clinical evaluation of removable partial denture frameworks fabricated traditionally or with selective laser melting: A randomized controlled trial. *J. Prosthet. Dent.*, 2024, 131(1):42–49.

[14] C. Ohkubo, Y. Sato, Y. Nishiyama, and Y. Suzuki. Titanium removable denture based on a one-metal rehabilitation concept. *Dent Mater. J.*, 2017, 36:517–523.

[15] W. J. O'Brien, *Dental Materials and Their Selection* (Quintessence Publishing Co., USA, 2002).

[16] R. Adell, U. Lekholm, B. Rockler, and P. Branemark, A 15-year study of osseointegrated implants in the treatment of the edentulous jaw, *Int. J. Oral. Surg.*, 1981, 10:387–416.

[17] T. Sakai, M. Kaga, and H. Oguchi, Two-year clinical observation of gallium alloy in pediatric patients, *Trans. Acad. Dent. Mat.*, 1993, 191:53–54.

Chapter 6

Bioceramics: An Introduction

Besim Ben-Nissan[*,‡] **and Giuseppe Pezzotti**[†]

Department of Chemistry, Materials and Forensic Science,
University of Technology, Sydney,
PO BOX 123 Broadway, 2007 NSW Australia
†*Department of Materials, Kyoto Institute of Technology,*
Sakyo-ku, Matsugasaki, Kyoto, 606-8585, Japan
‡*besim.ben-nissan@uts.edu.au*

An improved understanding of currently used bioceramics in human implants and bone replacement materials could contribute significantly to the design of new-generation prostheses and post-operative patient management strategies. Overall, the benefits of advanced ceramic materials in biomedical applications have been universally appreciated — specifically in terms of their strength, biocompatibility, and wear resistance. However, the supporting data is not sparse. Against this background, continuous development of new methods is pertinent — if not imperative — for a better understanding of the microstructure–property relationship as well as obtaining new directives to further improve ceramics as biomaterials. This chapter gives an overview of and reexamines key issues that concern both the processing and applications of ceramics as biomaterials.

6.1 Introduction

Trauma, degeneration, and diseases often make surgical repair or replacement necessary. When a person suffers from joint pain, the main priorities are the relief of pain and the prompt return to a healthy and functional lifestyle. These concerns usually require the replacement of skeletal parts that include the knees, hips, finger joints, elbows, vertebrae, and teeth, and the repair of the mandible. The worldwide biomaterials market is valued at close to US\$24,000M. Orthopedic and dental applications represent approximately 55% of the total biomaterials market. Orthopedic products worldwide exceeded US\$13 billion in the year 2000 — an increase of 12% over 1999 revenues. Expansion in these areas is expected to continue due to a number of factors. These include an aging population, increasing preference by younger- to middle-aged candidates to undertake surgery, improvements in technology and lifestyle, better understanding of body functionality, availability of improved aesthetics, and the need for better function [1].

A biomaterial, by definition, is "a non-drug substance suitable for inclusion in systems which augment or replace the function of bodily tissues or organs." As early as a century ago, artificial materials and devices had been developed to a point where they could replace various components of the human body. These materials were capable of being in contact with bodily fluids and tissues for prolonged periods of time, while eliciting little — if any — adverse reaction [2].

Some of the earliest biomaterial applications date as far back as ancient Phoenicia where loose teeth were bound together with gold wires to tie artificial ones to neighboring teeth. In the early 1900s, bone plates were successfully implemented to stabilize bone fractures and accelerate their healing. By the 1950s to 1960s, blood vessel replacements were in clinical trials and artificial heart valves and hip joints were in development.

Even in the preliminary stages of this field, surgeons and engineers identified materials and design problems that resulted in premature loss of implant function — such as through mechanical failure, corrosion, or inadequate biocompatibility of the component. Key factors in biomaterial usage are its biocompatibility, biofunctionality, and availability (to a lesser extent). Ceramics are ideal candidates with respect to all the above-mentioned criteria, except for their brittle behavior.

In this chapter, we shall revisit the presently available and currently investigated bioceramics, their preparation methods, properties, and their applications in comparison to biogenic, metallic, and polymeric biomaterials.

6.2   General Concepts of Bioceramics

It has been accepted that no foreign materials placed within a living body can be completely compatible. The only substances that conform completely are those manufactured by the body itself (autogenous). Any other substance that is recognized as foreign initiates some kind of reaction (host-tissue response). Figure 6.1 shows four response types of bioceramics. Each response type then determines the means of attaching the implant to the musculoskeletal system.

When a man-made material is placed within the human body, tissue reacts toward the implant in a variety of ways depending on the material type. The mechanism of tissue interaction (if any) depends on the tissue response to the implant surface. In general, tissue responses to a biomaterial may be described or classified as bioinert, bioresorbable, or bioactive as explained in the following. These responses have been well covered in a range of excellent review papers [3–5].

1. **Bioinert** refers to any material that once placed within the human body has minimal interaction with its surrounding tissue. Examples of bioinert materials are stainless steel, titanium,

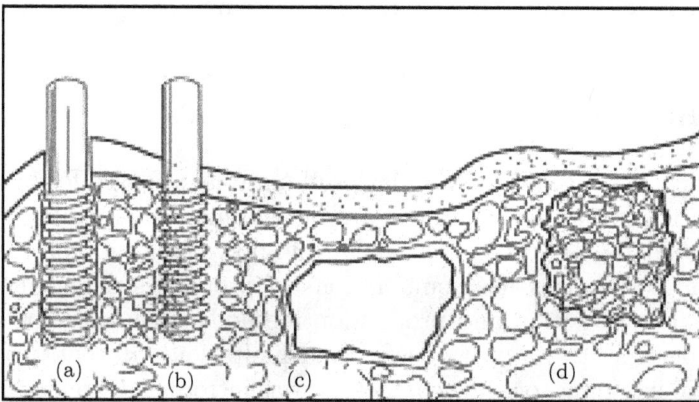

Figure 6.1. Classification of bioceramics according to their responses at the bone–implant interface: (a) bioinert alumina dental implant; (b) bioactive hydroxyapatite $(Ca_{10}(PO_4)_2(OH)_2)$ coating on a metallic dental implant; (c) surface active bioglass; (d) bioresorbable tricalcium phosphate implant $(Ca_3(PO_4)_2)$.

alumina, partially stabilized zirconia, and ultra-high-molecular-weight polyethylene. Generally, a fibrous capsule forms around a bioinert implant. Hence, the implant's biofunctionality relies on tissue integration through the capsule (Figure 6.1(a)).

2. **Bioactive** refers to a material which upon being placed within the human body interacts with the surrounding bone and, in some cases, even with the soft tissue. This occurs through a time-dependent kinetic modification of the surface, triggered by its implantation within the living bone. An ion exchange reaction between the bioactive implant and surrounding body fluids results in the formation of a biologically active carbonate apatite (CHAp) layer on the implant that is chemically and crystallographically equivalent to the mineral phase of bone. Prime examples of bioactive materials are synthetic hydroxyapatite [6,7] $[Ca_{10}(PO_4)_6(OH)_2]$, glass-ceramic $A-W$ [8,9], and Bioglass$^®$ [10] (Figure 6.1(b,c)).

3. **Bioresorbable** refers to a material that upon placement within the human body starts to dissolve (resorbed) and is slowly replaced by advancing tissue (such as bone). Common examples of bioresorbable materials are tricalcium phosphate $[Ca_3(PO_4)_2]$ and polylactic–polyglycolic acid copolymers. Calcium oxide, calcium carbonate (coral), and gypsum are other common materials that have been used during the last three decades (Figure 6.1(d)).

6.3   Bioceramics and Production Methods

In clinical practice, four basic classes of material are used for biomedical implants and devices. They are bioceramics, bio-metals (metals that could be used as biomaterials), bio-polymers, and composites. Each material class has combinations of properties determined by material composition and production methods used, while each set of properties has its own benefits and limitations. Recently, a fifth group of inorganic–organic composites was introduced, appropriately named hybrids since some natural materials are used.

Ceramics are the hardest of solids. Table 6.1 gives some of the mechanical properties of natural and synthetic biomaterials.

When a material yields under load such as in mechanical testing, line defects (dislocations) move through its structure. Metals

Table 6.1. Mechanical properties of biomaterials. Reprinted with permission from Lutton and Ben-Nissan [1].

	Young's Modulus GPa	Compressive Strength MPa	Tensile Strength MPa	Density g/cm^3	Fracture Toughness MPam$^{1/2}$
METALS					
Titanium (Ti–6Al–4V)	114	450–1850	900–1172	4.43	44–66
Cr–Co–Mo	210	480–600	400–1030	8.3	120–160
Stainless Steel (316L)	193	—	515–620	8.0	20–95
CERAMICS					
Alumina	420	4400	282–551	3.98	3–5.4
Zirconia (TZP)	210	1990	800–1500	5.74–6.08	6.4–10.9
Silicon Nitride (HPSN)	304	3700	700–1000	3.3	3.7–5.5
Hydroxyapatite (3% porosity)	7–13	350–450	38–48	—	3.05–3.15
HUMAN TISSUE					
Cortical Bone	3.8–11.7	88–164	82–114	1.7–2.0	2–12
Cancellous Bone	0.2–0.5	23	10–20	—	—
Cartilage	0.002–0.01	—	5–25	—	—
OTHERS					
Bone Cement (PMMA)	2.24–3.25	80	48–72	—	1.19
UHMWHD Polyethylene	0.69	20	38–48	0.94	—

are intrinsically soft and ductile due to their appropriate slip systems, which allow yielding and metallic bonding and where electrons are free to move around the ion cores. Metals can be shaped easily by machining or by casting from a molten state without any major difficulties. However, most ceramics are intrinsically hard due to their ionic, covalent, and/or mixed bonding, which presents an enormous lattice resistance to the motion of dislocations. Hence, ceramics cannot be shaped by melting and casting. These properties of hardness and strength of ceramics are exploited in areas where wear resistance is required.

In general, crack tip plasticity gives metals their high toughness. Energy is absorbed in the plastic zone, generating a tortuous path that makes crack propagation much more difficult. Although some plasticity can occur at the tip of a crack in a ceramic too, the energy absorption is relatively small and the fracture toughness is low. As a result (with the exception of partially stabilized zirconia (PSZ)), most ceramics have values of fracture toughness (K_{IC}) roughly one-fiftieth of those of ductile materials.

Due to their strong bonding, ceramics have very high melting — or more appropriately, dissociation — temperatures. Hence, ceramics can be produced only through high-temperature sintering. Sintering is a process of densification where powders are heated up usually to two-thirds of their melting temperature, and with the aid of a driving force such as diffusion, they consolidate (Figure 6.2). During densification, particles bond together to form necks between the particles, thereby causing the surface area to reduce and the powders to consolidate.

Full density is not achieved in normal pressureless sintering without the incorporation of sintering additives. Some porosity is usually retained in the sintered final products. The higher densities and small-grain structures required by bioceramics can be achieved by hot

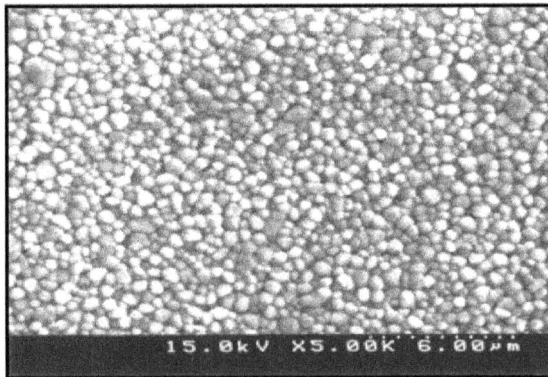

Figure 6.2.   Scanning electron microscopy (SEM) of a sintered bioceramic.

pressing (HP) where temperature and uniaxial pressure are applied simultaneously, or by hot isostatic pressing (HIP) where the powder is isostatically pressurized within a gaseous environment and heated to a high temperature (Figure 6.3).

Sintering rate is controlled by diffusion. However, a large driving force shortens the sintering time and increases the final density. Various methods used in producing advanced ceramics are given in Table 6.2. Hot isostatic pressing is most commonly used.

In the sintering of engineering advanced ceramics, the density could be further improved by adding sintering aids. However, for bioceramics where high purity is important, additives need to be kept to a minimum or must be totally avoided.

To produce high-purity alumina ceramic, the raw materials are bauxite and native corundum. However, alumina can be easily prepared by calcining alumina trihydrate. Alumina is commercially available either as a raw powder (up to purities > 99.99%) or as tabular sintered bodies that have been sintered without adding permanent binders. Sintering temperatures depend on the processes used.

Single crystals of alumina (i.e., sapphire rods) can be prepared by feeding fine alumina powders onto the surface of a seed crystal — which is slowly withdrawn from an electric arc or oxyhydrogen flame — as the fused powder builds up. Alumina single crystals up to 100 mm in diameter have been grown by this method. Since the late 1970s, alumina single crystals named Bioceram® produced by Kyocera, Japan, have been used as sapphire dental implants.

6.4 Bioinert Ceramics in Articulation

Ceramics are considered hard, brittle materials with relatively poor tensile properties. Other characteristics include excellent compressive strength, high resistance to wear, and favorably low frictional property in articulation. The low frictional property is enhanced by the fact that ceramics are hydrophilic with good wettability (Figure 6.4). They can be highly polished, thus providing a superior load-bearing surface with themselves or against polymeric materials in a physiological environment. Bioceramics used singularly or with additional natural, organic, or polymeric materials are among the most promising of all biomaterials for hard and soft tissue applications.

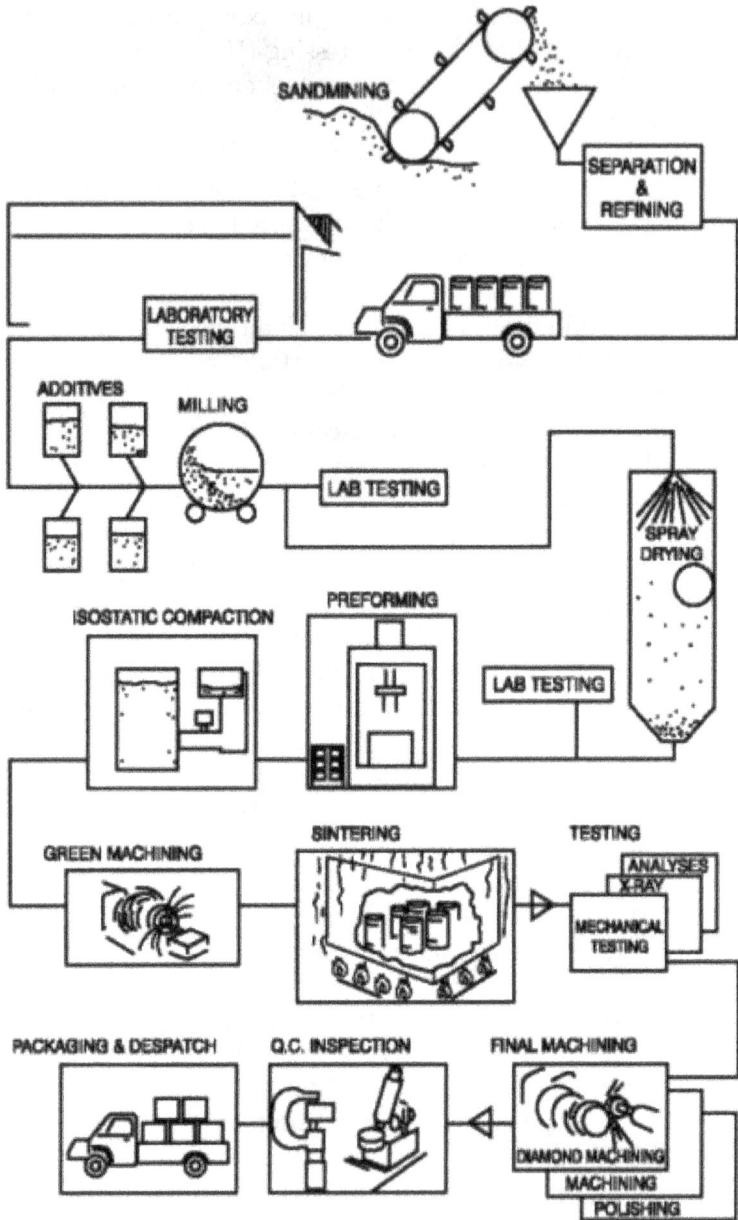

Figure 6.3. Schematic representation of one of the high-density bioceramic oxide fabrication steps.

Table 6.2. Some common bioceramic production methods.

PRESSING	CASTING
Uniaxial	Slip Casting
Cold Isostatic Pressing (CIP)	Thixotropic Casting
Hot Pressing (HP)	Gel Casting
Hot Isostatic Pressing (HIP)	Soluble Mold Casting

PLASTIC FORMING	COATINGS
	Sol-Gel Coating
Extrusion	Electrodeposition
Injection Molding	Flame/Plasma Spray
Compression Molding	SBF
	PVD/CVD

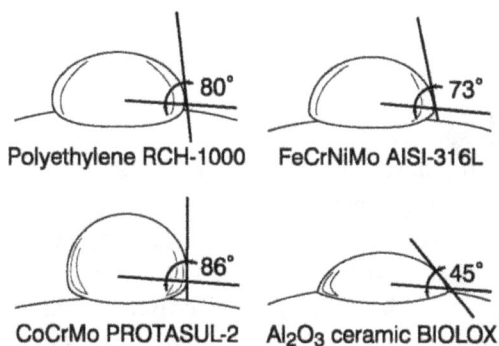

Figure 6.4. Hydrophilic/hydrophobic behavior shown by wetting angles of different orthopedic biomaterials: (a) Polyethylene (RCH–1000); (b) FeCrNiMo, AISI–316L stainless steel; (c) CoCrMo alloy (Protasul–2); (d) Alumina ceramic (Biolox).

Interest in ceramics for biomedical applications has increased over the last 30 years. Ceramics that are used in implantation and for clinical purposes include aluminum oxide (alumina), partially stabilized zirconia (PSZ) (both yttria [Y–TZP] and magnesia stabilized [Mg–PSZ]), Bioglass®, glass-ceramics, calcium phosphates (hydroxyapatite and β-tricalcium phosphate), and crystalline or glassy forms of carbon and its compounds.

During the 1960s and 1970s in Europe, Charnley, Scales, McKee, and Muller had already developed either metal–polyethylene (M–PE) bearings for total hip replacements (THR) or all metal (M–M) cobalt–chromium–molybdenum (CoCr) heads and cups [11]. During the same period, an alternative concept was introduced by Boutin in France: an alumina ceramic cup combined with an alumina femoral head (A–A). Boutin was concerned about tissue reactions to both metal and plastic debris and was therefore intrigued by the reputation of alumina ceramic as a highly wear-resistant bearing surface for extreme conditions.

Sir John Charnley proposed employing metal-on-plastic total hip replacement (THR) in 1962. Most total joint prostheses consist of an articulation of a metal alloy on UHMWPE. The latter material does not have the strength required by the stem of weight-bearing joint replacements, or for intermedullary nails or bone plates. Both the cobalt–chrome alloy and stainless steel are used for the bearing surface of joints. They can likewise be used for the entire femoral component of hips and knees, as well as for other joints such as the shoulder and the ankle. Metal-on-metal articulation in a total joint prosthesis has a high coefficient of friction and poor wear resistance — unless it has a very high surface finish. A good example of the use of HDPE is the total hip replacement carried out in 1962 by Charnley, where HDPE was used for the acetabular cup [11]. This particular design continued, and in the early 1970s, a metal alloy stem was employed with an alumina femoral head on a UHMWPE acetabular cup. For the last 25 years, this design has reportedly reduced wear rates by as much as 10 to 20 times as compared to wear rates of metal-on-metal alone. UHMWPE and the recently developed Highly Crosslinked Polyethylene (HCPE) are at present the preferred materials for use in conjunction with a metal or ceramic prosthesis. Creep in PE remains a problem. Wear of the polyethylene component of these prostheses does occur, and these wear particles can sometimes cause a severe tissue reaction and eventual loosening of the implant. UHMWPE is being improved in both strength and wear characteristics. It is essential that the bearing surface in contact with the polyethylene be very highly polished. The quality of the bearing surface finish is critical to the wear characteristics of UHMWPE. HCPE has proved to be a better material for articulating surfaces.

Alumina, to a lesser extent zirconia ceramics, and in recent times their composites have been currently used in THR as the femoral head and liners. As a result, the use of wear particles from ultra-high-molecular-weight polyethylene in various other combinations has greatly reduced [12].

6.4.1 *Alumina Ceramics*

High-purity alumina bioceramics have been developed as an alternative to surgical metal alloys for total hip prostheses and tooth implants. The high hardness, low friction coefficient, and excellent corrosion resistance of alumina offer a very low wear rate as the articulating surface in orthopedic applications. Medical-grade alumina has a very low concentration of sintering additives ($<0.5\,wt\%$), a relatively small grain size ($<7\,\mu m$), and a narrow grain size distribution. Such a microstructure is capable of inhibiting static fatigue and slowing crack growth while the ceramic is under a load. The average grain size of current medical-grade alumina is $1.4\,\mu m$ and the surface finish is usually controlled to a roughness of less than $0.02\,\mu m$. However, unless its surface is modified or used directly in articulating areas, alumina has a fundamental limitation as an implant material in that, like other "inert" biomaterials, a non-adherent fibrous membrane may develop at the interface. In certain circumstances, interfacial failure can occur, leading to loosening — as was observed in some dental implant designs.

Currently, alumina is used for orthopedic and dental implants, and can be polished to a high surface finish and high hardness. It has been used in wear-bearing environments [13], such as in total hip arthroplasties (THA) as the femoral head to help reduce wear particles from ultra-high-molecular-weight polyethylene (UHMWPE). Other applications for alumina include porous coatings for femoral stems or as porous alumina spacers (Huckstep nails) in revision surgeries. In the past, alumina — in polycrystalline and single-crystal forms — was also used in tooth implants in dental applications [3, 14–16].

The mechanical behavior of alumina ceramics in simulated physiological environments has led to long-term survival predictions for these materials when they were subjected to sub-critical stresses. At a 112-MPa stress level, the probability for medical-grade alumina to survive 50 years is 99.9%. Considering the tensile stresses encountered in many implants (such as in a ceramic hip joint ball), alumina ceramics can therefore be reliably employed. In a recent work by Oonishi *et al.* [17], hip simulator tests and clinical studies indicated that wear on alumina/UHMWPE THA was decreased by 25–30% when compared to that of metal/UHMWPE. Wear on THR of alumina/alumina was observed to be near zero in a similar hip simulator test. In knee simulator tests, UHMWPE wear against alumina decreased to one-tenth of that against metal. They further reported that during the last 23 years, no revisions were required due to PE or other wear problems. In retrieved cases, the UHMWPE surface against alumina was very smooth. However, in a comparative study on the UHMWPE surface against metal, many fibrils and scratches were found, illustrating the extremely good performance of alumina ceramics against UHMWPE. Recently, several *in vitro* and *in vivo* studies using femoral heads larger than 28 mm demonstrated the advantage of using an alumina–alumina pairing in young patients or patients with high-demand bodily function [17–19].

6.4.2   *Partially Stabilized Zirconia (PSZ)*

Compared to alumina, PSZ has a high Weibull modulus and hence better reliability, higher flexural strength and fracture toughness, lower Young's modulus (Table 6.1), and the ability to be polished to a superior surface finish [20, 21]. The higher fracture toughness is of particular importance in femoral heads due to the tensile stresses induced by the taper fit onto the femoral stem.

Following the production of particulate wear debris from implant materials, the consequential osteolysis has been pinpointed as the major cause of long-term failure in total hip replacements. The basic strategy to address the osteolysis problem is to reduce the number of polyethylene particles generated. This is done by improving the material at the articulating surface. For young active patients, the ceramic femoral head is strongly advocated because it produces less polyethylene wear compared to a conventional metal femoral head. On the other hand, attempts were also made to eliminate the use of polyethylene through metal-on-metal or ceramic-on-ceramic couples [17].

Partially stabilized zirconia femoral heads make up about 25% of the total number of operations per year in Europe and eight percent of the hip implant procedures in the USA. It has been reported that over 400,000 zirconia hip joint femoral heads have been implanted from 1985 until 2001. Most of the zirconia femoral heads (tetragonal zirconia polycrystal, TZP) consist of $97mol\%ZrO_2$ and $3mol\%Y_2O_3$.

Although not quite as hard as alumina, PSZ still possesses excellent wear resistance and has been used for similar orthopedic applications as alumina. Wear rates of UHMWPE against partially stabilized zirconia have been found to be low enough such that tribological debris would not be a problem in clinical applications [21, 22]. Preliminary results indicate that a ceramic-on-ceramic femoral head/acetabular cup system is preferred over ceramic/UHMWPE systems as polymeric wear debris is avoided [23]. In fact, Chevalier and co-workers in 1997 [24] reported that not only was the friction coefficient between an alumina cup and zirconia head much lower than that of ceramic against UHMWPE but the resultant wear between the two components was almost zero. Clarke *et al.* (2000) conducted a recent study [21, 22, 25] on the articulation of the femoral head in total hip replacement (THR), using hip simulators with alpha-calf serum as a lubricant. In this study, wear rates of alumina/alumina, zirconia/alumina, and zirconia/zirconia couples were investigated. Results revealed that wear rates using zirconia/zirconia exhibit a mild run-in phase, as compared to a more evident run-in phase for alumina/alumina articulation.

Following the run-in phase, weight changes of all couple samples were observed. Zirconia/zirconia wear offered little observable weight change. Alumina/alumina wear (although very low) revealed a steady weight loss trend after the run-in phase. In the case of zirconia/alumina (where the head was made of zirconia and the liner made of alumina), the zirconia head showed little weight loss but the alumina liner revealed a typical run-in phase followed by a steady state weight loss. The study thus revealed promise for hard-on-hard THR systems where wear rates were three times less in order of magnitude when compared to PE cups. The study employed alpha-calf serum at 50% concentration, while most other published studies used either water or saline solution, which can be quite detrimental to the performance of the zirconia ceramics.

Zirconia ceramic implants have had a somewhat controversial history regarding their longevity, phase-metastability, tetragonal to monoclinic transformations, degradation in water lubricant in simulation studies, and the influence of lubricants on their frictional and wear properties. At a Japanese orthopedic meeting in 1988, an orthopedic group from Bologna, Italy, reported that the wear of zirconia-on-zirconia is 5,000 times worse than that of alumina-on-alumina. While the zirconia samples used in these studies came from four different sources, the common denominator in these studies appeared to be the use of water as the test lubricant.

It has been shown that when evaluating total hip joint replacements (THR), the lubricant used in these laboratory evaluations significantly influences the wear results. Various studies have been conducted successfully when alumina-on-alumina bearings were lubricated using water, saline, and serum. However, zirconia-on-zirconia tests in water have consistently shown catastrophic results while those in serum have demonstrated good results. One such study by Oonishi and co-workers [13] showed that Y–TZP balls transformed from the tetragonal to monoclinic phase when tested with saline in a hip simulator.

A number of clinical studies have shown excellent short-term results when zirconia balls have been combined with alumina cups [24]. However, contemporary clinical studies of zirconia on polyethylene have shown mixed results. Given these somewhat contradictory results between laboratory and clinical studies, Clarke *et al.* studied [22, 25] the wear of zirconia-on-zirconia bearings in both water and serum. The debris and zirconia implants were then analyzed using Raman Microprobe Spectroscopy. The water lubrication test resulted in a wear about 10,000 times greater than with serum lubrication. The wear of both zirconia femoral head and cup in water lubrication showed a high weight loss of 28 mg after only 6,100 cycles. In contrast, the zirconia wear with serum lubrication had a weight loss of only 0.74 mg after 20 million cycles. This difference between the two lubricants was also distinct in the micro-wear of the ball surfaces. With serum, there were still some original machine tracks to be seen; with water, there was total surface deterioration (Figure 6.5).

The size of the wear debris ranged from 0.38 to 16.78 microns, with an average size of 1.80 microns. Analysis of the debris by Raman spectroscopy showed that the debris was almost exclusively in the monoclinic phase [26]. Therefore, it was proposed that the simulator with water lubrication created extensive zirconia transformation. However, under serum lubricant conditions, this transformation did

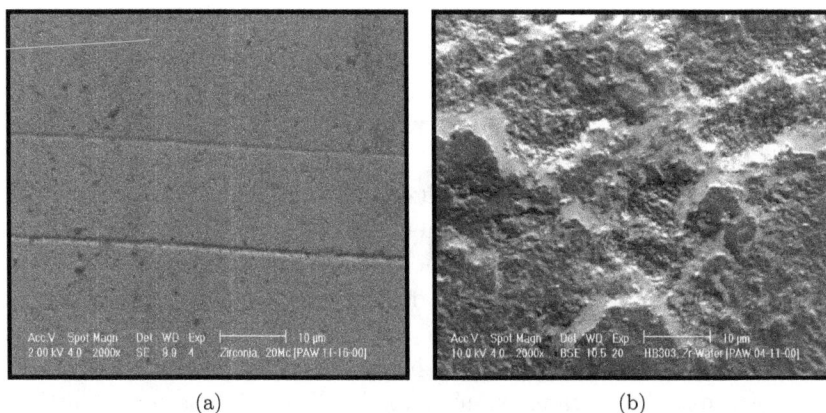

(a) (b)

Figure 6.5. SEM images of zirconia (TZP) femoral head deterioration in hip simulator studies showing comparative wear surfaces: (a) zirconia with serum lubrication; (b) zirconia with water lubrication. Reprinted with permission Williams *et al.* [26].

not occur; hence, the wear surface showed very little wear evidence even at 20 Mc. This phenomenon illustrated that an appropriate joint analogue fluid was of paramount importance for satisfactory wear tests. The metastability of Y–TZP ceramic is greatly affected by moisture and high temperature, and it can also be stress activated. Based on this difference in lubricant performance, Clarke *et al.* [25] postulated that the serum proteins either formed an effective solid lubricant film between the zirconia surfaces or acted to trap an adequate supply of moisture that effectively reduced the friction between opposing zirconia surfaces. Their study revealed the dramatic effect that serum proteins had at the bearing surface, thus greatly reducing the wear rate of zirconia.

It has been widely accepted that to improve THA longevity, it is also necessary to solve the late complications associated with implant fixation and polyethylene wear. It was reported by Woolson *et al.* [27] that the average wear rate of polyethylene against a 28-mm Co–Cr head was 0.14 mm/year at the mean follow-up of 5.7 years in cementless Harris–Galante prostheses (THA) [28]. Although the present wear rate (0.139 mm/year) is almost equal to the reported value, the present zirconia-on-polyethylene combination is in effect superior to the CoCr-on-polyethylene one in terms of volumetric wear because of the different head size used. Since the wear rate of metal-backed polyethylene tends to be influenced greatly by the polyethylene creep in the acetabular metal shell (particularly at the short follow-up duration), the present wear rate may become lower at a longer follow-up duration.

Despite these promising results, concerns remain regarding the above-mentioned degradation phenomenon — which is associated with the tetragonal-to-monoclinic phase transformation — when under long-term aqueous conditions such as an *in vivo* environment. One of the current zirconia femoral head manufacturers has improved conventional zirconia, leading to increased strength and high resistance against phase transformation. In addition, it was reported that in hip simulator testing, polyethylene wear against the improved zirconia head was lower than that against the Co–Cr head. When articulated with highly crosslinked polyethylene, very low wear rates were shown not only by zirconia heads but also by Co–Cr heads. However, because zirconia is more scratch resistant than Co–Cr, the former is a more suitable implant material for long-term clinical use [29].

Yttrium-stabilized tetragonal polycrystalline zirconia (Y–TZP) has a fine grain size and offers the best mechanical properties. Low-temperature degradation of TZP is known to occur due to the spontaneous phase transformation of tetragonal zirconia to the monoclinic phase, which occurs during aging at 130–$300°C$ and possibly within a water environment. It has been reported that this degradation leads to a decrease in strength because, alongside phase transformation, microcracks are formed.

6.4.3   *New Modified Zirconia Implants*

Recently, a new degradation-free zirconia–alumina composite has been reported: TZP/alumina composite (80%TZP of [90mol% ZrO_2–6mol%Y_2O_3–4mol%Nb_2O_5 composition] and $20\%Al_2O_3$) [12]. Another potential composite — which comprises 70vol%TZP (stabilized with 10mol%CeO_2), 30vol%Al_2O_3, and 0.05mol5TiO$_2$ — is currently being investigated in Japan.

Implant stability is critical in ensuring good long-term success of total joint replacements. Loss of either biological or cement fixation can lead to accelerated wear, pain, loss of function, or even fracture of the implant — each of which could potentially necessitate revision surgery. Fixation strength can be improved by using a macrotextured (porous or textured) surface, which enhances the potential for mechanical interlock at the implant–bone interface.

Oxidized zirconium, a material recently introduced for orthopedic bearing applications (Oxinium™, Smith & Nephew Inc., Memphis, TN), is reported to have beneficial wear and abrasion resistance [30,31]. However, it cannot be easily processed using traditional coating techniques. Therefore, an alternative chemical surface texturing method was used. The chemical texturing process has been used clinically on Ti–6Al–4V total hip replacement components to create a surface morphology suitable for bone ingrowth [32].

This texturing method (known commercially as ChemTex® 5-5-5 (CYCAM Inc., Houston, PA)) and a newly developed chemical texturing process (known commercially as Tecotex® I–103 (Tecomet, Woburn, MA)) were used to produce macrotextured surfaces ($R_{max} > 0.4$ mm) on a zirconium alloy (Zr–2.5Nb). These textured surfaces were subsequently oxidized to form a hard ceramic layer, uniformly about 5 μm thick, over the entire surface, which consists predominantly of monoclinic zirconia (Figure 6.6) [33].

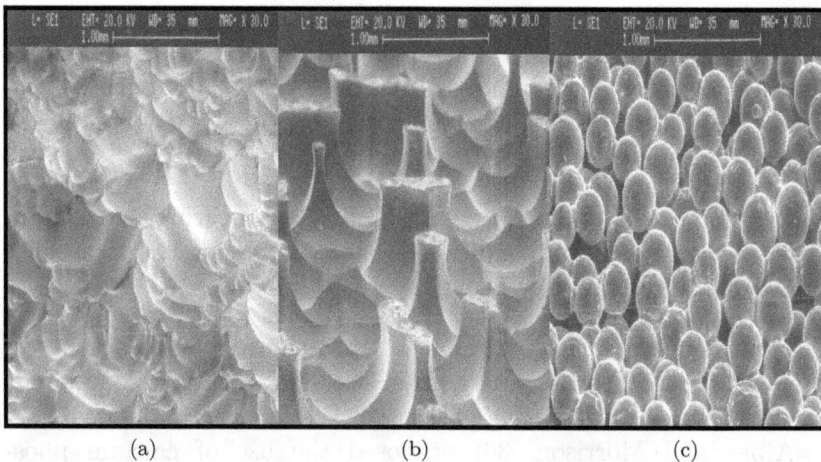

Figure 6.6. Surface texture SEM images of (a) ChemTex® textured (CT) surface; (b) Tecotex® textured (TT) surface; and (c) porous sintered bead (SB) coating (30x). Reprinted with permission Heuer *et al.* [33].

6.5   Bioresorbable and Bioactive Ceramics

6.5.1   *Calcium Phosphates for Bone Replacement Applications*

In 1926, De Jong initiated the first X-ray diffraction study of the bone [34]. In this study, apatite was identified as the only recognizable mineral phase. He also reported marked broadening of the diffraction lines of bone apatite, which he attributed to small crystal size. Following this study, numerous other studies have suggested the existence of other mineral phases in the bone. These include amorphous calcium phosphate (ACP), brushite, and octacalcium phosphate (OCP). The presence of substantial amounts of ACP or brushite has not been experimentally proved yet, and nuclear magnetic resonance studies support the conclusion that bone is composed essentially of carbonate-substituted hydroxyapatite (CHAp).

It was not until the 1970s that synthetic hydroxyapatite $[Ca_{10}(PO_4)_2(OH)_2]$ was accepted as a potential biomaterial. Synthetic hydroxyapatite forms a strong chemical bond with bone *in vivo*, and it is also able to remain stable under the harsh conditions encountered in the physiologic environment.

Bone-like carbonated apatite $Ca_{(10-x)}(PO_4)_{6-y}(OH)_{2-z}A_xB_yC_z$ (where A, B, and C are substitutional elements) is a non-stoichiometric mineral found in the hard tissues of all mammals. Synthetic hydroxyapatite $Ca_{10}(PO_4)_6(OH)_2$ has been an attractive material for chromatographic separation catalysis, ion exchange, and bone and tooth implants [35]. Since its inception, two common and easy methods have been used to produce synthetic HAp:

- Solid state reaction between Ca^{2+}- and PO_4^{3-}-bearing compounds;
- When under solution conditions, powders are sintered to a dense polycrystalline body by firing.

It must be noted that parameters that control the bioactivity of HAp include Ca/P ratio, purity, grain size, and secondary compounds that could be formed during production.

Albee and Morrison [36] proposed the use of calcium phosphate ceramics for biomedical applications, after observing accelerated bone growth when tricalcium phosphate was injected into bone defects. Pure tricalcium phosphate (TCP) $Ca_3(PO_4)_2$ is more soluble in the physiological environment than other phosphate ceramics (bioresorbable). Consequently, it can be used in situations where accelerated bone growth is desired. β-tricalcium phosphates have been used successfully as fillers for bone defects to stimulate new bone formation [37]. A study showed that after a 12-month period, β-tricalcium phosphate was totally absorbed. It was stated that these materials will be used to fill voids in bone structure since they dissolve over a period of time. It was also found that while the dissolution takes place, bone regrowth or advancement takes place at a similar rate.

The dissolution rates of some materials under simulated physiological conditions have been investigated, with particular emphasis on hydroxyapatite, β-tricalcium phosphate, and tetracalcium phosphate. Under *in vitro* conditions, the solubility of these materials has been shown to decrease in the following order [4, 38]:

Tetracalcium phosphate $>\beta$-Tricalcium Phosphate $>$ Hydroxyapatite.

It has been stated that hydroxyapatite is "scarcely resorbable," thus justifying the use of hydroxyapatite for osseous implants [39, 40].

It was proposed by various investigators that the initial formation of an amorphous calcium phosphate (ACP) at high pH could be followed by its transformation to hydroxyapatite (HA). The latter transformation could be via the formation of a precursor in the form of octacalcium phosphate (OCP). This chain of reactions has been proposed to be one of the templates that form HA. It has also been stated that as the pH decreases, other precursor phases such as dicalcium phosphate dihydrate (DCPD) may form [35]. Therefore, it has been accepted that other calcium phosphate phases (Table 6.3) could actively participate in the crystallization reaction of biological (biogenic) apatites.

Hydroxyapatite powders can be synthesized using a range of production methods [35]. However, one of the most commonly used methods [7, 41, 42] is from an aqueous solution of $Ca(NO_3)_2$ and NaH_2PO_4. After filtering and drying in this method, the product is calcined for about three hours at 1173 K to promote crystallization. Upon cold-press forming, the desired shape can be obtained by sintering for about one hour at about 1500 K to obtain full densification. Once sintering reaches above 1523 K, hydroxyapatite shows second-phase precipitation along grain boundaries and at multiple

Table 6.3. Calcium phosphate phases. Reprinted with permission from Ben-Nissan *et al.* [35].

Calcium phosphate phases	Mineral	Empirical formulas	Ca/P ratio	JCPDS
Dicalcium phosphate dihydrate	Brushite	$CaHPO_4.2H_2O$	1.00	11–293
Dicalcium phosphate	Monetite	$CaHPO_4$	1.00	
Octacalcium phosphate		$Ca_8H_2(PO_4)_6.5H_2O$	1.33	26.1056
β-Tricalcium phosphate	Whitlockite	β-$Ca_3(PO_4)_2$	1.50	9–169
Hydroxyapatite		$Ca_{10}(PO_4)_6(OH)_2$	1.67	9–432
Tetracalcium phosphate monoxide		$Ca_4(PO_4)_2O$	2.00	25–1137
Defect apatites		$Ca_{10-x}(HPO_4)_x$ $(PO_4)_{6-x}(OH)_{2-x}$ $0 < x < 2$	$(10-x){:}6$	

grain junctions with the formation of grain boundary microcracks, indicating significant degradation of mechanical properties.

6.5.2 *Simulated Body Fluid (SBF)*

Introduced by Kokubo and co-workers [43, 44], the simulated body fluid (SBF) is welcomed as a promising method in bioceramics production. This synthetic body fluid is highly supersaturated in calcium and phosphate — in relations to apatite formation — even under normal conditions. Therefore, if a material has a functional group effective for apatite nucleation on its surface, apatite can be formed spontaneously. For an artificial material to bond to the living bone, it is widely accepted that a bone-like apatite layer must form on its surface. The formation of the bone-like apatite layer on bioactive materials can be produced in a simulated body fluid (SBF) which has ion concentrations almost equal to those of human blood plasma. Currently, most bioceramics research studies use this solution to measure an artificial material's bioactivity by examining the apatite-forming ability on its surface when immersed in SBF.

Hydroxyapatite layers can be easily produced on various organic or inorganic substrates in SBF. Kokubo *et al.* in 1989 showed that after immersion in SBF, a wide range of biomaterial surfaces showed very fine crystallites of carbonate ion-containing apatite [43]. Osteoblasts have also been shown to proliferate and differentiate on this apatite layer.

SBF is a metastable solution. If an apatite-nucleating functional group is present on a substrate which is immersed in the fluid, the apatite spontaneously nucleates. It has been reported that this nucleation rate increases whenever excessive amounts of Ca^{2+} ions, PO_4H_2, Si–OH, Ti–OH, Zr–OH, Ta–OH, Nb–OH, or similar functional groups are present [44]. For example, it has been shown that highly porous gels of SiO_2, TiO_2, ZrO_2, Nb_2O_5, and Ta_2O_5 could form apatite layers on their surfaces in SBF. All these observations indicate that the above-mentioned functional groups with a specific structure are effective for apatite nucleation in the body environment [44].

6.5.3 *Coralline Apatites*

Coralline apatites can be derived from sea coral. Coral is composed of calcium carbonate in the form of aragonite. As coral is a naturally occurring structure, it has optimal strength and structural characteristics. The pore structure of coralline calcium phosphate produced by certain species is similar to human cancellous bone, making it a suitable material for bone graft applications (Figure 6.7). Coral and converted coralline hydroxyapatite have been used as bone grafts and orbital implants since the 1980s. This is because the porous nature of the structure allows the ingrowth of blood vessels to supply blood to the bone, which eventually infiltrates the implant.

The size and interconnectivity of pores are of utmost importance when hard and soft tissue ingrowth is required. Kühne *et al.* [45] showed that implants with an average pore size of around $260\,\mu m$ had the most successful ingrowth as compared to no implants (that is, simply leaving the segment empty). It was further reported that the interaction of the primary osteons between the pores via the interconnections allows the propagation of osteoblasts.

The hydrothermal method was first used by Roy and Linnehan [46] in 1974 to form hydroxyapatite directly from coral. It was reported that the complete replacement of aragonite ($CaCO_3$) by phosphatic material — via the hydrothermal process — was achieved

500μm

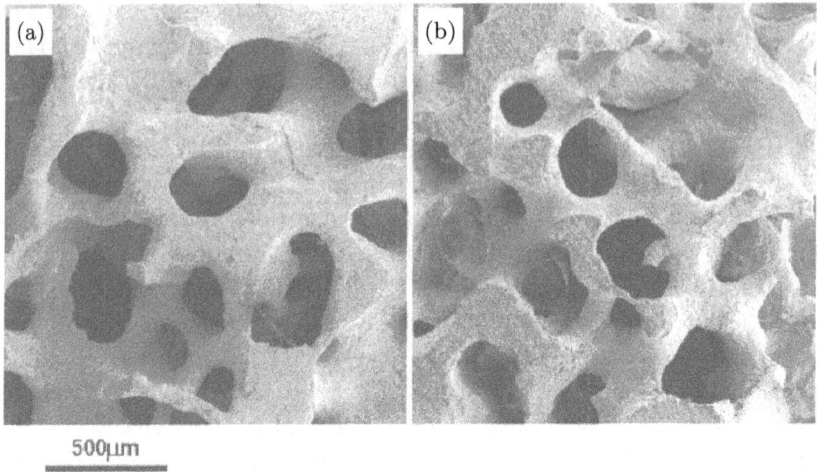

Figure 6.7. Comparison of the Australian coral: (a) in original state; and (b) after hydrothermal conversion.

using less than 533 K and 103 MPa. In 1996, HAp derived from Indian coral using the hydrothermal process was reported [47]. However, the resultant material was in powder form and it required further forming and sintering.

During the hydrothermal treatment, hydroxyapatite replaces the aragonite while preserving the porous structure. The following exchange takes place:

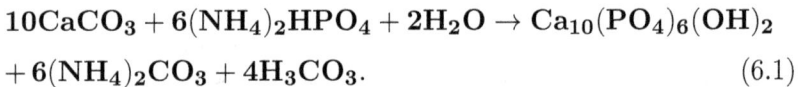

$$10CaCO_3 + 6(NH_4)_2HPO_4 + 2H_2O \rightarrow Ca_{10}(PO_4)_6(OH)_2$$
$$+ 6(NH_4)_2CO_3 + 4H_3CO_3. \tag{6.1}$$

The resulting material is known as coralline hydroxyapatite, be it in the porous coralline structure or in powdered form.

Alternatively, aragonite can be converted to carbonate hydroxyapatite using a microwave processing technique. Higher extents of conversion were reported [48].

Hu *et al.* [49] succeeded in converting a high-strength Australian coral (Porites) to monophasic hydroxyapatite using a two-stage process where the hydrothermal method was followed by a patented hydroxyapatite sol-gel coating process based on alkoxide chemistry. They reported a 120% increase in the biaxial strength of the double-treated coral as compared to one that is merely converted.

6.5.4 Calcium Phosphate Coatings

Due to its unfavorable mechanical properties, it has been accepted that porous hydroxyapatite cannot be used under load-bearing conditions. Instead, hydroxyapatite has been used as thin film coating on metallic alloys. Of the metallic alloys investigated, titanium-based alloys have shown to be the preferred material for thin film coatings [50]. Being lightweight and with high strength-to-weight ratios, titanium alloys possess good mechanical strength and fatigue resistance under load-bearing conditions.

Of the coating techniques utilized, thermal spraying (plasma, and to a lower extent flame spraying) tends to be the most commonly used and analyzed. This technique has faced the challenge of producing a controllable resorption response in clinical situations. While striving toward this target, thermally sprayed coatings are being improved continuously by using different compositions and post-heat treatments which convert amorphous phases to crystalline calcium phosphates. Currently, plasma coating of macrotextured orthopedic implants is used commercially, and other techniques involving less soluble fluorapatite compositions are also being investigated. Techniques that are capable of producing thin coatings include pulsed laser deposition [51] and sputtering [52] which, like thermal spraying, involve high-temperature processing. Other techniques such as electrodeposition [53, 54] and sol-gel [55] use lower temperatures and avoid the challenge associated with the structural instability of hydroxyapatite at elevated temperatures [56].

The advantages of the sol-gel technique are as follows:

- It results in a stoichiometric, homogeneous, and pure coating due to mixing on a molecular scale;
- Firing temperatures are reduced due to small particle sizes with high surface areas;
- It is able to produce uniform fine-grained structures (Figure 6.8);
- It uses different chemical routes (alkoxide or aqueous);
- It is easy to be applied to complex shapes using a range of coating techniques such as dip, spin, and spray coating;
- Due to its lower processing temperature, it avoids the phase transition ($\sim$1156 K) observed in titanium-based alloys used for biomedical devices.

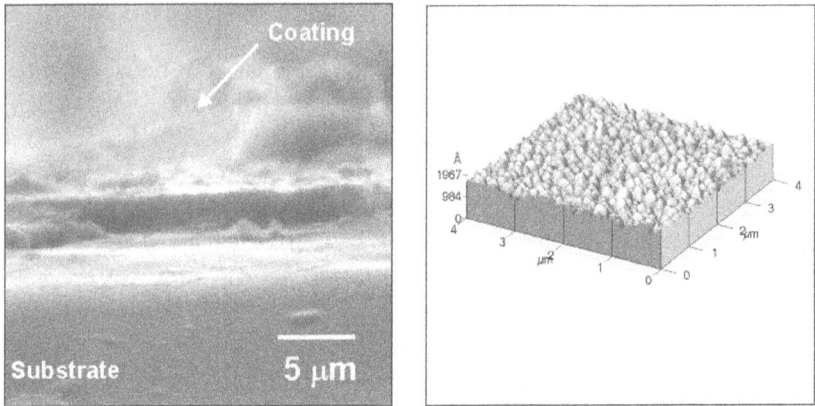

Figure 6.8. SEM and AFM images of sol-gel (alkoxide) derived hydroxyapatite coatings.

6.5.5 Synthetic Bone Graft Ceramics

Bone grafting is currently used in orthopedic and maxillofacial surgeries for these treatments: diaphyseal defects bridging, non-union, metaphyseal defect filling, and mandibular reconstruction.

Autogenous bone graft has the following characteristics:

- Osteogenic (that is, able to form bone due to living cells such as osteocytes or osteoblasts);
- Osteoconductive (that is, no capacity to induce or form bone but provides an inert scaffold upon which osseous tissue can regenerate bone);
- Osteoinductive (that is, able to stimulate cells to undergo phenotypic conversion to osteoprogenitor cell types capable of bone formation).

There are no substitutes for autogenous bone; there are, however, synthetic alternatives. Allografts have been used as an alternative; however, they offer low or no osteogenicity, increase immunogenicity, and resorb more rapidly than autogenous bone. In clinical practice, fresh allografts are rarely used because of unfavorable immune responses and the risk of disease transmission. The frozen and freeze-dried types are osteoconductive but are considered, at best, to be only weakly osteoinductive. Freeze-drying diminishes the structural strength of the allograft and renders it unsuitable for use in situations where structural support is required. Allograft bone is a useful material for patients who require bone grafting of a non-union but have inadequate autograft bone. Bulk allografts can be utilized to treat segmental bone defects [57]. Their use in reconstruction after bone tumor resection is well documented. However, they are not commonly used in post-trauma reconstruction in which bone lengthening and transport are usually required.

Calcium sulfate (plaster of Paris) and its composites are some of the oldest osteoconductive materials available. They have been used to fill bony defects. However, their main drawback is the chemical reaction that occurs during setting, which results in a non-homogeneous structure with anisotropic properties.

Demineralized bone matrix (DBM) was first observed by Urist in 1965 to induce heterotopic bone [58]. The active components of DBM are a series of glycoproteins that belong to a group of the transforming growth factor beta family (TGF-β). The members of this group are responsible for the morphogenic events involved in tissue and organ development. Urist also isolated a protein from the bone matrix, which was termed bone morphogenic protein (BMP) [58]. DBM is commercially available and is used in the management of non-union fractures. DBM is not suitable where structural support is required. To date, the main delay in developing clinical products has been the need to find a suitable carrier to deliver BMP to the site where its action is required. New-generation ceramic composites/hybrids could fill this gap. Experimentally, BMP-2 and OP-1® (BMP-7) have been shown to stimulate new bone formation in diaphyseal defects in rats, rabbits, dogs, sheep, and non-human primates [59]. BMPs as well as collagen with new calcium phosphate derivatives or composites could be used for bone remodeling where bone regeneration is required (such as therapeutic applications in osteoporosis).

Bovine collagen mixed with hydroxyapatite is marketed as a bone graft substitute, which can be combined with bone marrow aspirated from the fracture site. Although no disease transmissions have been recorded, its use will continue to be a source of concern. This material is osteogenic, osteoinductive, and osteoconductive, but it lacks the structural strength required.

6.5.6 *Bioglasses and Glass-Ceramics*

Since Hench and Wilson [60] discovered bioglasses that bond to living tissue (Bioglass®), various kinds of bioactive glasses and glass-ceramics with different functions — such as high mechanical strength, high machinability, and fast setting ability — have been developed. The glasses that have been investigated for implantation are primarily based on silica (SiO_2), which may contain small amounts of other crystalline phases. The most prominent and successful application of this is Bioglass®, which can be found in detail in various comprehensive reviews [5, 9, 61, 62]. Bioactive glass compositions lie in the CaO–P_2O_5–SiO_2 system. The first development of such a bioglass began in 1971 when 45S5 Bioglass® was proposed with a composition of 45%SiO_2, 24.5%CaO, 24.5%NaO_2, and 6%P_2O_5 by weight [10]. Hench [5] and Vrouwenvelder *et al.* [63] suggested that 45S5 Bioglass® has greater osteoblastic activity as compared to hydroxyapatite. The reasoning behind this is a rapid exchange of alkali ions at the surface, which then leads to the formation of a silica-rich layer over a period of time. This paves the way for Ca^{2+} and PO_4^{3-} ions to migrate to the silica-rich surface where they combine with soluble calcium and phosphate ions from the solution, eventually forming an amorphous CaO–P_2O_5 layer. This layer undergoes crystallization upon interacting with OH^-, CO_2^{3-}, and F^- from the solution. A similar phenomenon has been observed by other researchers of bioglass with similar compositions [64]. Li *et al.* [65] prepared glass-ceramics from a similar composition with different degrees of crystallinity. They found that the amount of remaining glassy phase directly influenced apatite layer formation and that total inhibition occurred when the glassy phase constituted less than about 5 wt%.

Due to the surface-active response of these materials, they have been accepted as bioactive (or surface-active) biomaterials and have been used in middle ear and other non-load-bearing applications. Bioglasses® have been used successfully in clinical applications as artificial middle ear bone and in alveolar ridge maintenance implants [60].

Bioglass®, when subjected to heat treatment, will result in reduced alkaline oxide content and precipitated crystalline apatite in the glass. The resultant glass-ceramic is named Ceravital®, which exhibits fairly high mechanical strength but lower bioactivity than Bioglass®.

Kokubo *et al.* in 1982 [8] produced a glass-ceramic which contained oxyfluorapatite $Ca_{10}(PO_4)_6(OH, F_2)$ and wollastonite $(CaO.SiO_2)$ in a MgO–CaO–SiO_2 glassy matrix. It was named A–W glass-ceramic. It was reported that this A–W glass-ceramic spontaneously bonds to living bone without forming any fibrous tissue around it.

A bioactive and machinable glass-ceramic named Bioverit® has also been developed. It contains apatite and phlogophite $(Na, K)Mg_3(AlSi_3O_{10})(F)_2$, and is used in clinical applications as an artificial vertebra.

6.6 Nano-bioceramics, Composites, and Hybrids

6.6.1 *Nanoapatite-polymer Fiber Composites*

Bone is a composite in which nanosized apatite platelets are deposited on organic collagen fibers. If three-dimensional synthetic organic fibers can be fabricated into a composite structure and then modified with functional groups effective for apatite nucleation, morphologically similar bone structures could perhaps be prepared in such a manner. The resultant composite could be expected to exhibit bioactivity as well as mechanical properties analogous to those of the living bone.

Quite recently, ethylene–vinyl alcohol copolymer (EVOH) fibers constituting two-dimensional fabrics were subjected to a silane coupling treatment and subsequent soaking in a calcium silicate solution with a molar ratio of $Si(OC_2H_5)_4/H_2O/C_2H_5OH/Ca(NO_3)_2$ of 1.0/4.0/4.0/0.014/0.2. In this investigation, Kim *et al.* [66] and Kokubo *et al.* [67] have shown that after soaking in SBF for two days, nanosized apatite particles can be deposited uniformly on individual fibers constituting a fabric. The same fibers were also modified with an anatase-type titania on their surfaces after silane coupling treatment. This was done by soaking the fibers in a titania solution, $Ti(OiC_3H_7)_4/H_2O/C_2H_5OH/HNO_3$, with a molar ratio of 1.0/1.0/9.25/0.1, followed by soaking them in 0.1M-HCl solution at 80°C for eight days.

These pioneering works thus show that if these techniques were to be successfully applied to three-dimensional fabrics, then bioactive materials somehow similar to those of the living hard and soft tissues could possibly be produced.

6.6.2   *Bioceramics in In Situ Radiotherapy and Hyperthermia*

One of the most common approaches in cancer treatment is the removal of the diseased parts. Unfortunately, recovery of or return to full function is seldom achieved. Non-invasive treatment techniques — where only the cancer cells are destroyed — were introduced in the mid-1980s. In 1987, microspheres of $17Y_2O_3$–$19Al_2O_3$–$64SiO_2$ (mol%) glass, 20–30 μm in diameter, were shown to be effective for *in situ* radiotherapy of liver cancer [68,69]. [89]Yttrium in this glass is non-radioactive but can be activated by neutron bombardment to become ^{90}Y, which is a β-emitter with a half-life of 64.1 hours. The glass microspheres are usually injected into the diseased liver through the hepatic artery. Once entrapped in small blood vessels, they block the blood supply to the cancer and directly irradiate the cancer with β-rays. Since the β-ray transmission is only 2.5 mm in diameter on living tissue, and since the glass microspheres have high chemical durability, the surrounding normal tissue is hardly damaged by the β-rays.

These glass microspheres are already used clinically in Australia, Canada, and the U.S.A. The content of Y_2O_3 in the microspheres is, however, limited to only 17 mole% as they are prepared by conventional glass melting techniques. Recently, Kokubo *et al.* successfully prepared pure Y_2O_3 polycrystalline microspheres — which are 20 to 30 μm in diameter — using a high-frequency induction thermal plasma melting technique [70] (Figure 6.9). It was reported that they observed higher chemical durability than the Y_2O_3-containing glass microspheres. It was further reported that these ceramic microspheres are more effective for *in situ* radiotherapy of cancer.

Oxygen is known to be poorly supplied to cancer cells to produce lactic acid. Hence, cancer cells can be destroyed at around 43°C, whereas normal living cells are kept alive even at 48°C. If ferrimagnetic or ferromagnetic materials are implanted around cancer cells and placed under an alternating magnetic field, it is expected that,

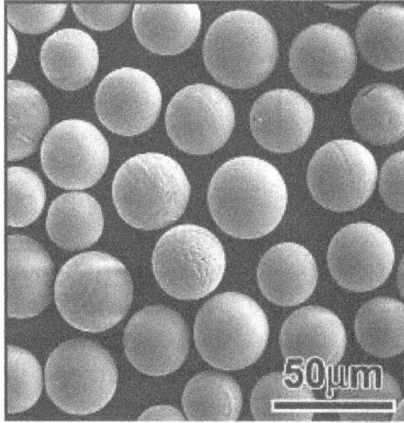

Figure 6.9. SEM image of Y_2O_3 microspheres for radiotherapy applications. Reprinted with permission from Kokubo *et al.* [67].

through magnetic hysteresis loss of the ferri- or ferromagnetic materials, locally heated cancer cells can be destroyed.

Kokubo and co-workers prepared ferrimagnetic glass-ceramic compositions containing 36 wt% of 200-nm-sized magnetite (Fe_3O_4) within a CaO–SiO_2 matrix. It was reported that cancer cells in the medullary canal of rabbit tibia were completely destroyed when this glass-ceramic was inserted into the tibia and placed under an alternating magnetic field of 300 Oe with 100 kHz [71]. This kind of invasive treatment, however, cannot be applied to humans since cancer cells metastasize. In the case of humans, ferri- or ferromagnetic materials must be injected into the cancer in microspheric form of 20 to 30 μm in diameter through blood vessels — an approach similar to that used for radioactive microspheres. For this purpose, the heat-generating efficiency of the ferrimagnetic material must be further increased. Recently, microspheres of 20 to 30 μm in diameter, with magnetite particles of 50 nm in size, were deposited on silica microspheres of 12 μm in diameter. The technique involved first of all the deposition of $FeO(OH)$ from a solution, followed by its transformation into Fe_3O_4 by a specific heat treatment at 600°C under a CO_2–H_2 gas atmosphere [72]. It was reported that the heat-generating efficiency of this material was about four times that of the above-described glass-ceramic.

6.6.3 Bone Cement Composites

During the last five years, bone cement materials have grown in popularity and are slated to be the osteoconductive substitutes for bone graft. They are prepared like acrylic cements, where a range of powders such as monocalcium phosphate, tricalcium phosphate, and calcium carbonate are mixed in a sodium phosphate solution. These cements are produced without polymerization, and the reaction is nearly non-exothermic. The final compounds are reported to have a strength of 10–100 MPa in compression. However, the strength is only 1–10 MPa in tension they are very weak under shear forces. These composites are currently used in orthopedics for fracture management. It has been suggested that these materials could improve the compressive strength of vertebral bodies in osteoporosis. Injection of calcium phosphate cement has been shown to be feasible and effective: The cement indeed improved compressive strength [73].

Attempts have been made to prepare hydroxyapatite/ceramic composites by adding various ceramic reinforcements: metal fibers [74], Si_3N_4 or hydroxyapatite whiskers [75], Al_2O_3 platelets [76], and ZrO_2 particles [77]. In many cases, the composites could not be successfully prepared due to problems related to poor densification.

Hydroxyapatite/metal and hydroxyapatite/polymer composites are two typical classes of materials that have been examined for improving the toughness characteristics of synthetic hydroxyapatite. In both cases, improvement in toughness can be detected by studying the crack-face-bridging mechanism in operation during plastic stretching of metallic or polymeric ligaments. Zhang *et al.* [78] proposed a toughened composite consisting of hydroxyapatite dispersed with silver particles. This material was obtained by a conventional sintering method. It was reported that the toughness of these composites increased to 2.45 MPa m$^{1/2}$ upon loading the mixture with 30 vol% of silver. Silver is used not only because of its ductility in terms of fracture toughness but also because it is inert and has antibacterial properties [79]. Attempts to supersede metal alloys with carbon-fiber-reinforced plastics and various composites to stabilize fractures have met with limited success. To date, the only exception is a new titanium metal core composite hip implant which has been clinically assessed in Europe with promising results [76, 77].

6.6.4 *Biomimetic Hybrid Composites*

The conventional way to synthesize an inorganic material-based composite is to subject one of the mixture constituents to a specifically designed heat treatment. This process is also commonly used to produce biomaterials. However, conceptually, it is far from the biomineralization process which occurs in nature. The natural process produces fine hybrid structures which are hardly reproducible by classic consolidation processes. The traditional sintering route is not directly applicable to produce ceramic/polymer composites because no polymers will withstand the densification temperature of any ceramic material. Hydroxyapatite/polyethylene (HAp/PE) composites have been obtained by loading the polymeric matrix with an inorganic filler. In recent years, several research groups have demonstrated the feasibility of *in vitro* techniques to synthesize biomimetic material structures [43, 77–83]. Currently, a range of HAp/PE-based composites is being produced and marketed by a UK based company. The sophistication of the biomimetic route has not been paired yet, and these techniques, so far, have not proved to be fully applicable to clinical applications [82]. It can be easily predicted that more and more dense bioceramic-based hybrid materials will be introduced, thus opening up new horizons in biomaterial production and application methods.

A new alternative route has been proposed recently [79]. It is based on an *in situ* polymerization process carried out in an inorganic scaffold (which has submicrometer-sized open porosity). This is an intermediate method between conventional sintering and *in vitro* biomineralization, because it still employs sintering for the preparation of the inorganic scaffold; however, the subsequent hybridization of the scaffold with an organic phase is carried out through a chemical route. While this method is targeted at relatively complex structural designs, it enables the synthesis of biomimetic (hybrid) inorganic/organic composites in rather simple and easily reproducible ways. A schematic representation of this efficient synthesis route is given in Figure 6.10.

A common characteristic of natural biomaterials — such as bone, nacre, sea urchin tooth, and other tough hybrid materials in nature — is the strong microscopic interaction between the inorganic and organic phases. This characteristic allows the organic phase to act

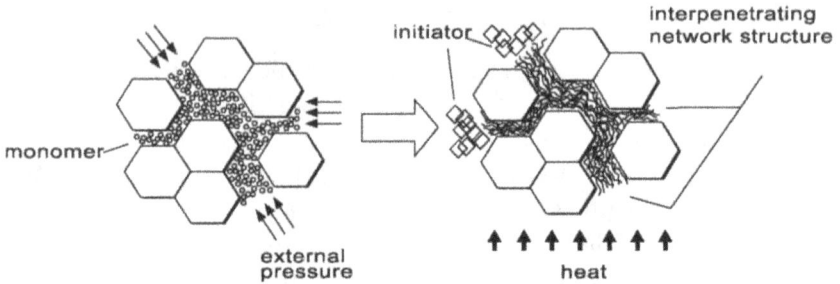

Figure 6.10. Schematic representation of the *in situ* polymerization synthesis route of new-generation hybrid materials.

as a plastic energy-dissipating network, where stretching (bridging) ligaments are formed across the surfaces of a propagating crack on a nanoscale level. Such complexity has led to the common perception that, to mimic the natural designs, *in situ* synthesis techniques should be adopted. Precipitation of calcium carbonate or hydroxyapatite into a polymeric matrix, for example, has been proposed as a novel synthetic route to biomimetic composites [81–84]. Despite significant advances in understanding biological mineralization and developing new fabrication processes, the composites to date obtained by these methods are by far in the embryonic stage for actual biomedical applications due to their low structural performance.

Fracture tests were carried out on two natural biomaterials — bovine femur and Japanese nacre (*Crassostrea Nippona*). Their results were then compared with a synthetic hydroxyapatite/nylon–6 composite obtained by *in situ* polymerization of caprolactam infiltrated into a porous apatite scaffold. The comparison showed that the level of fracture incurred was about two orders of magnitude higher than that of monolithic hydroxyapatite, and it is due to the stretching of protein or polymeric ligaments across the crack faces during fracture propagation [79].

Nanoscale modeling of synthetically manufactured hybrids and composites is still in its infancy. However, mimicking natural microstructures by using strong synthetic molecules may lead to new-generation biomaterials, whose toughness characteristics will be comparable with those of the materials available in nature. A formidable challenge remains in the optimization of the morphology and bioactivity of these novel hybrid composites.

6.7 Design with Bioceramics

Five important factors should be considered in any implantation work:

1. Production method of the material used,
2. Biocompatibility, tissue–implant interface reactions, and choice of the material used,
3. Applied stresses and biomechanics of the joint,
4. Physical well-being and age of the patient, and
5. Surgical technique.

Various criteria exist when selecting a biomaterial for a particular biomedical application. After biocompatibility, mechanical properties are the second decisive criterion when it comes to selecting a material for a particular orthopedic or maxillofacial application. The selected mechanical properties of a range of synthetic and natural biomaterials are shown in Table 6.1.

In the context of mechanical properties, an important criterion involves scrutiny of the modulus of elasticity and Poisson's ratio. These are intrinsic material constants that describe a material's deformability, which therefore influence the stiffness of any structure made from this material. At a bone–implant load-carrying interface, the greater the stiffness of the implant material, the more load it will carry while less will be carried by the surrounding tissue. However, this issue can be detrimental due to stress shielding and the resultant bone resorption.

For example, evaluation of plate stiffness is crucial when it comes to choosing a material for a fracture plate. Woo [85] has experimentally verified this by comparing a rigid Co–Cr alloy and a flexible composite plate made of graphite, carbon fibers, and polymethylmetacrylate resin (GFMM). The latter material has an elastic modulus of approximately $1/10(10–40\,\text{GPa})$ that of the Co–Cr alloy ($250\,\text{GPa}$). Four-point bending tests were performed on the cortical bone adjacent to the fracture plate. These specimens were removed post-operatively after one year of implantation in dog femurs. The tests showed that the strength of the bone adjacent to less rigid GFMM-plated bone was much greater than that of the Co–Cr-plated bone. Although stiffness is not the only determining factor of this increase, its importance is nevertheless highlighted here.

Material failure can occur in tensile, compressive, and shear modes. Metals tend to have tensile and compressive strengths that do not differ greatly; ceramics tend to be weak in tension and strong in compression. The lack of crystallographic slip systems in ceramics and glasses prevents dislocation motion and generation, resulting in a material that is hard and brittle. To determine if a class of materials is appropriate for a particular application, it is mandatory to carefully assess the nature of loading that this application demands. For example, if an application requires the selected material to withstand tensile stress, then the material's tensile strength must be improved by making surface layers compressive relative to the interior. After all, applied force should overcome the compressive force before the tensile force takes over. Depending on the bioceramics used, surface compression can be introduced by various surface modification techniques such as ion exchange, quenching, and surface crystallization. The ion exchange in glass and glass-ceramics can be accomplished by diffusion or electrical migration techniques. Larger ions are exchanged with smaller ions (e.g., K^+ for Na^+), making the surface compressive due to lattice straining.

As for a material's resistance to fracture, it is determined by an extrinsic property named fracture toughness. This tends to be high for metals and low for ceramics. This is an important parameter because it more appropriately reflects a material's performance than its tensile strength data. Fracture toughness data of ceramics and metals show that resistance to crack propagation and failure is much higher for metals, which means that tensile failures would occur more readily in ceramics.

Strength and fracture toughness testing procedures usually involve short-term assessments and are prone to statistical scatter. In addition, they neglect the effects of dynamic fatigue on metals or static fatigue (slow crack growth) on ceramics. Therefore, results from these assessments can be considered only as upper limits to a material's performance. Given the complex overlapping of various degradation phenomena, mechanical analyses have to be carefully performed according to case-by-case testing procedures. For example, the fatigue behavior of a vapor-deposited pyrolytic carbon film of about 500 nm thickness onto a stainless steel substrate showed that the film did not break until the substrate underwent plastic deformation (deformation of 0.0013 strain after 10^6 cyclic loading) [86].

This case illustrated that the fracture of thin films strongly depends on the behavior of the substrates used.

Microhardness and nanohardness indicate a material's ability to resist wear and impact. Wear performance is a very important consideration in the selection of an implant material, as wear is the result of the removal and relocation of matter through the contact of two surfaces. However, both plastic and elastic deformations involve many different types of wear as described in the following:

- Corrosive wear is due to chemical activity on one of the sliding materials. The sliding action promotes the removal of corrosion products (that otherwise protect the surface from further corrosive attack), resulting in faster corrosion rates.
- Surface fatigue wear is due to the formation of subsurface microcracks followed by the breaking off of large chunks under repeated loading and sliding cycles.
- Abrasive wear is a process in which particles are pulled off from one surface and adhere to the other during sliding. This type of wear is the most important process in biomaterials and can be minimized with particular care regarding smoothing the sliding surfaces.
- Wear related to phase transformation is a kind of wear process peculiar to zirconia implants. It arises from the metastability of some polycrystalline zirconia materials and from the tendency of the tetragonal phase to transform into the monoclinic polymorph. Since the tetragonal-to-monoclinic transformation occurs with volume expansion, hard monoclinic particles tend to detach from the sliding surface and, being trapped in between the sliding surfaces, strongly accelerate surface degradation. The resistance to transformation wear of a zirconia material is remarkably affected by the kind of lubricant between the sliding surfaces as explained in previous sections [17].

In summary, mechanical property data of any potential implant material must be considered with care because many extrinsic factors dominate the properties, particularly in the case of bioceramics. A material's microstructure and testing environment are the main controlling factors among the variables. In all cases, published data can be considered only as guidelines for the behavior of materials in use.

6.8   Future of Bioceramics

As discussed in this chapter, the properties of bioceramics are strongly influenced by these factors: raw materials selected for preparation, the method used to fabricate, processes used to consolidate, and the final machining processes. All these factors contribute to their final structure and hence to their long-term performance as bioceramics. The optimization of bioceramics in medical applications can be achieved by further studies of the effects of processing conditions on their structures and hence their long-term properties.

In particular, the nature and effect of additives — whether to improve biological performance or to ease processing — on the local and systemic responses need further investigation. Sometimes, the improvement of one property could be detrimental to the other properties.

In the early 1970s, bioceramics were employed to perform singular, biologically inert roles, such as to provide parts for bone replacement. The realization that cells and tissues in the body perform many other vital regulatory and metabolic roles has highlighted the limitations of synthetic materials as tissue substitutes. The demands of bioceramics have changed from maintaining an essentially physical function without eliciting a host response to providing a more integrated interaction with the host. This is accompanied by increasing demands for medical devices to improve the quality of life as well as extend its duration. Bioceramics potentially can be used as body interactive materials — helping the body to heal or promoting regeneration of tissues, thus restoring physiological functions. This approach is being explored in the development of a range of new-generation bioceramics which incorporate biogenic materials with a widened selection of applications.

Tissue engineering has been directed to take advantage of the combined use of living cells and tri-dimensional ceramic scaffolds to deliver vital cells to the damaged site in a patient. To date, strategies that combine a relatively traditional approach (such as bioceramic implants) with the acquired knowledge have been found to be feasible and productive when applied to the fields of cell growth and differentiation of osteogenic cells. A stem cell is a cell from the embryo, fetus, or adult that has the ability to reproduce for long periods. It also can give rise to specialized cells that make up the tissues and organs of the body. An adult stem cell is an undifferentiated (unspecialized) cell that occurs in a differentiated (specialized) tissue. It is able to renew itself and become specialized to yield all of the specialized cell types of the tissue from which it originates. Cultured bone marrow cells can be regarded as a mesenchymal precursor cell population derived from adult cells. They can differentiate into different lineages (osteoblasts, chondrocytes, adipocytes, and myocytes) and undergo limited mitotic divisions without expressing any telomerase activity. When implanted into immuno-deficient mice, these cells can combine with mineralized tri-dimensional scaffolds to form a highly vascularized bone tissue. Cultured cells/bioceramic composites can be used to treat full-thickness gaps of bone diaphysis with excellent integration of the ceramic scaffold with bone and good functional recovery. Excellent innovative work is in progress, and clinical applications are becoming quite common.

Ultimately, the field of bioceramics is fundamental to advances in the performance and function of medical devices and is a critical part of medicine and surgery. Bioceramics science is truly interdisciplinary. Therefore, the development of improved bioceramics hinges on the outcome of advances in materials, physical, and biological sciences, engineering, and medicine. The correlations between material property and biological performance will be useful in the design of improved bioceramics, particularly to overcome the problems of implant rejection and related infections.

The challenge remains to provide safe and efficacious bioceramics with the required properties and an acceptable biocompatibility level. As the field of biomaterials finds increasing applications in cellular and tissue engineering [87,88], it will continue to be used in new ways as part of the most innovative therapeutic strategies.

References

[1]   P. P. Lutton and B. Ben-Nissan, Biomaterials in the marketplace: Focus on orthopedic and dental applications, *Materials Technology*, 1997, 12(3–4):121–126.

[2]   R. H. Doremus, Review — Bioceramics, *J. Mater. Sci.*, 1992, 27:285–297.

[3]   J. W. Boretos, Advances in bioceramics, *Adv. Ceram. Mater.*, 1987, 2:15–24.

[4] R. Z. LeGeros, Calcium phosphate materials in restorative dentistry: A review, *Adv. Dent. Res.*, 1988, 2:164–183.

[5] L. L. Hench, Molecular design of bioactive glasses and ceramics for implants, in *Ceramics: Towards the 21st Century*, eds. W. Soga and A. Kato, (Ceram. Soc. of Japan, 1991) pp. 519–534.

[6] H. Aoki, CaO–P$_2$O$_5$ Apatite, *Japanese Patent JP*, 78110999 (1978).

[7] M. Jarcho, C. H. Bolen, M. B. Thomas, J. F. Bobick, J. F. Kay, and R. H. Doremus, Hydroxylapatite synthesis and characterization in dense polycrystalline form, *J. Mater. Sci.*, 1976, 11:2027–2035.

[8] T. Kokubo, M. Shigematsu, Y. Nagashima, M. Tashiro, T. Nakamura, T. Yamamuro, and S. Higashi, Apatite–Wollastonite containing glass-ceramic for prosthetic application, in *Bulletin of Institute for Chemical Research*, (Kyoto University, 1982) 60:260–268.

[9] T. Kokubo, Novel biomaterials derived from glasses, in *Ceramics: Towards the 21st Century*, eds. W. Soga and A. Kato, (J. Ceramic. Soc. Japan, 1991) pp. 500–518.

[10] L. L Hench, R. J. Splinter, W. C. Allen, and T. K. Greenlee, Bonding mechanisms at the interface of ceramic prosthetic materials, *J. Biomed. Mater. Res. Symp.*, 1972, 2:117–141.

[11] I. C. Clarke, Role of ceramic implants — design and clinical success with total hip prosthetic ceramic-to-ceramic bearings, *Clinical Orthopedics and Related Research*, 1992, 282:19–30.

[12] D. J. Kim, D. Y. Lee, and J. S. Han, Low temperature stability of zirconia/alumina hip joint heads, in Key Engineering Materials, 240–242, in *Bioceramics 15*, eds. B. Ben-Nissan, D. Sher, and W. Walsh, (Trans. Tech. Publications, Switzerland, 2003) pp. 831–834.

[13] H. Oonishi, Y. Takayaka, I. C. Clarke, and H. Jung, Comparative wear studies of 28-mm ceramic and stainless steel total hip joints over two to seven year period, *J. Long-Term Effects Med. Implants*, 1992, 2:37–47.

[14] S. F. Hulbert, J. C. Bokros, L. L. Hench, J. Wilson, and G. Heimke, Ceramics in clinical applications: past, present and future, in *Ceramics in Clinical Applications*, ed. P. Vincenzini, (Elsevier Sci. Publ., Amsterdam, 1997) pp. 3–27.

[15] K. Hayashi, N. Matsuguchi, K. Uenoyama, T. Kanemaru, and Y. Sugioka, Evaluation of metal implants coated with several types of ceramics as biomaterials,*J. Biomed. Mater. Res.*, 1989, 23: 1247–1259.

[16] R. L. Huckstep and P. P. Lutton, New concepts in stabilization and replacement of bones and joints, *Mater. Forum*, 1991, 15:253–260.

[17] H. Oonishi, I. C. Clarke, V. Good, H. Amino, M. Ueno, S. Masuda, K. Oomamiuda, H. Ishimaru, M. Yamamoto, and E. Tsuji, Needs of bioceramics to longevity of total joint arthroplasty, in Key

Engineering Materials, 240–242, in *Bioceramics 15*, eds. B. Ben-Nissan, D. Sher, and W. Walsh, (Trans. Tech. Publications, Switzerland, 2003) pp. 735–754.

[18] L. Sedel, Tribology and clinical experience of alumina–alumina articulations, in *Proceeding of the 66th Annual Meeting of the American Academy of Orthopedic Surgeons*, (USA, 1999) pp. 120.

[19] G. Willmann, The evolution of ceramics in total hip arthroplasty, *Hip International*, 2000, 10:193–203.

[20] O. C. Standard, K. Schindhelm, B. K. Milthorpe, C. R. Howlett, and C. C. Sorrell, Biocompatibility of zirconia ceramics, in *Proc. of Int. Ceram. Conf. Austceram*, 92, Vol. 2, ed. M. J. Bannister, (CSIRO Pub., Melbourne, Australia, 1992) pp. 611–616.

[21] V. Saikko, Wear of polyethylene acetabular cups against zirconia femoral heads studied with a hip joint simulator, *Wear*, 1994, 176:207–212.

[22] I. C. Clarke, V. Good, P. Williams, D. Schroeder, L. Anissian, A. Stark, H. Oonishi, J. Schuldies, and G. Gustafson, Ultra-low wear rates for rigid-on-rigid bearings in total hip replacements, in *Proc. Inst. Mech. Engrs.*, 2000, Vol. 214, Part H:331–347.

[23] A. Pizzoferrato, S. Stea, and G. Ciapetti, Alternative articulating surfaces for total hip replacement, *Current Opinion in Orthop.*, 1995, 6:42–47.

[24] J. Chevalier, B. Cales, J. M. Drouin, and Y. Stefani, Ceramic–Ceramic bearing systems compared on different testing configurations, in *Bioceramics 10*, eds. L. Sekel and C. Rey, (University Press, Cambridge, UK, 1997) pp. 271–274.

[25] I. C. Clarke, Clinical and tribological perspectives of wear in alumina–alumina THR, in Key Engineering Materials, 240–242, *Bioceramics 15*, eds. B. Ben-Nissan, D. Sher, and W. Walsh, (Trans. Tech. Publications, Switzerland, 2003), pp. 755–764.

[26] P. A. Williams, I. C. Clarke, G. Pezzotti, D. D. Green, and B. Ben-Nissan, Water lubrication effects on zirconia debris production in hip-joint simulators, in Key Engineering Materials, 240–242, *Bioceramics 15*, eds. B. Ben-Nissan, D. Sher, and W. Walsh, (Trans. Tech. Publications, Switzerland, 2003) pp. 835–838.

[27] S. T. Woolson and M. G. Murphy, Wear of the polyethylene of Harris–Galante acetabular components inserted without cement, *J. Bone Joint Surg.*, 1995, 77(9):1311–1314.

[28] K. Tanaka, J. Tamura, K. Kawanabe, M. Shimizu, and T. Nakamura, Effect of alumina femoral heads on polyethylene wear in cemented total hip arthroplasty: old versus current alumina, *J. Bone Joint Surg. Br.*, 2002, 85B(5):655–660.

[29] T. Nakamura, Novel zirconia/alumina composites for TJR, in Key Engineering Materials, 240–242, *Bioceramics 15*, eds. B. Ben-Nissan, D. Sher, and W. Walsh, (Trans. Tech. Publications, Switzerland, 2003) pp. 765–768.

[30] M. Spector, M. D. Ries, R. B. Bourne, W. S. Sauer, M. Long, and G. Hunter, Wear performance of Ultra High Molecular Weight Polyethylene on oxidized zirconium total knee femoral components, *J. Bone Joint Surg.* AM, 2001, 83A, Supp. 2, Part 2:80–86.

[31] G. Hunter and M. Long, Abrasive wear of oxidized Zr–2.5Nb, CoCrMo and Ti–6Al–4V against bone cement, in Trans. of 6th Biomater. Congress, (Soc. Biomat., Hawaii, 2000), p.835.

[32] D. D. D'Lima, S. M. Lemperle, P. C. Chen, R. E. Holmes, and C. W. Colwell, Bone response to implant surface morphology, *J. Arthrop.*, 1998, 13(8):928–934.

[33] D. Heuer, A. Harrison, H. Y. Gupta, and G. Hunter, Chemically textured and oxidized zirconium surfaces for implant fixation, in Key Engineering Materials, 240–242, *Bioceramics 15*, eds. B. Ben-Nissan, D. Sher, and W. Walsh, (Trans. Tech. Publications, Switzerland, 2003) pp. 789–792.

[34] W. F. De Jong, La Substance Material darts lesos, *Rec. Tav. Chim.*, 1997, 45:415–448.

[35] B. Ben-Nissan, C. Chai, and L. Evans, Crystallographic and spectroscopic characterization and morphology of biogenic and synthetic Apatites, in *Encyclopedic Handbook of Biomaterials and Bioengineering Vol. 1, Part B: Applications*, eds. D. L. Wise, D. J. Trantolo, D. E. Altobelli, M. J. Yaszemski, J. D. Gresser, and E.R. Schwartz, (Marcel Dekker Inc., New York, 1995) pp. 191–221.

[36] F. H. Albee and H. F. Morrison, Bone graft surgery, *Ann. Surg.*, 1920 (reprinted in Clin. Orthro. & Rel. Res., 1996, 324:5–12) 71:32–39.

[37] A. M. Gatti, D. Zaffe, and G. P. Poli, Behavior of tricalcium phosphate and hydroxyapatite granules in sheep bone defects, *Biomaterials*, 1990, 11:513–517.

[38] C. P. A. T. Klein, A. A. Driessens, and K. de Groot, Relationship between the degradation behavior of calcium phosphate ceramics and their physical chemical characteristics and ultrastructural geometry, *Biomaterials*, 1984, 5:157–160.

[39] W. Den Hollander, P. Patka, C. P. A. T. Klein, and G. A. K. Heidendal, Macroporous calcium phosphate ceramics for bone substitution: a tracer study on biodegradation with ^{45}Ca tracer, *Biomaterials*, 1991, 12:569–573.

[40] M. M. A. Ramselaar, F. C. M. Driessens, W. Kalk, J. R. de Wijn, and P. J. van Mullen, Biodegradation of four calcium phosphate ceramics;

in vivo rates and tissue interactions, *J. Mater. Sci.: Mater. Med.*, 1991, 2:63–70.

[41] E. Hayek and H. Newesely, Pentacalcium Monohydroxyorthophosphate, *Inorg. Synth.*, 1963, 7:63–65.

[42] D. J. Greenfield and E. D. Eanes, Formation chemistry of amorphous calcium phosphates prepared from carbonate-containing solutions, *Calcif. Tissue Res.*, 1972, 9:152–162.

[43] T. Kokubo, H. Kushitani, Y. Ebisawa, T. Kitsugi, S. Kotani, K. Ohura, and T. Yamamuro, Apatite formation on bioactive ceramics in body environment, in *Bioceramics Vol. 1*, eds. H. Oonishi, H. Aoki, and K. Sawai, (Ishiyaku Euro America, 1989) pp. 157–162.

[44] T. Kokubo, H. M. Kim, M. Kawashita, and T. Nakamura, Novel ceramics for biomedical applications, *J. Aust. Ceram. Soc.*, 2000, 36(1):37–46.

[45] J. H. Kuhne, R. Bartl, B. Frisch, C. Hammer, V. Jannson, and M. Zimmer, Bone formation in coralline hydroxyapatite — effects of pore size studied in rabbits, *Acta Orthopedica Scandinava*, 1994, 65(3):246.252.

[46] D. M. Roy and S. K. Linnehan, Hydroxyapatite formed from coral skeletal carbonate by hydrothermal exchange, *Nature*, 1974, 247:220–222.

[47] M. Sivakumar, T. S. Kumar, K. L. Shantra, and K. P. Rao, Development of hydroxyapatite derived from Indian coral, *Biomaterials*, 1996, 17:1709–1714.

[48] J. Pena, R. Z. Le Geros, R. Rohanizadeh, and J. P. Leros, $CaCO_3$/Ca–P biphasic materials prepared by microwave processing of natural aragonite and calcite, in Key Engineering Materials, 192–195, *Bioceramics 13*, eds. S. Giannini and A. Moroni, (Trans Tech Publications, Switzerland, 2001) pp. 267–270.

[49] J. Hu, J. J. Russell, B. Ben-Nissan, and R. Vago, Production and analysis of hydroxyapatite from Australian corals via hydrothermal process, *J. Mater. Sci. Letters*, 2001, 20:85–87.

[50] C. S. Chai and B. Ben-Nissan, Interfacial reactions between hydroxyapatite and titanium, *J. Aust. Ceram. Soc.*, 1993, 29:81–90.

[51] C. M. Cottel, D. B. Chrisey, K. S. Grabowski, J. A. Sprague, and C. R. Rossett, Pulsed laser deposition of hydroxyapatite thin films on Ti–6Al–4V, *J. Appl. Biomater.*, 1992, 3:87–93.

[52] J. L. Ong, L. C. Lucas, W. R. Lacefield, and E. D. Rigney, Structure, solubility and bond strength of thin calcium phosphate coatings produced by ion beam sputter deposition, *Biomaterials*, 1992, 13(4):249–254.

[53] P. Ducheyne, W. van Raemdock, J. C. Heughebaert, and M. Heughe-baert, Structural analysis of hydroxyapatite coatings on titanium, *Biomaterials*, 1986, 7:97–103.

[54] I. Zhitomirsky and L. Gal-Or, Electrophoretic deposition of hydrox-yapatite, *J. Biomed. Mater. Res.*, 1997, 21:1375–1381.

[55] B. Ben-Nissan, D. D. Green, G. S. K. Kannangara, and A. Milev, ^{31}P NMR studies of diethyl phosphite derived nanocrystalline hydroxya-patite, *J. Sol-Gel Sci. Tech.*, 2001, 21:27–37.

[56] W. Van Raemdonck, P. Ducheyne, and P. DeMeester, Calcium phos-phate ceramics, in *Metal and Ceramic Biomaterials Vol. II*, eds. P. Ducheyne and G. W. Hastings, (CRC Press, 1984) pp. 143–162.

[57] G. E. Friedlaender, D. M. Strong, W. W. Tomford, and H. J. Mankin, Long term follow-up of patients with osteochondral allografts: a corre-lation between immunogenic responses and clinical outcome, *Orthop. Clin. North. Am.*, 1999, 30:583–585.

[58] M. R. Urist, Bone: Formation by autoinduction, *Science*, 1965, 12:893–899.

[59] S. D. Cook, M. W. Wolfe, S. L. Salkeld, and D. C. Rueger, Effect of recombinant human osteogenic Protein-1 on healing of segmental defects in non-human primates, *J. Bone Joint Surg.*, 1996, 77-A:734–750.

[60] L. L. Hench and J. Wilson, Surface active materials, *Science*, 1984, 226:630–636.

[61] L. L. Hench, Bioactive ceramics, in *Bioceramics: Materials Charac-teristics* vs. *in vivo* Behavior, Vol. 523, eds. P. Ducheyne and J. E. Lemons, (Ann. of the New York Academy of Science, New York, 1988) pp. 54–71.

[62] T. Kokubo, Recent progress in glass-based materials for biomedical applications, *J. Ceramic. Soc.* Japan, 1991, 99:965–973.

[63] W. C. A. Vrouwenvelder, C. G. Groot, and K. de Groot, Histological and biochemical evaluation of osteoblasts cultured on bioactive glass, hydroxyapatite, titanium alloy, and stainless steel, J. Biomed. Mater. Res., 1993, 27:465–475.

[64] O. H. Andersson and I. Kangasniemi, Calcium phosphate formation at the surface of bioactive glass *in vitro*, *J. Biomed. Mat. Res.*, 1991, 25:1019–1030.

[65] P. Li, Q. Yang, F. Zhang, and T. Kokubo, The effect of residual glassy phase in a bioctive glass-ceramic on the gormation of its surface apatite layer *in vitro*, *J. Mater. Sci.: Mater. Med.*, 1992, 3:452–456.

[66] H. M. Kim, Y. Sasaki, J. Suzuki, S. Fujibayashi, T. Kokubo, T. Matsushita, and T. Nakamura, Mechanical properties of bioactive titanium metal prepared by chemical treatment, in Key Engineering

Materials, 192–195, *Bioceramics 13*, eds. S. Giannini and A. Moroni, (Trans. Tech. Pub., Switzerland, 2000) pp. 227–230.

[67] T. Kokubo, Novel inorganic materials for biomedical applications, in Key Engineering Materials, 240–242, *Bioceramics 15*, eds. B. Ben-Nissan, D. Sher, and W. Walsh, (Trans. Tech. Publications, Switzerland, 2003) pp. 523–528.

[68] H. M. Kim, F. Miyaji, T. Kokubo, S. Nishiguchi, and T. Nakamura, Graded surfaces structure of bioactive titanium prepared by chemical treatment, *J. Biomed. Mater. Res.*, 1999, 45(2):100–107.

[69] G. J. Ehrhardt and D. E. Day, Therapeutic use of ^{90}Y microspheres, *Int. J. Radiation Appl. & Inst., Part B, Nucl. Med. & Biol.*, 1987, 14(3):233–242.

[70] M. Kawashita, T. Kokubo, and Y. Inoue, Preparation of Y_2O_3 microspheres for *in situ* radiotherapy of cancer, in *Bioceramics Vol. 12*, eds. H. Ohgushi, G. W. Hastings, and T. Yoshikawa, (World Scientific, Singapore, 1999) pp. 555–558.

[71] M. Ikenaga, K. Ohura, T. Yamamuro, Y. Kotoura, M. Oka, and T. Kokubo, Localized hyperthermic treatment of experimental bone tumors with ferromagnetic ceramics, *J. Orthop. Res.*, 1993, 11(6):849–855.

[72] M. Kawashita, M. Tanaka, T. Kokubo, T. Yao, S. Hamada, and T. Shinjo, Preparation of magnetite microspheres for hyperthermia of cancer, in Key Engineering Materials, 218–220, *Bioceramics 14*, eds. S. Brown, I. Clarke, and P. Williams, (Trans Tech Pub., Switzerland, 2002) pp. 645–648.

[73] K. D. Kuhn, *Bone Cements*, (Springer, New York, 2000).

[74] A. J. Ruys, K. A. Zeigler, A. Brandwood, B. K. Milthorpe, S. Morrey, and C. C. Sorrell, Reinforcement of hydroxyapatite with ceramic and metal fibers, in *Bioceramics Vol. 4*, eds. W. Bonfield, G. W. Hastings, and K. E. Tanner, (Butterworth–Heinemenn Ltd, London, UK, 1991) pp. 281–286.

[75] K. Ioku, T. Noma, N. Ishizawa, and M. Yoshimura, Hydrothermal synthesis and sintering of hydroxyapatite powders dispersed with Si_3N_4 whiskers, *J. Ceram. Soc. Jpn. Int. Ed.*, 1990, 98:48–53.

[76] S. Gautier, E. Champion, and D. Bernache-Assollant, Effect of processing on the characteristics of a $20vol\%Al_2O_3$ platelet reinforced hydroxyapatite composite, in *Bioceramics Vol. 10*, eds. L. Sedel and C. Rey, (University Press, Cambridge, UK, 1997) pp. 549–552.

[77] W. Bonfield, M. D. Grynpas, A. E. Tully, J. Bowman, and J. Abram, Hydroxyapatite reinforced polyethylene: a mechanically compatible implant material for bone replacement, *Biomaterials*, 1981, 2: 185–186.

[78] X. Zhang, G. H. M. Gubbels, R. A. Terpstra, and R. Metselaar, Toughening of calcium hydroxyapatite with silver particles, *J. Mater. Sci.*, 1997, 32:235–243.

[79] G. Pezzotti and S. M. F. Asmus, Fracture behavior of hydroxyapatite/polymer interpenetrating network composites prepared by *in situ* polymerization process, *Mater. Sci. Eng.*, 2001, 316:231–237.

[80] M. Sarikaya, J. Liu, and I. A. Aksay, Nacre: Properties, Crystallography, and formation, in *Biomimetics: Design and Processing of Materials*, eds. M. Sarikaya and I. A. Aksay, (American Institute of Physics, New York, 1995) pp. 34–90.

[81] P. Calvert and S. Mann, Review: Synthetic and biological composites formed by *in situ* precipitation, *J. Mater. Sci.*, 1988, 23:3801–3806.

[82] N. H. Ladizesky, I. Ward, and W. Bonfield, Hydrostatic extrusion of polyethylene filled with hydroxyapatite, *Polymers Adv. Tech.*, 1997, 8:496.504.

[83] R. L. Reis, A. M. Cunha, and M. J. Bevis, Load bearing and ductile hydroxyapatite polyethylene composites for bone replacement, in *Bioceramics Vol. 10*, eds. L. Sedel and C. Rey, (University Press, Cambridge, UK, 1997) pp. 515–518.

[84] N. Almqvist, N. H. Thomson, B. L. Smith, G. D. Stucky, D. E. Morse, and P. K. Hansma, Methods for fabricating and characterizing a new generation of biomimetic materials, *Mater. Sci. Eng.*, 1999, C7:37–43.

[85] S. L. Y. Woo, The relationships of changes in stress levels on long bone remodeling, in *Mechanical Properties of Bone*, ed. S. C. Cowin, (American Society of Mechanical Engineers, New York, 1981) pp. 107–129.

[86] J. C. Bokros, Deposition structure and properties of pyrolytic carbon, in *Chemistry and Physics of Carbon Vol. 5*, ed. P. L. Walker, (Marcel Dekker Inc., New York, 1969) pp. 70–81.

[87] M. J. Zafar, D. Zhu, and Z. Zhang, 3D printing of bioceramics for bone tissue engineering. *Materials (Basel).* 2019 Oct 15;12(20):3361. doi: 10.3390/ma12203361. PMID: 31618857; PMCID: PMC6829398.

[88] G. L. Koons, M. Diba, and A. G. Mikos, Materials design for bone-tissue engineering. *Nat Rev Mater*, 5, 584–603 (2020). https://doi.org/10.1038/s41578-020-0204-2.

Chapter 7

Polymeric Hydrogels

Xia Song and Jun Li*

*Department of Biomedical Engineering,
College of Design and Engineering, National University of Singapore,
Lower Kent Ridge Road, Singapore 119276, Singapore
bielj@nus.edu.sg; jun-li@nus.edu.sg

Polymeric hydrogels are of special importance to polymeric biomaterials because of their favorable biocompatibility. Hydrogels are crosslinked macromolecular networks formed by hydrophilic polymers swollen in water or biological fluids. The crosslinks can be formed by either covalent bonds or physical cohesion forces that exist between the polymer segments. Polymeric hydrogels are primarily classified into chemical and physical hydrogels (based on the bonding type of the crosslinks), although they can also be classified in many other ways. Chemical hydrogels can be prepared by copolymerization of a monomer with a crosslinker or by crosslinking water-soluble polymers. Physical hydrogels can be made of natural biopolymers, thermosensitive synthetic polymers, amphiphilic triblock copolymers, or many other copolymers. Furthermore, polyelectrolyte complexes and polymer-cyclodextrin inclusion complexes can likewise form hydrogels. All chemical and physical hydrogels described in this chapter are of biomedical significance. The biomedical applications of these materials in drug delivery and tissue engineering are hence discussed.

7.1 Introduction

Among many polymeric biomaterials, hydrogels are of special interest because of their favorable biocompatibility and the many unique advantages that accompany them [1–8]. For example, hydrogels play an important role in controlled drug delivery: They are able to deliver delicate bioactive agents such as proteins and peptides. In addition, hydrogels have been reported to promote tissue repair and regeneration. In this chapter, a general overview of polymeric hydrogels — in terms of their definition and classification — is first presented. This is followed by a discussion of both chemical and physical hydrogels with biomedical significance — in terms of their structures and preparation methods. On the note of biomedical significance, the biomedical applications of different types of hydrogels — such as controlled drug delivery and tissue engineering — are also discussed.

7.2   Definition and Classification of Hydrogels

7.2.1   *Definition of Hydrogels*

Hydrogels are crosslinked macromolecular networks formed by hydrophilic polymers swollen in water or biological fluids [1]. Their three-dimensional networks can retain large volumes of water in crosslinked structures. The extent of swelling and the content of water retained depend on two factors: the hydrophilicity of the polymer chains and the crosslinking density. The crosslinks can be formed by covalent bonds. Alternatively, they can be formed by physical cohesion forces that exist between the polymer segments — such as ionic bonding, hydrogen bonding, van der Waals forces, or forces that arise due to hydrophobic interactions (Figure 7.1) [2].

Hydrogels can also be described in a rheological way [9]. Aqueous solutions of hydrophilic polymers without crosslinking at low concentrations (where no significant chain entanglements occur) normally exhibit Newtonian behavior. However, the crosslinked polymer networks — either chemically or physically — show viscoelastic and sometimes pure elastic behavior upon swelling in water.

7.2.2   *Classification of Hydrogels*

Polymeric hydrogels can be classified in two different ways as follows [3]:

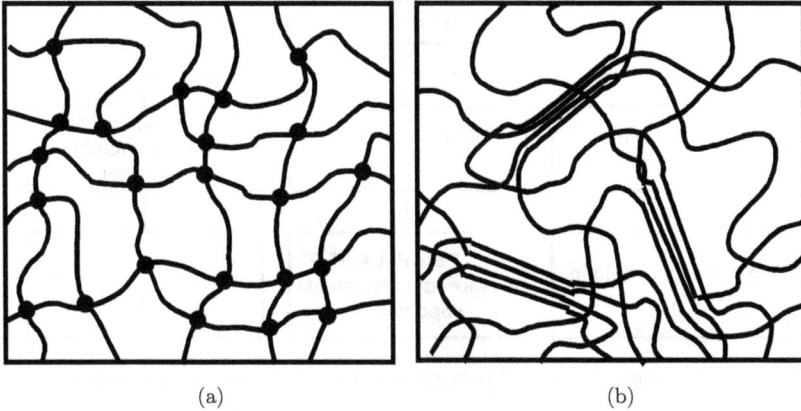

(a)   (b)

Figure 7.1. Schematic presentation of (a) a chemically crosslinked hydrogel; (b) a physical hydrogel with multiple interaction zones. Reprinted with permission from reference [6].

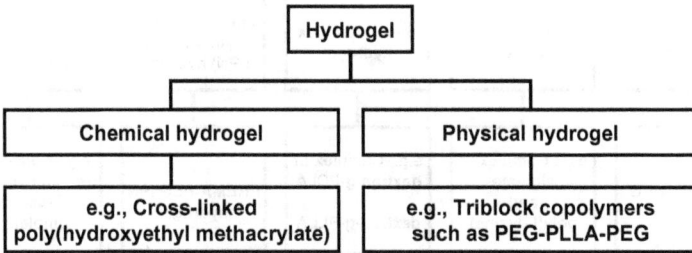

Figure 7.2. Classification of polymeric hydrogels based on the bonding type of the crosslinks.

- Based on the bonding type of the crosslinks, hydrogels are divided into chemical and physical hydrogels (Figure 7.2).
- Based on the sources of the polymers, hydrogels are classified into natural hydrogels, synthetic hydrogels, and natural and synthetic combination hydrogels (Figure 7.3).

In addition to these classifications, Figures 7.4 to 7.6 show other forms of classification based on polymer structures, physical properties, and biodegradability. (Examples of each hydrogel type are also given in Figures 7.2 to 7.6.)

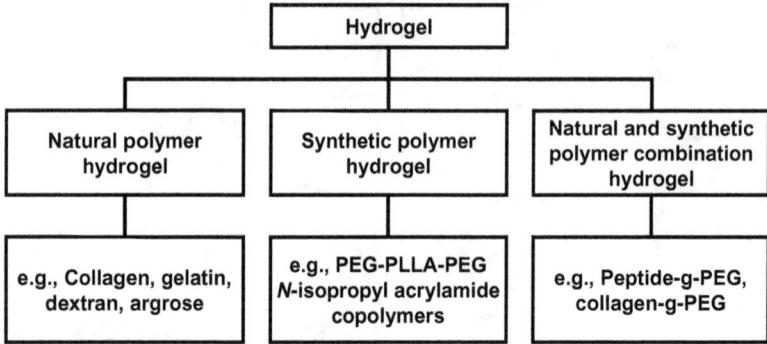

Figure 7.3. Classification of polymeric hydrogels based on the sources of the polymers.

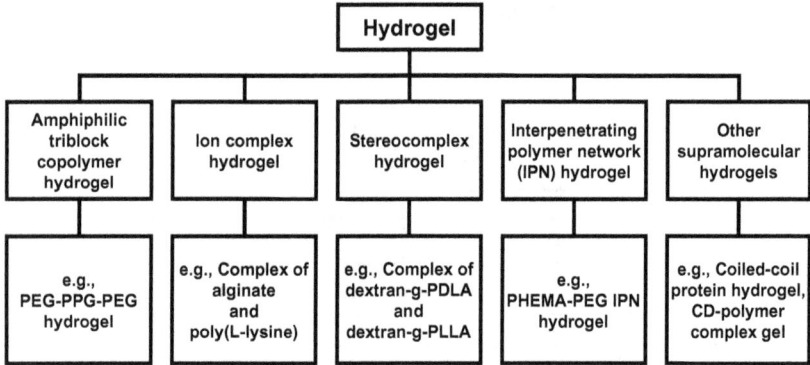

Figure 7.4. Classification of polymeric hydrogels based on the chemical and higher structures of the polymer.

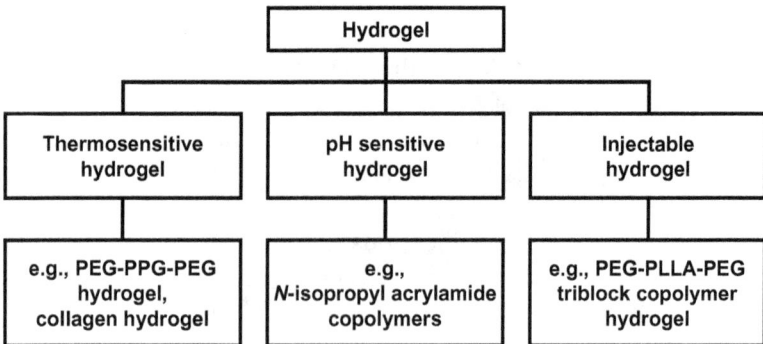

Figure 7.5. Classification of polymeric hydrogels based on their physical properties.

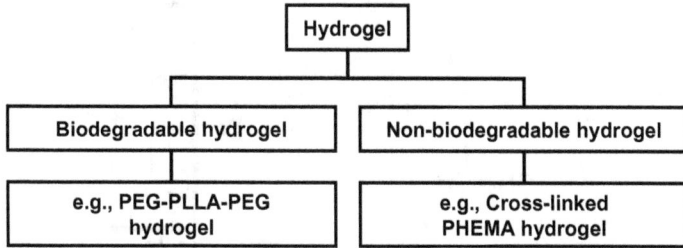

Figure 7.6. Classification of polymeric hydrogels based on the biodegradability of the polymer.

7.3 Chemical Hydrogels and their Biomedical Applications

The polymer networks of chemical hydrogels are formed by chemical crosslinking through covalent bonding. Chemical hydrogels are also called permanent hydrogels. They cannot be dissolved in water or other solvents unless the covalent crosslinks are cleaved. Chemical hydrogels are mainly prepared using one of the following approaches [1–3]:

- Copolymerization of a monomer with a crosslinker;
- Crosslinking of water-soluble polymers with crosslinkers;
- Crosslinking of water-soluble polymers with irradiation.

7.3.1 *Copolymerization of Monomers with Crosslinkers*

Free radical polymerization of water-soluble monomers in the presence of a crosslinker results in chemically crosslinked hydrogels (Figure 7.7) [3]. An example is shown in Figure 7.8(a), where hydrogels based on copolymers of N–(2–hydroxypropyl)–methacrylamide (HPMA) and N,O–dimethacryloylhydroxylamine (DMHA) were synthesized [10]. The hydrolytic stability of these hydrogels was studied in buffers with a pH range of 2 to 8. The hydrogels were stable at acidic pH (below 5), but were hydrolyzed at neutral and mildly alkaline pH (Figure 7.8(b)). This study showed that although

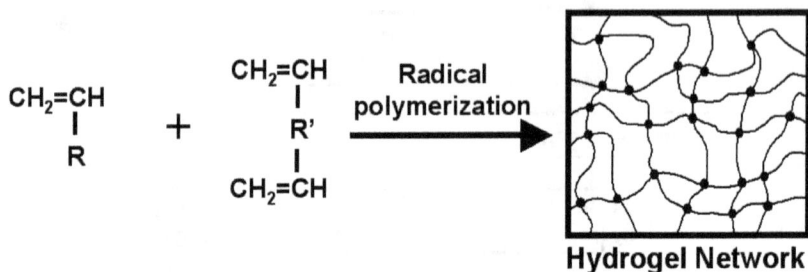

Figure 7.7. Formation of chemical hydrogels by copolymerization of a monomer with a crosslinker.

the hydrogels were chemically crosslinked, they were biodegradable because the crosslinker could be hydrolyzed under physiological conditions.

For the controlled release of the anticancer drug, doxorubicin was chemically bonded to the water-soluble poly(HPMA) segments. The release rate of the anticancer drug was then examined (Figure 7.9). The rate at which the Dox-polymer conjugate was released from the hydrogel depended on the pH of the incubation medium:

- At pH 5.0, the conjugate release could occur only by diffusion since the hydrogel matrix remained stable at this pH, and the drug was released slowly.
- At pH 6.5, the conjugate was released faster: The rate of release was controlled both by the rate of diffusion and the rate of matrix degradation.
- At pH 7.4 and 8.0, the conjugate release rates were the highest: The release rates were comparable to those of gel degradation, which meant that conjugate release was controlled mainly by the rate of matrix degradation.

7.3.2 *Crosslinking of Water-Soluble Polymers*

The crosslinking of water-soluble multifunctional polymers by reactions between functional groups results in chemical hydrogels

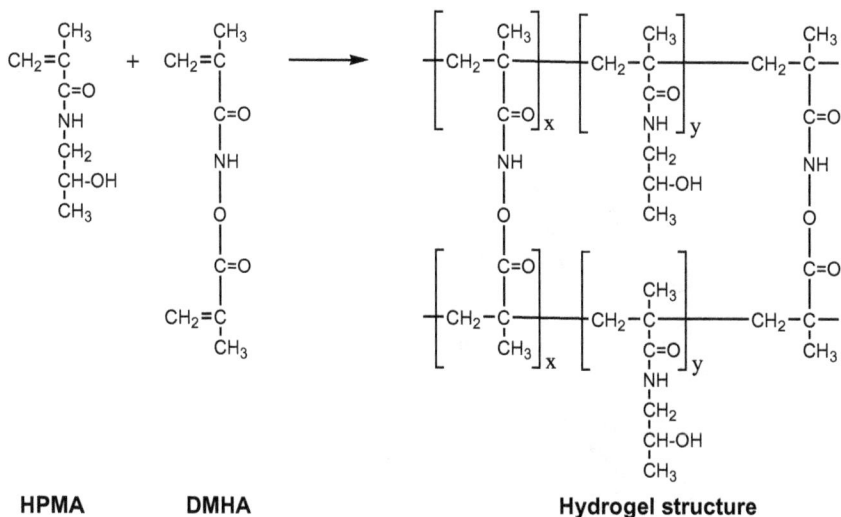

HPMA   DMHA   **Hydrogel structure**

(a)

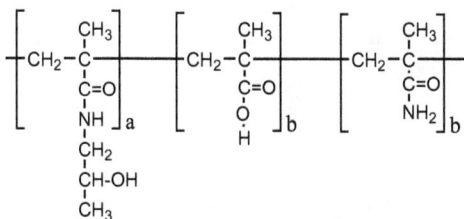

Polymeric product of hydrolysis

(b)

Figure 7.8. (a) Synthesis and structure of the HPMA hydrogel; (b) structure of its hydrolysis products Reprinted with permission from reference [5].

(Figure 7.10(a)). In addition to this approach, crosslinking of water-soluble multifunctional polymers by the addition of bifunctional or multifunctional reagents also results in chemical hydrogels (Figure 7.10(b)). Figure 7.11 shows some examples of the

X. Song & J. Li

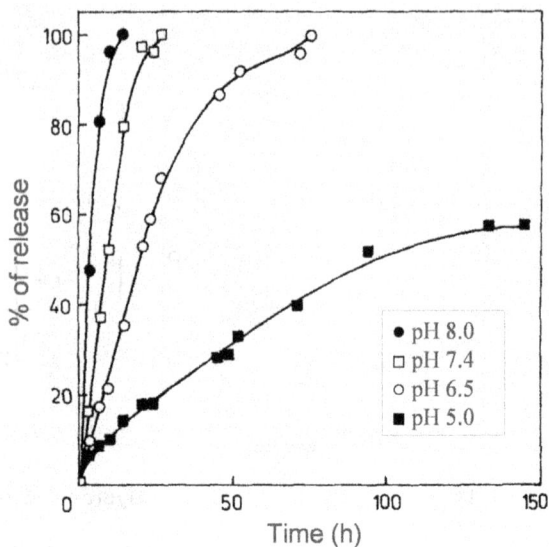

Figure 7.9. *In vitro* release of Dox-polymer conjugates from HPMA–DMHA hydrogels in phosphate at pH 5.0, 6.5, 7.4, and 8.0. Reprinted with permission from reference [5].

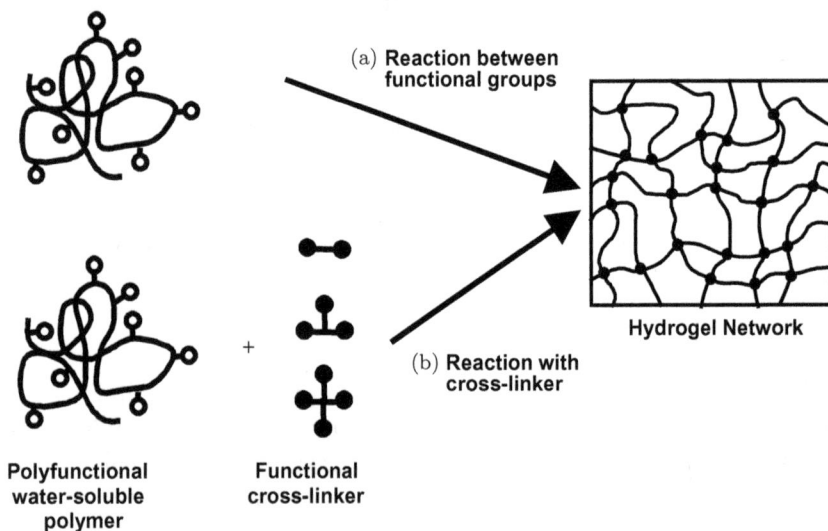

Figure 7.10. Preparation of hydrogels by crosslinking water-soluble polymers: (a) reaction between functional groups; (b) reaction with a crosslinker.

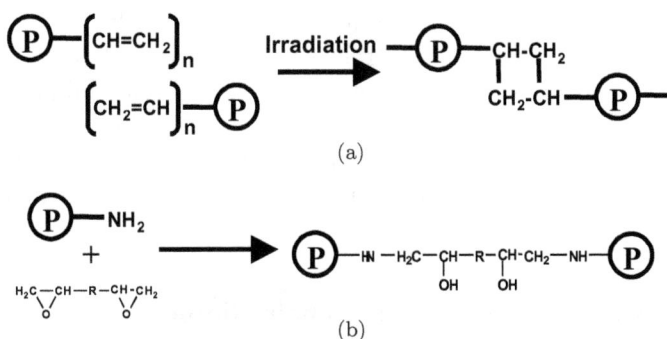

(a)

(b)

Figure 7.11. Examples of crosslinking reactions to prepare hydrogels from water-soluble polymers: (a) addition reaction of vinyl groups; (b) reaction of amino groups with bisepoxy compounds. Reprinted with permission from reference [2].

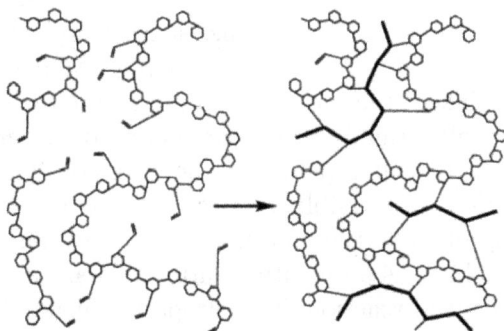

Figure 7.12. Schematic representation of the formation of dextran hydrogel by a radical addition reaction. Reprinted with permission from reference [6].

crosslinking reactions:

- Figure 7.11(a) shows that water-soluble polymers modified with vinyl groups can be polymerized to produce hydrogels once the radical reaction is started by chemical initiation or UV-/γ-irradiation. Polysaccharides such as dextran are crosslinked in this way (Figure 7.12) [11].
- Figure 7.11(b) shows that water-soluble polymers with amino groups are crosslinked by bisepoxy compounds. Many natural biopolymers, such as collagen and gelatin, have been crosslinked in this way to produce chemical hydrogels [12, 13].

The release of proteins from the dextran hydrogel shown in Figure 7.12 was studied. The release rate depended on and could be manipulated by the initial water content and crosslinking density of the gel. By incorporating dextranase, degradation systems were obtained: The degradation rate of the gel was dependent on the concentration of dextranase in the gel and the crosslinking density of the gel.

7.4 Physical Hydrogels and Their Biomedical Applications

Physical hydrogels are continuous, disordered three-dimensional hydrophilic polymer networks formed by cohesive forces capable of forming non-covalent crosslinks [2]. The cohesion forces include ionic bonding, hydrogen bonding, van der Waals forces, and forces that arise due to hydrophobic interactions, stereocomplexation, crystallization, and other weak interactions. Since physical hydrogels are not covalently crosslinked, the formation of physical crosslinks is largely dependent on the thermodynamic parameters of the medium, such as temperature, pH, salt type, and ionic strength. This also means that the formation is reversible, and the gelation can be induced by a change in any of these thermodynamic parameters. This makes a physical hydrogel act as an in situ gelation system in water without needing any chemical reaction. This property thus makes it feasible to utilize physical hydrogels in macromolecular drug delivery and tissue engineering applications because of their simplicity and safety *in vivo*.

7.4.1 *Natural Biopolymer Hydrogels*

Typical natural biopolymers that form physical hydrogels include proteins, such as collagen and gelatin, and polysaccharides, such as agarose, amylose, and cellulose derivatives [14]. Renaturation to the triple helical conformation in proteins and the double helical conformation in polysaccharides induces physical crosslinking during gel formation [2, 14].

For example, type I collagen is predominant in higher-order animals, especially in the skin, tendon, and bone where extreme forces are transmitted [15]. Figure 7.13 shows the chemical, secondary,

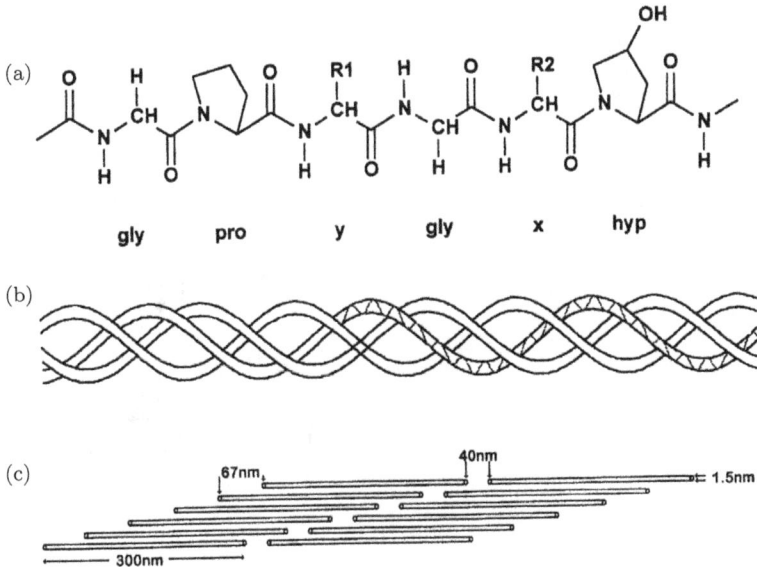

Figure 7.13. Chemical structure of type I collagen: (a) primary amino acid sequence; (b) secondary left-handed helix and tertiary right-handed triple-helix structure; (c) staggered quaternary structure. Reprinted with permission from reference [10].

tertiary, and quaternary structures of type I collagen. Helix formation followed by aggregation of the helices results in a junction point, which acts as physical crosslinking for the gelation of the biopolymer aqueous solution (Figure 7.14).

The attractiveness of collagen and gelatin as biomaterials stems from the view that they are natural materials with low immunogenicity. As such, they are perceived by the body as normal constituents rather than as foreign matter [15]. Therefore, collagen and gelatin hydrogels have been proposed for the controlled release of protein drugs via polyion complexation [16]. Figure 7.15 shows a conceptual scheme of the release system. A positively charged protein drug is electrostatically complexed with negatively charged polymer chains, constituting a carrier matrix. If an environmental change — such as increased ionic strength — occurs, the complexed drug will be released from the drug–carrier complex. Even if such an environmental change does not occur, degradation of the polymer carrier itself will also lead to drug release. Since the latter is more likely to

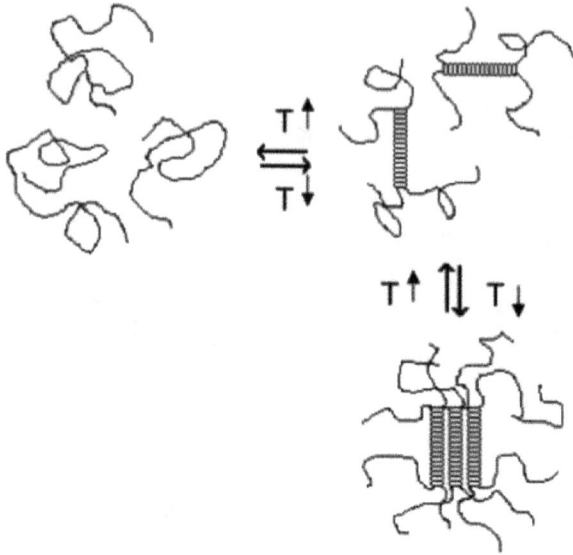

Figure 7.14. Gelation mechanism of biopolymers in water: random coils become helices, which subsequently aggregate to form the junction zones of a gel. Reprinted with permission from reference [9].

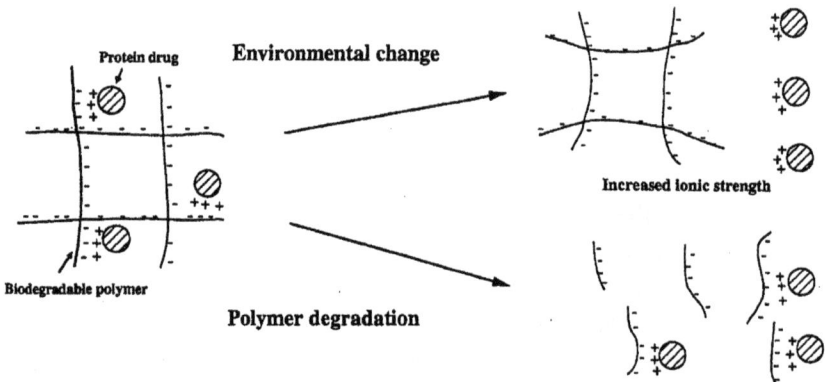

Figure 7.15. Release of protein drugs from biodegradable polymer carriers on the basis of polyion complexation. Reprinted with permission from reference [11].

occur *in vivo* than the former, it is preferable that the drug carrier be prepared from biodegradable polymers. The biodegradation behavior of the carrier then shapes the drug release profile in this drug–carrier system.

7.4.2 *Thermoshrinking Hydrogels*

Aqueous solutions of some polymers, such as poly(N–isopropyl-acrylamide) (PNIPAAm), as shown in Figure 7.16), precipitate with increasing temperature. The temperature at which a polymer solution precipitates is called the lower critical solution temperature (LCST). Below the LCST, the enthalpy term — which is mostly contributed by hydrogen bonding between polymer polar groups and water molecules — leads to the dissolution of the polymer. Hydrogels made of such polymers or their copolymers accordingly shrink with increasing temperature. Hence, they are known as thermoshrinking hydrogels. Thermoshrinking hydrogels undergo thermally reversible swelling and deswelling [2, 14].

An aqueous solution of high-molecular-weight NIPAAm/acrylic acid copolymer (2–5 mol%) showed reversible gelation above a critical concentration ($\sim 4\,\text{wt\%}$), without noticeable hysteresis at approximately 32°C [14]. This resulted in an opaque, loose gel that was deformable under shear stress. It was proposed that such properties could be used for the design of a refillable macrocapsule-type biohybrid artificial pancreas. Isolated islets of Langerhans suspended in the polymer solution were effectively entrapped in the gel when the

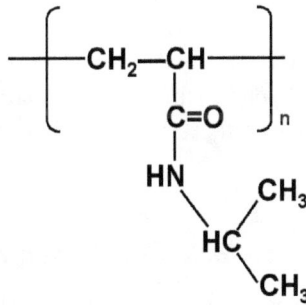

Figure 7.16. Chemical structure of poly(N–isopropyl acrylamide). Reprinted with permission from reference [9].

solution temperature was raised from 25°C to body temperature, and the gel showed no cytotoxicity. Moreover, as opposed to a traditional cell-entrapping matrix of alginate [17], another significant advantage of the gel was its higher permeability (brought about by the heterogeneous character of the gel), which then helped to facilitate insulin secretion from the entrapped islets. Compared with those cultured in a two-dimensional matrix (culture dish), chondrocytes immobilized in a thermoreversible NIPAAm/acrylic acid copolymer gel exhibited better phenotypic expression with a round shape [18].

Another study developed a thermoresponsive reversible "smart" supramolecular hydrogel based on PNIPAAm [19]. This novel star–star supramolecular architecture was formed by the self-assembly of a star-shaped PNIPAAm host polymer and a star-shaped adamantyl-PEG guest polymer through inclusion complexation. Rheological studies have proven that the pseudo-block copolymer mixture was in a sol state at lower temperatures. Upon reaching temperatures above the LCST, the PNIPAAm chains collapsed and aggregated, forming physical crosslinks in the supramolecular hydrogel. The hydrogel turned completely back into a clear and free-flowing solution upon cooling. The thermoreversible sol-gel transition endows this supramolecular hydrogel with great potential for injectable drug delivery applications.

In recent work, a thermoresponsive alginate–g–PNIPAAm copolymer was synthesized, which formed micelles at low copolymer concentrations and injectable hydrogels at high copolymer concentrations at temperatures above the LCST [20]. For this interesting system, an anticancer drug, doxorubicin (DOX), was easily mixed with the copolymer solution at room temperature. A self-assembled hydrogel was then formed when the temperature was raised to body temperature. It was shown that the hydrogel could slowly release self-assembled micelles with encapsulated DOX in the release medium for enhanced therapeutic effects in multidrug-resistant cancer cells (Figure 7.17).

7.4.3 Amphiphilic Triblock Copolymer Hydrogels

Recently, physical hydrogels formed from synthetic amphiphilic triblock copolymers have attracted special attention due to their potential applications in drug delivery. As an illustration, the

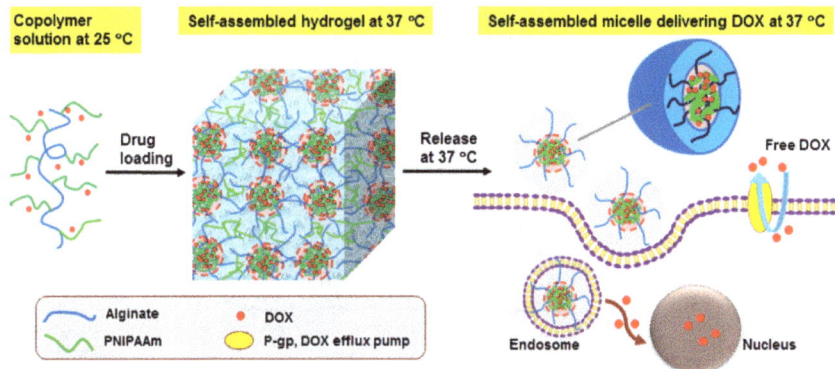

Figure 7.17. Schematic illustration of the alginate-*g*-PNIPAAm copolymer solution at 25°C and the self-assembled hydrogel at 37°C. The hydrogel could release self-assembled micelles with encapsulated drugs for enhanced therapeutic effects on multidrug-resistant cancer cells. Reprinted with permission from reference [15].

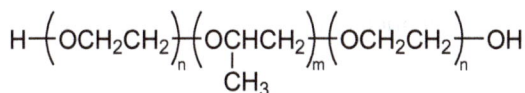

$$H\left(OCH_2CH_2\right)_n\left(OCHCH_2\atop CH_3\right)_m\left(OCH_2CH_2\right)_n OH$$

Figure 7.18. Chemical structure of the PEG–PPG–PEG triblock copolymer.

temperature-induced sol-gel transition behavior of block copolymers of poly(ethylene glycol)–poly(propylene glycol)–poly(ethylene glycol) (PEG–PPG–PEG, as shown in Figure 7.18) has been extensively studied and utilized to deliver drugs such as polypeptides and proteins [21, 22].

Another well-studied triblock copolymer that undergoes temperature-induced gelation is poly(ethylene glycol)–poly(L-lactide)–poly(ethylene glycol) (PEG–PLLA–PEG, as shown in Figure 7.19) [23,24]. However, PEG–PLLA–PEG differs from PEG–PPG–PEG in that it is biodegradable owing to the PLLA block. Furthermore, the length of the middle PLLA block affects the gelation concentration and temperature (as shown in Figure 7.20). In terms of the drug release profile, a model drug — FITC-labeled dextran (MW 20,000) — was mixed with an aqueous solution of the 5000–2040–5000 triblock copolymer above the critical gelation temperature at a given polymer concentration. The mixture was then gelled by cooling to body temperature. Over the next 10 days,

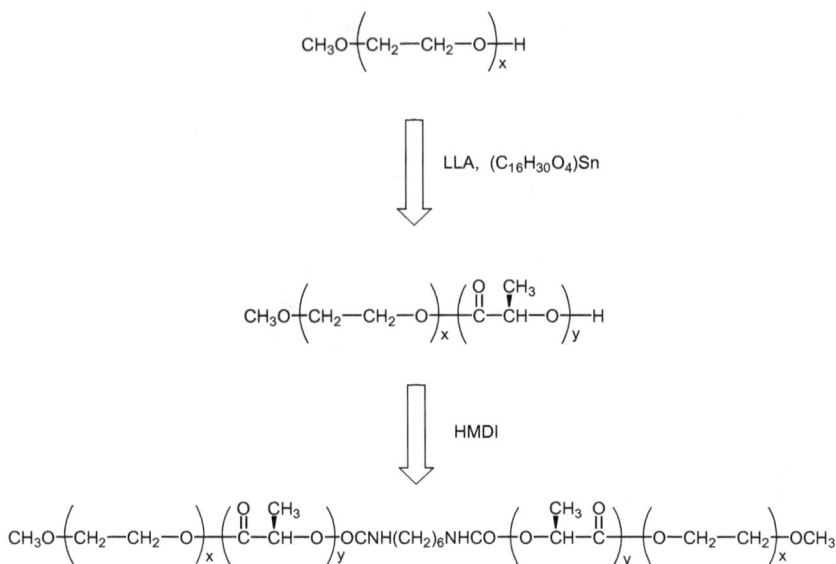

Figure 7.19. Preparation of the PEG–PLLA–PEG triblock copolymer.

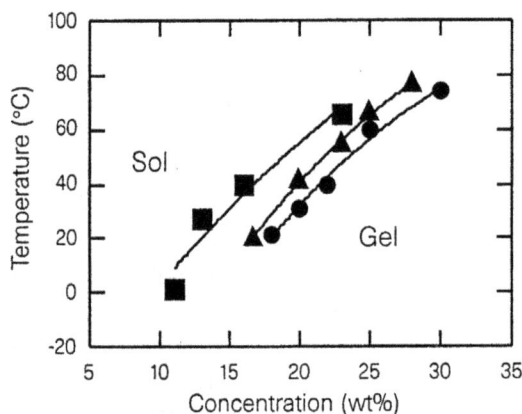

Figure 7.20. Gel-sol transition curves of PEG–PLLA–PEG triblock copolymers: (■) 5000–2040–5000; (▲) 5000–3000–5000; (•) 5000–5000–5000. Reprinted with permission from reference [18].

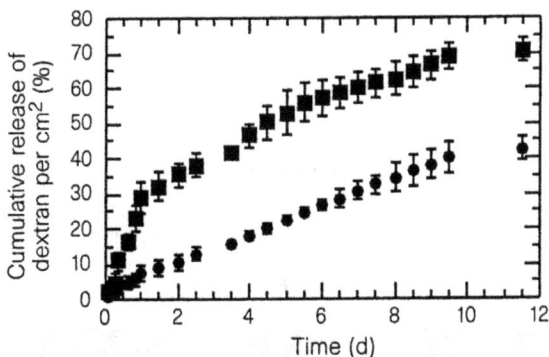

Figure 7.21. *In vitro* release of FITC-labeled dextran (MW 20,000) from PEG–PLLA–PEG (MW 5000–2040–5000) triblock copolymer; FITC-labeled dextran (5.4 mg) was mixed with 0.5 ml of aqueous polymer solution ((■) 23 wt%; (•) 35 wt% polymer). Reprinted with permission from reference [18].

dextran was released at a constant rate with or without a burst effect depending on the polymer concentration (Figure 7.21).

7.4.4 *Other Novel Synthetic Copolymer Physical Hydrogels*

More novel physical hydrogel systems formed with temperature- or pH-sensitive copolymers or based on the complexation of enantiomeric polymers or polypeptide segments have also been reported recently. Graft copolymers of poly(N–isopropyl acrylamide)–poly(acrylic acid) were synthesized and found to undergo temperature-induced sol-gel phase transitions over a wide pH range [25]. Self-assembled hydrogels have been reported to be induced by stereo complexation of enantiomeric lactic oligomers grafted to dextran [26,27], as well as by coiled-coil aggregation of artificial protein domains in polymer backbones [28] or side chains [29].

Novel physical hydrogels with more than one desirable property have been developed by using different synthetic copolymers. One example is polyurethane (PU) copolymers consisting of temperature-sensitive Pluronic F127 and PPG segments and a biodegradable poly(3-hydroxybutyrate) (PHB) segment [30]. The hydrogels formed by these components were both thermogelling and biodegradable. PU copolymers with varying PPG contents were synthesized and

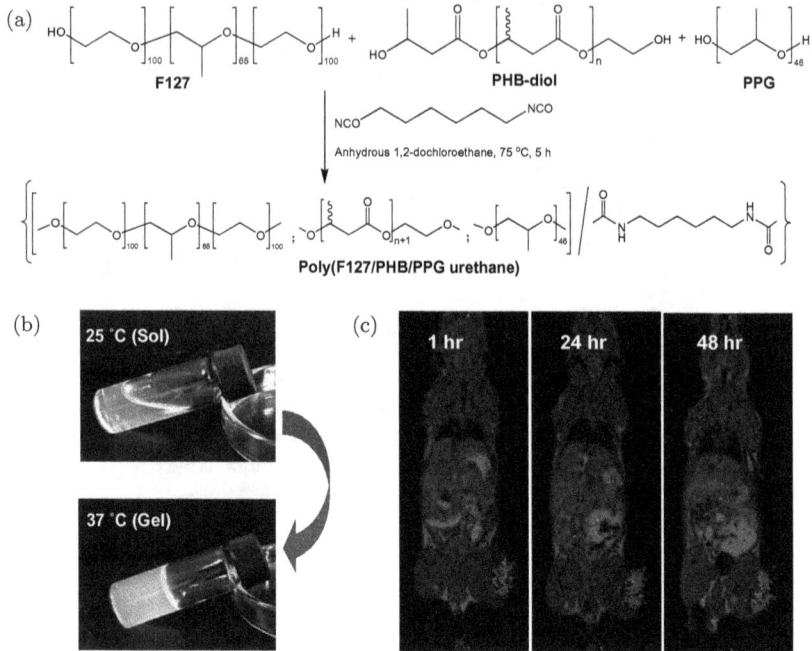

Figure 7.22. (a) Synthetic of poly(F127/PHB/PPG urethane) thermogelling copolymers; (b) photos of the copolymer solutions and hydrogels at different temperatures; and (c) micro-PET images of mice after injection of ^{90}Y-loaded hydrogels into tumors. Reprinted with permission from reference [25].

used as injectable hydrogels for local delivery of the radionuclide ^{90}Y for tumor radio-brachytherapy. The hydrogel formed by the PU copolymer containing 34 wt% PPG showed excellent injectability and could retain ^{90}Y at the tumor site for a prolonged period of time in a mouse tumor model (Figure 7.22). A degradation test was also carried out and significant degradation of the copolymer was observed after 14 weeks, indicating that the hydrogels could eventually be removed from the injection site after treatment.

Another PU copolymer system containing both thermogelling PPG segments and biodegradable PHB segments was analyzed for injectable hydrogel formation to achieve prolonged delivery of plasmid DNA (pDNA) [31]. The *in vitro* release study revealed that the release of pDNA micelleplexes in the hydrogel was prolonged to more than 4 weeks as compared to that of free pDNA, which was completely released in 2 weeks.

7.4.5 *Polyelectrolyte Complex Hydrogels*

Some water-soluble polyelectrolyte copolymers can form hydrogels with metal ions or with another countercharged polyelectrolyte polymer. We reported hydrogel formation between positively charged modified collagen and negatively charged synthetic polyelectrolyte terpolymers containing poly(methacrylic acid) at certain pH values, ionic strengths, and concentrations of the polymers (Figure 7.23) [32]. This hydrogel system has been applied in tissue engineering for the microencapsulation of hepatocytes that are used in bioartificial liver assist devices. As shown in Figure 7.24, the cells were suspended in a solution of modified collagen and added to a solution of HEMA–MMA–MAA terpolymers to form microcapsules through a complex coacervation reaction. The membrane of the capsules is a hydrogel permeable to nutrients required to maintain the metabolic functions of the cells. On the other hand, products secreted by the cells diffuse out of the capsules, thereby providing immunological protection to the cells by restraining the migration of antibodies and cells across the membrane.

Alginate-based microencapsulation systems based on an alginate hydrogel core coated with a polycation layer and an alginate outer

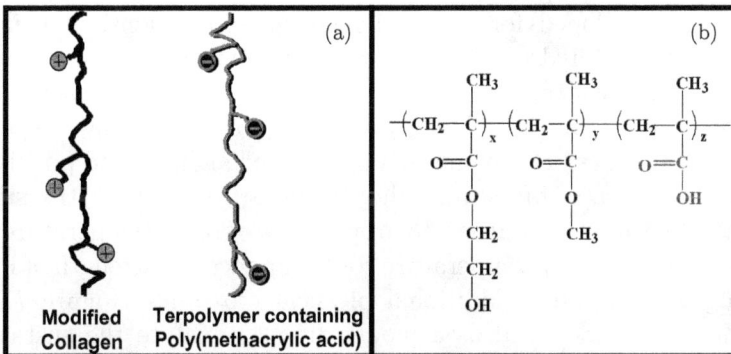

Figure 7.23. (a) Gel formation between modified collagen and a terpolymer containing poly(methacrylic acid) by ionic complexation; (b) chemical structure of the polyelectrolyte terpolymer.

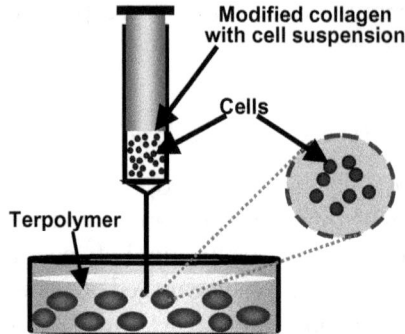

Figure 7.24. Schematic representation of the microencapsulation process of rat hepatocytes.

membrane have been widely studied and reported for cell encapsulation, especially for diabetes treatment [33, 34]. Some examples include barium alginate microcapsules developed for the encapsulation of embryo-derived mouse embryo progenitor-derived insulin-producing-1 (MEPI-1) cells for hyperglycemia correction [35] and calcium alginate microcapsules developed for the encapsulation of human embryonic stem cells (hESCs) to prevent teratoma formation in hESCs during transplantation [36]. The encapsulation of embryonic stem (ES) cells in spherical alginate beads formed by extruding the cell–alginate mixture into a $CaCl_2$ bath for differentiation into insulin-producing cells was also investigated [37].

Alginate-based polyelectrolyte complex (PEC) hydrogels have also been developed for other biomedical applications. One novel and smart PEC hydrogel system was prepared using alginate-graft-poly(N-isopropylacrylamide) (Alg-g-PNIPAAm) and chitosan (Cts) in aqueous media [38]. The hydrogels were formed by polyelectrolyte complexes between negatively charged alginate and positively charged chitosan. Moreover, the temperature-induced transition of PNIPAAm chains from hydrophilic at room temperature to hydrophobic at body temperature could enhance the strength of PEC hydrogels by forming additional physical crosslinks (Figure 7.25). Rhodamine B was used as a model drug to analyze the sustained release behavior of the PEC hydrogel. These PEC hydrogels exhibited more sustained release of the model drug than did the corresponding non-PEC hydrogels. Moreover, they can respond to both

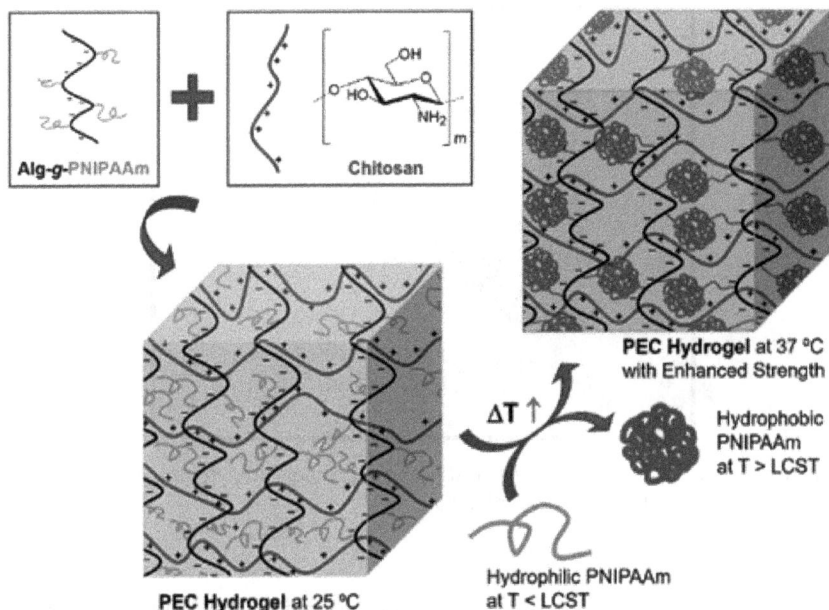

Figure 7.25. Schematic illustration of PEC hydrogels formed by Alg-*g*-PNIPAAm and chitosan and the temperature-induced transition of PNIPAAm blocks from hydrophilic to hydrophobic, which enhances the strength of PEC hydrogels. Reprinted with permission from reference [33].

temperature and pH changes, showing great potential as smart drug delivery systems.

7.4.6 Supramolecular Hydrogels Formed from Cyclodextrins and Polymers

In the past decade, there have been extensive studies on macro-molecular self-assembly between polymers and cyclodextrins — when cyclodextrins thread onto polymer chains [39–41]. These supramolecular structures are called polyrotaxanes. A new class of polymer hydrogels with novel supramolecular systems that are suitable for a wide range of biomedical applications has been developed based on the formation of polyrotaxanes (Figure 7.26). Since then, extensive studies have been carried out to explore this new type of supramolecular hydrogel for biomedical applications [42].

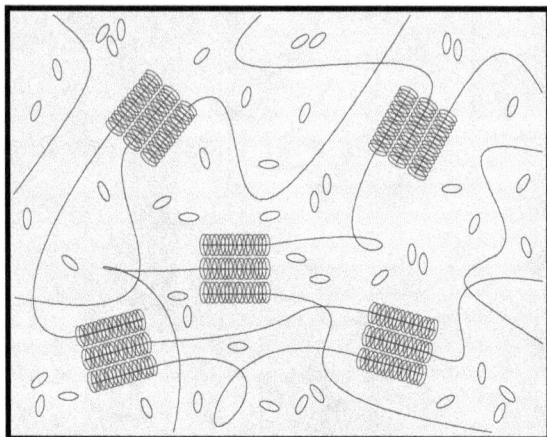

Figure 7.26. Schematic representation of supramolecular hydrogels formed by α-cyclodextrin and poly(ethylene glycol).

The supramolecular hydrogels were found to be thixotropic and reversible [43]. The viscosity of the hydrogel greatly decreased as it was agitated (Figure 7.27(a)). This property renders the hydrogel formula injectable even through the use of a fine needle. The diminished viscosity of the hydrogel eventually returned to its original value, in most cases within hours, when no further agitation occurred (Figure 7.27(b)). These thixotropic and reversible properties of the gel afford us a unique injectable hydrogel drug delivery system. Currently, bioactive agents (such as drugs, proteins, vaccines, or plasmid DNAs) can be incorporated in the gel — which is in a syringe at room temperature — without any contact with organic solvents. The drug-loaded hydrogel formula can then be injected into the tissue under pressure because of its thixotropic property. After gelling is restored *in situ*, the hydrogel serves as a depot for controlled release. Compared to implantable hydrogels, injectable hydrogels are definitely more appealing.

The drug delivery properties of injectable hydrogels formed with α-cyclodextrin (α-CD) and poly(ethylene glycol) (PEG or PEO) of different molecular weights have been evaluated *in vitro* using dextran-FITC (MW 20,000) as a model drug [8]. As shown in Figure 7.28, the release rate significantly decreased as the molecular weight of PEO increased to 35,000 Da. The hydrogels composed

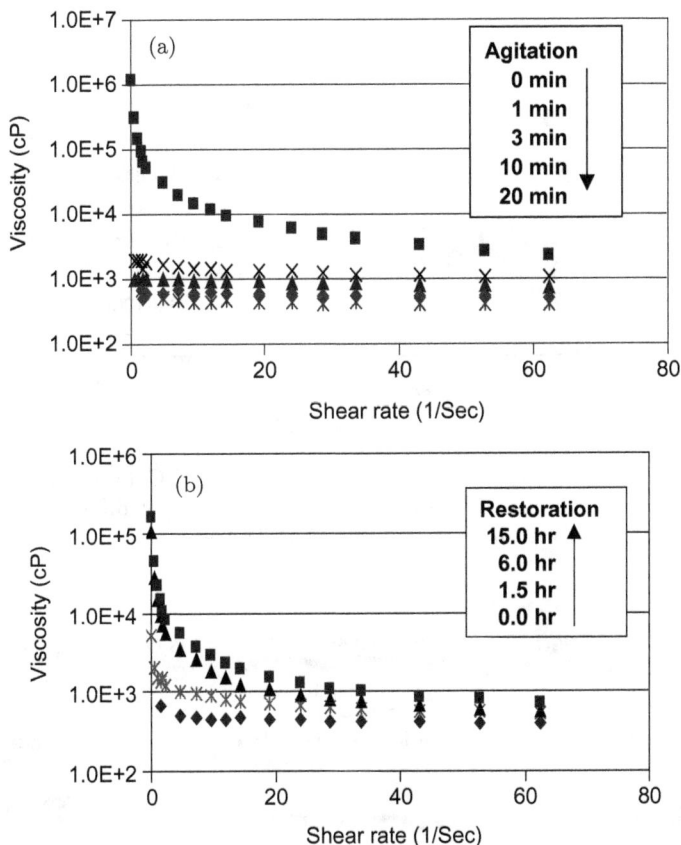

Figure 7.27. (a) Viscosity changes of Gel–20K–60 as a function of agitation time at a shear rate of $120 \, \mathrm{s}^{-1}$. (b) Restoration of gel viscosity after $20 \, \mathrm{min}$ of agitation at a shear rate of $120 \, \mathrm{s}^{-1}$.

of PEOs of 35,000 Da and 100,000 Da exhibited sustained and controlled release of dextran-FITC over time.

To further improve the release property of polyrotaxane-based supramolecular hydrogels, new designs of hydrogels formed with α-CD and different diblock or triblock copolymers have been developed [44]. The triblock copolymers consist of a hydrophobic middle block, such as poly(propylene glycol) (PPG or PPO) or poly(3-hydroxybutyrate) (PHB), flanked by PEO blocks at both ends (Figure 7.29). It was hypothesized that the intermolecular hydrophobic interactions between the middle blocks could further strengthen

X. Song & J. Li

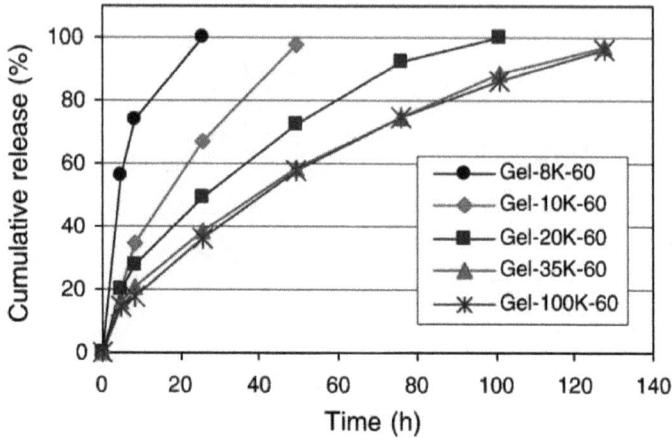

Figure 7.28. *In vitro* release profiles of dextran-FITC (MW 20,000) from supramolecular hydrogels formed with α-CD and PEO of different molecular weights. Reprinted with permission from reference [39].

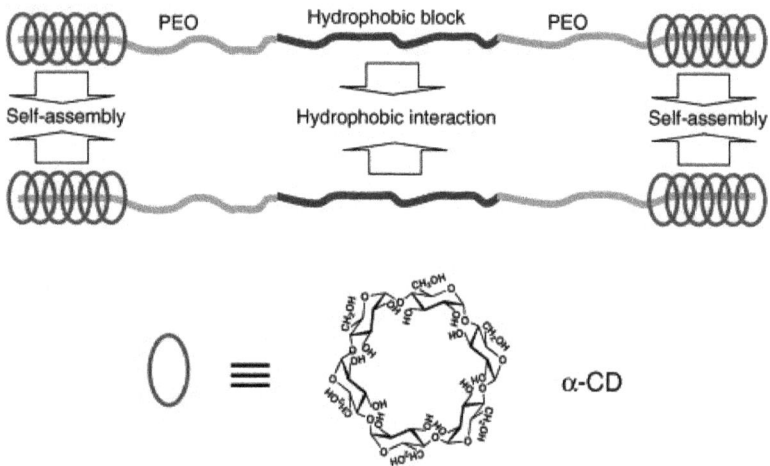

Figure 7.29. Schematic illustration of triblock copolymers consisting of a hydrophobic middle block flanked by PEO blocks at both ends. Reprinted with permission from reference [39].

and stabilize the hydrogels for long-term controlled release of therapeutic agents.

The supramolecular hydrogels developed from α-CD and PEO-PPO-PEO were both thermosensitive and thixotropic [41]. Compared with traditional hydrogels formed by thermosensitive PEO-PPO-PEO triblock copolymers alone [22], the addition of α-CD significantly reduced the gelation concentration, presumably attributed to the partial formation of inclusion complexes between the α-CD and PEO segments [45]. An *in vitro* release study of the supramolecular hydrogels with PEO-PPO-PEO triblock copolymers of different molecular weights and compositions was conducted using a model protein drug, FITC-labeled bovine serum albumin (BSA-FITC). This study revealed the importance of having a good balance between the block lengths of PEO and PPO segments for protein delivery [8].

Similarly, another triblock copolymer was synthesized and analyzed with poly((R)-3-hydroxybutyrate) (PHB) as the hydrophobic middle block flanked by two PEO blocks [46]. PHB, a natural and biodegradable biopolyester with high hydrophobicity and crystallinity, is an attractive polymer for biomedical applications. PEO-PHB-PEO triblock copolymers with different lengths of PHB blocks and PEO blocks have been investigated for inclusion complexation with α-CD for hydrogel formation [44, 47, 48]. The addition of α-CD also resulted in a very low gelation concentration of the PEO-PHB-PEO copolymers (Figure 7.30) [8, 44]. The gelation is attributed to the cooperative action of inclusion complexation between α-CD and the flanking PEO chains and the micellization of the middle PHB chains, leading to a strong hydrogel network. This cooperative action contributes to the excellent long-term sustained release of dextran-FITC for more than one month compared to that of pure PEO-PHB-PEO triblock copolymer or α-CD-PEO hydrogels.

Supramolecular hydrogels based on other biopolyester block copolymers, such as poly(ε-caprolactone) (PCL), have also been developed for drug delivery [49–51]. Again, the combination of the inclusion complexations between α-CD and the PEO chains and the hydrophobic interactions between the PCL chains cooperatively drove the gelation. An *in vitro* release study revealed that the α-CD-PEO-PCL hydrogels showed sustained and controlled release of dextran-FITC for more than one month, which was much longer

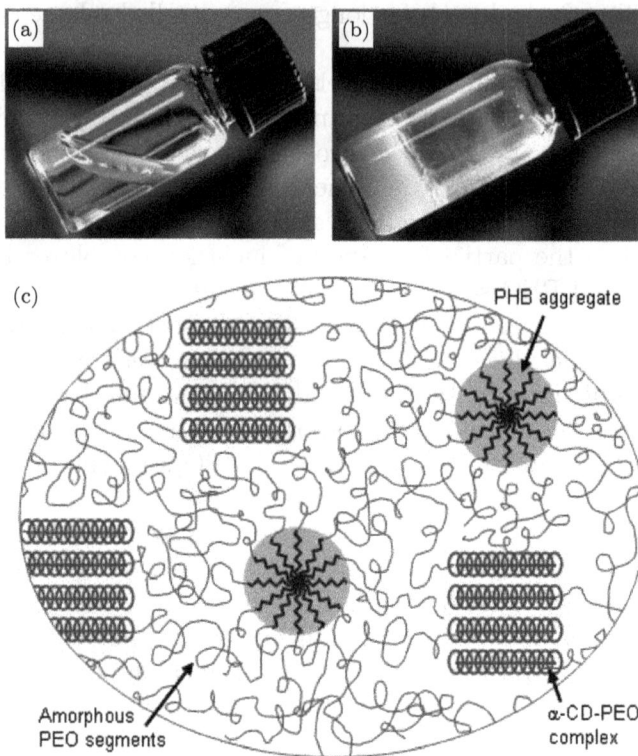

Figure 7.30. Photos of the (A) PEO-PHB-PEO triblock copolymer solution and (B) α-CD-PEO-PHB-PEO supramolecular hydrogel. (C) Schematic illustration of the proposed network structure of the supramolecular hydrogel. Reprinted with permission from reference [39].

than that of the α-CD-PEO control hydrogels. This was presumably attributed to the strong hydrophobic interactions between the PCL segments, resulting in the lower molecular weight of the PEO blocks required for long-term sustained release.

Additionally, supramolecular hydrogels formed by α-CD and biodegradable methoxy-poly(ethylene glycol)-b-poly(ε-caprolactone) -b-poly[2-(dimethylamino)ethyl methacrylate] (MPEG-PCL-PDMA EMA) triblock copolymers with anchored DNA nanoparticles have been developed for injectable sustained gene delivery [52]. This supramolecular hydrogels with PCL as the hydrophobic core exhibited a shorter gelation time and significantly greater stiffness and strength than the α-CD-PEO control hydrogels. The *in vitro* DNA release properties of the pDNA-encapsulated supramolecular hydrogels were analyzed by a hydrogel dissolution study. The results showed that compared with the α-CD-PEO control hydrogel, which released all the DNA in 3 days, the supramolecular hydrogels with PCL as the core could sustain DNA release for up to 6 days.

A more complicated and unique supramolecular hydrogels system involving two types of supramolecular self-assemblies between CDs and polymers has been developed for enhanced drug delivery properties (Figure 7.31) [53]. One supramolecular self-assembly mechanism involved host–guest complexation between the β-CD of the β-Cyclodextrin-PNIPAAm host polymer and the adamantyl groups of the Ad-PEG guest polymer to form pseudo-block copolymers. The other mechanism involved polypseudorotaxane formation between the α-CD and the PEG segments of the pseudo-block copolymers

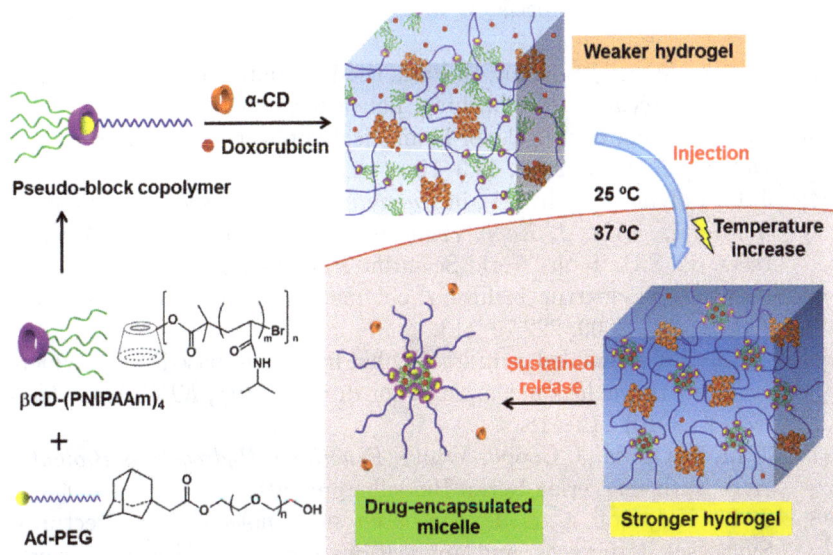

Figure 7.31. Schematic illustration of dual supramolecular hydrogels formed between α-CD and the βCD-PNIPAAm/Ad-PEG pseudo-block copolymer. A temperature increase from room temperature to body temperature enhances thermoresponsive hydrogels, which can release supramolecular micelles as anticancer drug carriers in a sustained manner for efficient cellular uptake and enhanced anticancer drug delivery in multidrug-resistant cancer cells. Reprinted with permission from reference [49].

to form the supramolecular hydrogel. More interestingly, the properties of the injectable hydrogel could be strengthened and enhanced by
increasing the temperature from room temperature to body temperature due to the hydrophobic interactions of the PNIPAAm chains.
Compared to the control hydrogels formed by the α-CD and PEG
polymers alone, the thermoresponsive hydrogel exhibited more controlled and sustained release of the anticancer drug DOX for up to
4 days at 37°C. In addition, the supramolecular hydrogel system
slowly released self-assembled supramolecular micelles, which could
further act as drug carriers of DOX. More efficient cellular uptake
and enhanced therapeutic effects have been demonstrated *in vitro* in
multidrug-resistant cells.

References

[1]   N.A. Peppas, *Hydrogels in Medicine and Pharmacy*, CRC Press,
       Florida, 1987.
[2]   K. Park, W.S.W. Shalaby, H. Park, Biodegradable Hydrogels for Drug
       Delivery, Technomic Publishing, Lancaster, 1993.
[3]   A.S. Hoffman, Hydrogels for biomedical applications, *Advanced Drug
       Delivery Reviews*, 2002, 43:3–12.
[4]   J. Li, Polymeric hydrogels, in *Biomaterials Engineering and Process-
       ing Series - Vol. 1, Engineering Materials for Biomedical Applica-
       tions*, ed. S.H. Teoh, World Scientific Pub, New Jersey, 2004.
[5]   J. Li, Cyclodextrin inclusion polymers forming hydrogels, *Adv.
       Polym. Sci.*, 2009, 222:79–113.
[6]   J. Li, Self-assembled supramolecular hydrogels based on polymer-
       cyclodextrin inclusion complexes for drug delivery, *NPG Asia Mate-
       rials* 2 (2010) 112–118.
[7]   J. Li, Y. Osada, J. Cooper-White, *Functional Hydrogels as Biomate-
       rials*, Springer-Verlag Berlin Heidelbergm, 2018.
[8]   J. Li, X.J. Loh, Cyclodextrin-based supramolecular architectures:
       Syntheses, structures, and applications for drug and gene delivery,
       Adv. Drug Deliv. Rev., 2008, 60(9):1000–1017.
[9]   W.E. Hennink, C.F. van Nostrum, Novel crosslinking methods to
       design hydrogels, *Advanced Drug Delivery Reviews*, 2002, 54(1):
       13–36.
[10]   K. Ulbrich, V. Šubr, L.W. Seymour, R. Duncan, Novel biodegrad-
       able hydrogels prepared using the divinylic crosslinking agent N,O-
       dimethacryloylhydroxylamine. 1. Synthesis and characterisation of

rates of gel degradation, and rate of release of model drugs, *in vitro* and *in vivo*, *Journal of Controlled Release*, 1993, 24(1):181–190.

[11] W.E. Hennink, O. Franssen, W.N.E. van Dijk-Wolthuis, H. Talsma, Dextran hydrogels for the controlled release of proteins, *Journal of Controlled Release*, 1997, 48(2):107–114.

[12] R. Tu, C.L. Lu, K. Thyagarajan, E. Wang, H. Nguyen, S. Shen, C. Hata, R.C. Quijano, Kinetic study of collagen fixation with polyepoxy fixatives, *Journal of Biomedical Materials Research*, 1993, 27(1): 3–9.

[13] J.M. Lee, C.A. Pereira, L.W.K. Kan, Effect of molecular structure of poly(glycidyl ether) reagents on crosslinking and mechanical properties of bovine pericardial xenograft materials, *Journal of Biomedical Materials Research*, 1994, 28(9):981–992.

[14] B. Jeong, S.W. Kim, Y.H. Bae, Thermosensitive sol–gel reversible hydrogels, *Advanced Drug Delivery Reviews*, 2002, 54(1):37–51.

[15] W. Friess, Collagen – biomaterial for drug delivery, *European Journal of Pharmaceutics and Biopharmaceutics*, 1998, 45(2):113–136.

[16] Y. Tabata, Y. Ikada, Protein release from gelatin matrices, *Advanced Drug Delivery Reviews*, 1998, 31(3):287–301.

[17] B. Vernon, S.W. Kim, Y.H. Bae, Insulin release from islets of Langerhans entrapped in a poly(N-isopropylacrylamide-co-acrylic acid) polymer gel, *Journal of Biomaterials Science*, Polymer Edition, 1999, 10(2):183–198.

[18] Y.H. An, V.A. Mironov, A. Gutowska, *Reversible Gelling Culture Media for in-vitro Cell Culture in Three-Dimensional Matrices*, US, 2000.

[19] Z.-X. Zhang, K.L. Liu, J. Li, A Thermoresponsive Hydrogel Formed from a Star–Star Supramolecular Architecture, *Angewandte Chemie International Edition*, 2013, 52(24):6180–6184.

[20] M. Liu, X. Song, Y. Wen, J.-L. Zhu, J. Li, Injectable thermoresponsive hydrogel formed by alginate-g-poly(n-isopropylacrylamide) that releases doxorubicin-encapsulated micelles as a smart drug delivery system, *ACS Applied Materials & Interfaces*, 2017, 9(41): 35673–35682.

[21] P. Alexandridis, T. Alan Hatton, Poly(ethylene oxide)-poly(propylene oxide)-poly(ethylene oxide) block copolymer surfactants in aqueous solutions and at interfaces: Thermodynamics, structure, dynamics, and modeling, *Colloids and Surfaces A: Physicochemical and Engineering Aspects*, 1995, 96(1):1–46.

[22] L.E. Bromberg, E.S. Ron, Temperature-responsive gels and thermogelling polymer matrices for protein and peptide delivery, *Advanced Drug Delivery Reviews*, 1998, 197–221.

[23] B. Jeong, Y.H. Bae, D.S. Lee, S.W. Kim, Biodegradable block copolymers as injectable drug-delivery systems, *Nature*, 1997, 388(6645):860–862.

[24] B. Jeong, Y.H. Bae, S.W. Kim, Drug release from biodegradable injectable thermosensitive hydrogel of PEG–PLGA–PEG triblock copolymers, *Journal of Controlled Release*, 2000, 63(1):155–163.

[25] G. Chen, A.S. Hoffman, Graft copolymers that exhibit temperature-induced phase transitions over a wide range of pH, *Nature*, 1995, 373(6509):49–52.

[26] S.J. de Jong, S.C. De Smedt, M.W.C. Wahls, J. Demeester, J.J. Kettenes-van den Bosch, W.E. Hennink, Novel self-assembled hydrogels by stereocomplex formation in aqueous solution of enantiomeric lactic acid oligomers grafted to dextran, *Macromolecules*, 2000, 33(10):3680–3686.

[27] S.J. de Jong, S.C. De Smedt, J. Demeester, C.F. van Nostrum, J.J. Kettenes-van den Bosch, W.E. Hennink, Biodegradable hydrogels based on stereocomplex formation between lactic acid oligomers grafted to dextran, *Journal of Controlled Release*, 2001, 72(1):47–56.

[28] W.A. Petka, J.L. Harden, K.P. McGrath, D. Wirtz, D.A. Tirrell, Reversible hydrogels from self-assembling artificial proteins, *Science*, 1998, 281(5375):389–392.

[29] C. Wang, R.J. Stewart, J. Kopeček, Hybrid hydrogels assembled from synthetic polymers and coiled-coil protein domains, *Nature*, 1999, 397(6718):417–420.

[30] J.-L. Zhu, S.W.-K. Yu, P.K.-H. Chow, Y.W. Tong, J. Li, Controlling injectability and in vivo stability of thermogelling copolymers for delivery of yttrium-90 through intra-tumoral injection for potential brachytherapy, *Biomaterials*, 2018, 180:163–172.

[31] W.W.M. Soh, R.Y.P. Teoh, J. Zhu, Y. Xun, C.Y. Wee, J. Ding, E.S. Thian, J. Li, Facile construction of a two-in-one injectable micelleplex-loaded thermogel system for the prolonged delivery of plasmid DNA, *Biomacromolecules*, 2022, 23(8):3477–3492.

[32] S.-M. Chia, K.W. Leong, J. Li, X. Xu, K. Zeng, P.-N. Er, S. Gao, H. Yu, Hepatocyte encapsulation for enhanced cellular functions, *Tissue Engineering*, 2000, 6(5):481–495.

[33] A. Murua, A. Portero, G. Orive, R.M. Hernandez, M. de Castro, J.L. Pedraz, Cell microencapsulation technology: Towards clinical application, *Journal of Controlled Release*, 2008, 132(2):76–83.

[34] S.T. Chua, X. Song, J. Li, Hydrogels for Stem Cell Encapsulation: Toward Cellular Therapy for Diabetes, in *Functional Hydrogels as Biomaterials*, eds., J. Li, Y. Osada, J. Cooper-White, (Springer Berlin Heidelberg, Berlin, Heidelberg, 2018), pp. 113–127.

[35] S. Shao, Y. Gao, B. Xie, F. Xie, S.K. Lim, G. Li, Correction of hyperglycemia in type 1 diabetic models by transplantation of encapsulated insulin-producing cells derived from mouse embryo progenitor, *Journal of Endocrinology*, 2011, 208:245–255.

[36] M. Chayosumrit, B. Tuch, K. Sidhu, Alginate microcapsule for propagation and directed differentiation of hESCs to definitive endoderm, *Biomaterials*, 2010, 31(3):505–14.

[37] N. Wang, G. Adams, L. Buttery, F.H. Falcone, S. Stolnik, Alginate encapsulation technology supports embryonic stem cells differentiation into insulin-producing cells, *Journal of Biotechnology*, 2009, 144(4):304–312.

[38] M. Liu, J. Zhu, X. Song, Y. Wen, J. Li, Smart Hydrogel Formed by Alginate-g-Poly(N-isopropylacrylamide) and Chitosan through Polyelectrolyte Complexation and Its Controlled Release Properties, Gels, 2022.

[39] A. Harada, J. Li, M. Kamachi, The molecular necklace: A rotaxane containing many threaded α-cyclodextrins, *Nature*, 1992, 356(6367):325–327.

[40] J. Li, A. Harada, M. Kamachi, Sol–Gel Transition during inclusion complex formation between α-cyclodextrin and high molecular weight poly(ethylene glycol)s in aqueous solution, *Polymer Journal*, 1994, 26(9):1019–1026.

[41] J. Li, X. Li, Z. Zhou, X. Ni, K.W. Leong, Formation of supramolecular hydrogels induced by inclusion complexation between pluronics and α-cyclodextrin, *Macromolecules*, 2001, 34(21):7236–7237.

[42] X. Song, J. Li, Recent advances in polymer-cyclodextrin inclusion complex-based supramolecular hydrogel for biomedical applications, in *Functional Hydrogels as Biomaterials* eds. J. Li, Y. Osada, J. Cooper-White (Springer Berlin Heidelberg, Berlin, Heidelberg, 2018), pp. 141–163.

[43] J. Li, X. Ni, K.W. Leong, Injectable drug-delivery systems based on supramolecular hydrogels formed by poly(ethylene oxide)s and α-cyclodextrin, *Journal of Biomedical Materials Research Part A*, 2003, 65A(2):196–202.

[44] J. Li, X. Li, X. Ni, X. Wang, H. Li, K.W. Leong, Self-assembled supramolecular hydrogels formed by biodegradable PEO–PHB–PEO triblock copolymers and α-cyclodextrin for controlled drug delivery, *Biomaterials*, 2006 27(22):4132–4140.

[45] X. Ni, A. Cheng, J. Li, Supramolecular hydrogels based on self-assembly between PEO-PPO-PEO triblock copolymers and α-cyclodextrin, *Journal of Biomedical Materials Research Part A*, 2009 88A(4):1031–1036.

[46] J. Li, X. Li, X. Ni, K.W. Leong, Synthesis and characterization of new biodegradable amphiphilic poly(ethylene oxide)-b-poly[(R)-3-hydroxy butyrate]-b-poly(ethylene oxide) triblock copolymers, *Macromolecules*, 2003, 36(8):2661–2667.

[47] X. Li, J. Li, K.W. Leong, Preparation and characterization of inclusion complexes of biodegradable amphiphilic poly(ethylene oxide)−poly[(R)-3-hydroxybutyrate]−poly(ethylene oxide) triblock copolymers with cyclodextrins, *Macromolecules*, 2003, 36(4): 1209–1214.

[48] X. Li, J. Li, K.W. Leong, Role of intermolecular interaction between hydrophobic blocks in block-selected inclusion complexation of amphiphilic poly(ethylene oxide)-poly[(R)-3-hydroxybutyrate]-poly(ethylene oxide) triblock copolymers with cyclodextrins, *Polymer*, 2004, 45(20):6845–6851.

[49] X.J. Loh, K.B.C. Sng, J. Li, Synthesis and water-swelling of thermo-responsive poly(ester urethane)s containing poly(epsilon-caprolactone), poly(ethylene glycol) and poly(propylene glycol), *Biomaterials*, 2008, 29(22):3185–3194.

[50] D.-Q. Wu, T. Wang, B. Lu, X.-D. Xu, S.-X. Cheng, X.-J. Jiang, X.-Z. Zhang, R.-X. Zhuo, Fabrication of supramolecular hydrogels for drug delivery and stem cell encapsulation, *Langmuir*, 2008, 24(18): 10306–10312.

[51] T. Wang, X.-J. Jiang, T. Lin, S. Ren, X.-Y. Li, X.-Z. Zhang, Q.-Z. Tang, The inhibition of postinfarct ventricle remodeling without poly-cythaemia following local sustained intramyocardial delivery of ery-thropoietin within a supramolecular hydrogel, *Biomaterials*, 2009, 30(25):4161–4167.

[52] Z. Li, H. Yin, Z. Zhang, K.L. Liu, J. Li, Supramolecular anchoring of DNA polyplexes in cyclodextrin-based polypseudorotaxane hydro-gels for sustained gene delivery, *Biomacromolecules*, 2012, 13(10): 3162–3172.

[53] X. Song, Z. Zhang, J. Zhu, Y. Wen, F. Zhao, L. Lei, N. Phan-Thien, B.C. Khoo, J. Li, Thermoresponsive hydrogel induced by dual supramolecular assemblies and its controlled release property for enhanced anticancer drug delivery, *Biomacromolecules*, 2020, 21(4):1516–1527.

Chapter 8

Biomedical Composites for Human Body Tissue Replacement and Regeneration

Qilong Zhao* and Min Wang[†,‡]

**Inst of Biomed & Health Eng, Shenzhen Inst of Adv Tech
Chinese Academy of Sciences, Shenzhen 518055, China
[†]Depart of Mech Eng, Univ of Hong Kong, Pokfulam Road, Hong Kong
[‡]memwang@hku.hk*

The performance of a biomedical composite is affected by many factors, including those in composite design and composite manufacture. Understanding the roles of major influencing factors is very important for successfully developing a biomedical composite from design to clinical applications. This chapter provides concise coverage of biomedical composites, from the rationale, fundamentals, templates from nature, design, and manufacture to their clinical applications. New technologies, such as 3D printing, have been increasingly used in making high-performance and customized biomedical composite products. Clinical applications of biomedical composites have also been expanding, from using non-porous non-biodegradable or biodegradable composites for human tissue replacement to employing porous biodegradable composites for human tissue regeneration. Beyond human body tissue repair, biomedical composites can be found in areas such as oncology where composite nanoparticles, the so-called theranostics, are very useful for early detection and effective treatment of cancer. Biomedical composites are fascinating biomaterials and more and more biomedical products will be made out of these materials.

8.1 Introduction

With the rapid increase in aging populations in developed as well as developing countries, treating the loss or dysfunction of tissues or organs in human bodies caused by aging, disease, and/or injury has become a major healthcare problem worldwide. There is an urgent need to develop effective strategies to assist human body tissue replacement or regeneration. The use of biomaterials for body tissue substitution has been one of the mainstream strategies to address these problems since ancient times. Within a long period of time, a variety of biomaterials, including biocompatible metallic, polymeric, and bioceramic materials, have been investigated and used for directly replacing or aiding the regeneration of human body tissues after tissue loss or dysfunction. Despite their success in modern medicine, these materials have their respective limitations. For example, metallic prostheses or implants made from Co-Cr alloy or Ti alloy have been widely used in clinics as bone or tooth substitutes. However, their stiffness (Young's modulus: normally over 100 GPa) is much higher than our most stiff tissues (Young's modulus of bone and tooth: 0.4–80 GPa) [1]. The stiffness mismatch will lead to tissue resorption or pathological remodeling at the implant–tissue interface with the metallic prosthesis/implant according to "Wolff's Law" [2]. Polymeric materials show excellent ductility and flexibility as well as tunable mechanical properties that are affected by polymer chains along with the capability of being adapted to the stiffness of specific human body tissues. Some of them further exhibit attractive biodegradability in physiological environments and desirable compatibility with target cells/tissues [3]. However, polymeric materials themselves cannot match the exceptional mechanical properties of some human body tissues that combine high rigidity with high toughness. Additionally, lacking bioactivity is a problem for polymer-based biomaterials, particularly those based on synthetic polymers. Ceramics such as calcium phosphate (Ca-P), bioglasses, carbon-based materials, and metal or non-metal oxides, have been widely used for repairing human body tissues, especially bone, where some of them exhibit attractive bioactivities (e.g., osteoconductivity and osteoinductivity) [4]. But most of the ceramic biomaterials are brittle and cannot bear high loads in tension. Therefore, it is often difficult to employ one type of mono-component material to fulfill the comprehensive requirements of "ideal" biomaterials to substitute or regenerate human body tissue.

To address materials challenges, composites, with a composite being defined as a mixture of two or more homogeneous phases that are bonded together, provide a solution as they can offer a combination of advantages arising from one or more component materials while circumventing the weaknesses of another component material, thereby providing desired, and sometimes unique, properties and functions over their original mono-composition component materials (i.e., metals, polymers, and/or ceramics). Although "composite" is not a new concept or material, and has been widely explored and employed in general engineering for thousands of years, suitable composites have been bringing new opportunities to biomedical engineering, particularly for tissue substitution or regeneration. Over the past several decades, composites for biomedical applications, termed "biomedical composites," have made remarkable advances in human body tissue repair. This chapter will present and discuss many aspects of biomedical composites, including biological templates, motivations, rationale, design, manufacture, and typical applications, aiming to inspire researchers and provide guidelines for developing next-generation biomedical composites with superior properties and functions.

8.1.1 *Biological Composites*

An "ideal" biomaterial for human body tissue replacement or regeneration is one that is as similar as possible to the native tissue, not only in physical properties (e.g., mechanical properties) but also in biological characteristics, based on the belief or assumption that the closest similarity will lead to the best clinical outcome. Similarity in mechanical characteristics is one of the important prerequisites for biomaterials with regard to their successful integration with the host tissues for long-term stability and reliability [5]. Investigating the structural and compositional characteristics of body tissues (which are "biological materials") that possess excellent mechanical properties (e.g., bone, which has both high rigidity and high toughness) is the first step toward developing biomaterials with tissue-mimicking mechanical properties.

Many body tissues are biological composites and for most biological composites, composites constituted by just a few commonly seen constituents offer the foundation for new biomaterials development. Even with these few commonly seen constituents ranging from polysaccharides, proteins, to minerals, biological composites exhibit a variety of properties and functions. It is therefore very important to understand the structure and properties of biological composites prior to embarking on developing new biomaterials for human body tissue repair. Bone is a typical biological composite, and in particular, a nanocomposite (Figure 8.1) whose structure has been widely investigated [6]. The main components of bone include a natural polymer, collagen (mainly collagen type I), stiff and brittle bone minerals (nanosized bone apatite, mainly calcium phosphate crystals), and multiple bone cell types. Crosslinked collagen fibrils, which are self-assembled into ordered structures such as sheets or fibers, constitute the extracellular matrix (ECM) of bone, offering

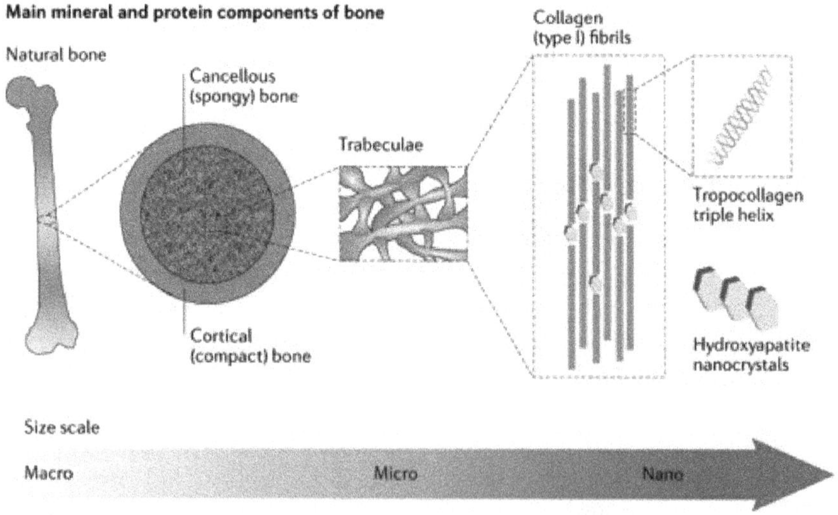

Figure 8.1. Schematic illustration showing the hierarchical composite structure of bone. Reprinted with permission [7] Copyright 2020 Springer Nature.

a structural framework for bone cells. Bone apatite crystals exist within or between collagen fibrils, resulting in a biological composite with a hierarchically arranged structure and hence an excellent combination of stiffness and toughness. In addition, bones exhibit gradient density in structure: dense cortical or compact bone in the outer region and cancellous or spongy bone in the interior (which shows a porous network of bony spicules, termed trabeculae). The composite nature and hierarchical structure together endow the bone with outstanding mechanical properties, including high load-bearing capacity and excellent fatigue resistance, which provide the benchmark for designing bone tissue analogues [7].

In addition to human body tissues, biological composites with excellent mechanical properties are also frequently encountered in various non-human living organisms, from plants to marine species. Investigations into the structure–property–function relationships of these biological composites have given us significant insights, assisting us in designing new biomaterials with superior mechanical properties for human body tissue repair. Wood is a typical plant-type biological composite that has been used as an engineering material for thousands of years owing to its outstanding mechanical properties. It can possess a very high Young's modulus of up to 30 GPa and a high compressive strength of up to 300 MPa in some dense forms [8]. It should be particularly noted that even with such high load-bearing capability, the structure of wood is porous, allowing highly efficient water and nutrient transport. The excellent mechanical properties and mass transport functions of wood are the direct results of its multiscale composite structure [9]. The basic building blocks in wood are anisotropic lignocellulosic compositions, i.e., cellulose, hemicelluloses, and lignin, forming a natural fibril-based composite. Aligned cellulose fibrils are embedded within lignin and hemicellulose matrix, and this composite structure is further assembled into bundles of cellulose microfibrils that offer the load-bearing mechanical strength, whereas the hierarchical porous structures within the composite matrix provide the paths for mass transport. The multiscale composite structure of wood provides not only inspirations for designing new man-made biomaterials but also the structural basis for constructing functional or mechanically reinforced structural materials via post-processing [10, 11], which can be very useful in the biomedical field.

The narce of mussels, which possess excellent mechanical properties arising from their composite nature, provides another fine example of a biological composite. It displays a combination of high ultimate strength and high fracture toughness. Numerous efforts in biomimicry have been made to develop man-made materials with comparable mechanical properties, following the accumulated structural/compositional insights into nacre. The major component (~91 wt%) of nacre is brittle inorganic aragonite platelet layers, where organic protein layers are alternately inserted between them, thereby forming a brick-cement-like multiscale composite architecture [12]. The inorganic and organic components within the composite architecture of nacre contribute to both high ultimate strength and high fracture toughness. Another part of a mussel that attracts much attention for designing biomedical composites is its hinge of bivalve shells, which provides exceptional fatigue resistance to thousands of repeated opening-and-closing motions. The composition of this hinge is similar to that of nacre, consisting of inorganic brittle aragonites (the major component) and organic proteins, where the rigid aragonites show radially aligned nanowire structures and are embedded within the resilient protein matrix [13]. The hard–soft multiscale composite structure can suppress stress concentration and increase resistance to bending fracture, which provides useful insights for designing engineering or biomedical materials that require high fatigue resistance. Notably, such strong and tough biological composites, even with complicated, ordered hierarchical structures, are normally formed via natural biomineralization under physiological environments which are very mild as compared to commonly encountered material manufacturing processes. Making man-made composites with similar outstanding mechanical properties to those of biological composites in mild conditions or through green synthesis routes is a great challenge.

8.1.2   Biomedical Composites

In the endeavor to develop biomaterials for human body tissue repair, natural biological systems, particularly biological composites, have provided many templates and much inspiration. One of the big questions in the context of designing new biomaterials is how to mimic the complex, hierarchical architecture and superior properties of biological composites. Over the past few decades, many biomedical composites have been made and investigated on the basis of lessons learned from the composition and structure of biological composites, achieving new and sometimes unexpected properties (e.g., a combination of high rigidity and high toughness) and functions [14, 15].

In general, a biomedical composite is composed of at least two different types of materials (which exist as different phases in composites), among which the interface (i.e., the boundary between different phases in composites) can be clearly distinguished. A typical two-phase composite usually has one dominant, continuous phase (>50% by volume, usually having relatively low stiffness and strength), termed "matrix material," and one discontinuous, normally well-dispersed minor phase (<50% by volume, usually having significantly higher stiffness and strength), termed "reinforcement." The regions of separation where the contact or interaction between the matrix material and reinforcement occurs are called "interface." Certainly, some composites exhibit bi-continuous phase structures with similar volume percentages for matrix and reinforcement, with the reinforcement still being the stiffer and stronger phase in the composite [16]. The properties and functions of a biomedical composite are generally determined by the properties of constituents, i.e., the matrix material and reinforcement, as well as the interface between them. Notably, rather than simple combinations of properties and functions of each constituting material, composites can exhibit new properties that are not offered by an individual constituting material [17].

By using different classification criteria, biomedical composites can be grouped into different sub-types. For example, according to the matrix material, composites are categorized as polymer–matrix composites, metal–matrix composites, and ceramic–matrix composites. Generally, the type of matrix material determines the mechanical characteristics of resulting composites. For instance, polymer–matrix composites usually show outstanding ductility and flexibility. According to the geometry of the reinforcement, composites can also be categorized as particle-reinforced composites (Figure 8.2(a)), fiber-reinforced composites (Figure 8.2(b)), and structural composites (Figure 8.2(c)). Particle-reinforced composites can be further classified into large-particle-reinforced composites (the average size of particulate reinforcement $> 100\,\text{nm}$) and dispersion-strengthened materials (the average size of particulate reinforcement

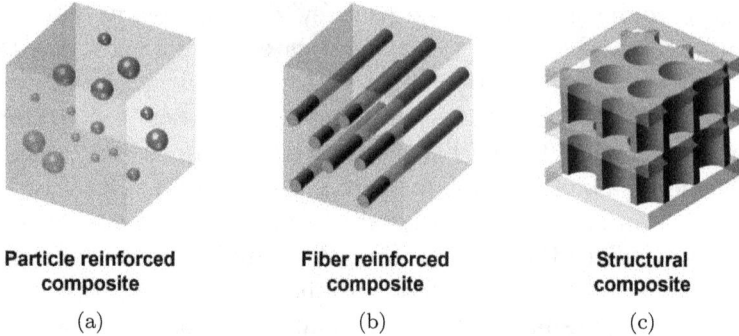

Particle reinforced
composite

Fiber reinforced
composite

Structural
composite

(a)   (b)   (c)

Figure 8.2. Schematic illustrations showing representative structures of (a) particle-reinforced composites, (b) fiber-reinforced composites, and (c) structural composites.

ranging from 10 to 100 nm). Particle-reinforced composites can be easily found in different engineering fields. Representative examples include spheroidite steel (ductile Fe-based matrix reinforced by stiff Fe_3C particles), automobile tires (compliant rubber matrix reinforced by stiff carbon particles), and concrete (aggregates bonded by cement). Varying in geometry and length of the fibrous reinforcement, fiber-reinforced composites are sub-divided into short-fiber-reinforced composites (non-continuous fibers dispersed in the matrix with aligned or random orientations) and long-fiber-reinforced composites (fibers running through the matrix usually in the continuous and aligned manner). Fiber-reinforced composites usually display excellent axial strength and stiffness, with mechanical properties being highly related to the density, length, and arrangement of the fiber reinforcement. Structural composites, which generally exhibit multi-layer structures, are divided into laminates and sandwich panels. Laminates commonly refer to structures of stacked anisotropic layers in a specific sequence, whereas sandwich panels usually refer to structures consisting of two stiff face sheets and one flexible interlayer between them. In the biomedical field, according to their biological properties, biomedical composites can also be categorized into bioinert composites, bioactive composites, and biodegradable composites. Each constituent material in a bioinert composite does not interact or react with cells or biological tissues, resulting in their high stability in the physiological environment. By contrast, at least one constituent material in a bioactive composite should possess bioactivity, having the capability of eliciting specific cellular responses and directing cellular behavior. For biodegradable composites, all constituent material should degrade in the biological environment into non-toxic species, which can be cleared or absorbed by human bodies subsequently without causing severe adverse effects. With modern technologies, biomedical composites with required mechanical, biological, and other properties should and can be designed and manufactured for human body tissue repair.

8.2 Materials for Biomedical Composites and Interface Control

For any material intended to be used in biomedical composites that will be implanted inside human bodies or be in contact with human body tissues or fluids, good biocompatibility is the paramount requirement. If a material is biodegradable, its degradation products in the human body environment should be biocompatible as well.

8.2.1 *Materials for the Matrix*

Commonly used materials for the matrix of biomedical composites include biomedical polymers (natural or synthetic, and in the solid state without water inclusion or in the form of hydrogels which are composed of polymer network(s) and large amounts of water), implantable metals, and bioceramics. For all these matrix materials, after meeting the first criterion on biocompatibility, other required or desirable properties will be considered and attained. The choice of a specific material as the matrix will be determined according to the specific clinical application requirements.

Polymers are by far the dominant matrix materials for biomedical composites. Most polymers are considered to be safe for cells or biological tissue unless incomplete removal of cytotoxic monomers, crosslinkers, or initiators occurs during the synthesis or synthesis/fabrication process. One major group of polymers for biomedical composite is bioinert polymers such as silicon rubber, poly(ethylene) (PE), poly(propylene) (PP), poly(urethane) (PU), poly(vinyl pyrrolidone) (PVP), poly(tetrafluoroethylene) (PTFE), poly(methyl methacrylate) (PMMA), polycarbonate (PC), poly(etheretherketone) (PEEK), poly(sulfone) (PSU), and ultra-high-molecular-weight polyethylene (UHMWPE). Representative composite examples include PTFE-/PU-based artificial vascular grafts and UHMWPE-based tendon/ligament/joint substitutes. Biodegradable polymers are now increasingly used for the matrix of biomedical composites. Polyesters such as poly (ε-caprolactone) (PCL), poly(lactic acid) (PLA), poly(glycolic acid) (PGA), and polyhydroxybutyrate (PHB), as well as their co-polymers such as poly(lactic-co-glycolic acid) (PLGA), poly(lactic acid-co-ε-caprolactone) (PLCL), and poly(hydroxybutyrate-co-hydroxyvalerate) (PHBV), are polymer matrices in either non-porous or porous biomedical composites. Many of these polymers have been approved by the US Food and Drug Administration (FDA) for medical uses [18]. Polymers with desired electrical properties, such as conductive poly(acrylonitrile) (PAN) and ferroelectric poly(vinylidene fluoride) (PVDF) [19], have also been used as the matrix of composites with electroactive properties. Apart from the above-mentioned synthetic polymers, natural polymers including polysaccharides (such as hyaluronic acid, alginate, and chitosan) and proteins (such as collagen, gelatin, elastin, silk fibroin, and ECM proteins) have also been widely used as the matrix of biomedical composites owing to their excellent biocompatibility and in particular bioactivity. Some of them such as gelatin and their derivates, collagen, and other ECM proteins possess bioactive domains of arginine-glycine-aspartic acid (RGD) sequences and matrix metalloproteinase (MMP)-sensitive degradation properties, facilitating integrin-mediated cellular focal adhesion and tissue remodeling [20]. When a polymer is used as the matrix in a biomedical composite, one obvious advantage is the ease of processing (as compared to metal or ceramic matrices), for either thermoplastic or thermosetting polymers, into various product geometries (wire, rod, plate, film, etc.) and designed micro-/nanostructures (micro-/nanoparticle, micro-/nanoplate, micro-/nanofiber, etc.).

Hydrogels are a specific group of polymers formed by hydrophilic polymer networks that can contain water and/or biological fluids that are thousands of times the weight of the polymer network [21]. Owing to the inherent high compatibility with cells and biological tissues, porous and water-rich hydrogels provide tissue-mimicking viscoelasticity and facilitate mass transport of nutrients and migration of cells, and hence hydrogels and their composites are increasingly used in tissue engineering and regenerative medicine [22]. In addition, hydrogels have also shown promise for long-term effective and reliable interfacing with soft and wet biological tissues [23]. Hydrogels are normally formed through polymerization of monomers or crosslinking (chemical or physical) of polymer chains. Commonly used monomers for forming hydrogels for biomedical applications include N-isopropylacrylamide (NIPAM), acrylic acid (AA), and hydroxyethyl methacrylate (HEMA), while polymers frequently used for forming biomedical hydrogels range from synthetic polymers such as poly(ethylene glycol diacrylate) (PEGDA) and poly(vinyl alcohol) (PVA) to natural or naturally derived polymers such as alginate, chitosan, collagen, gelatin, and gelatin methacryloyl (GelMA) [24]. Despite their unique advantages for biomedical applications, hydrogels have the inherent limitations of low strength and low stiffness. Reinforcing hydrogels and/or discovering stronger hydrogels are important areas for R & D of hydrogels and their biomedical composites.

Metallic biomaterials are also important matrix materials for biomedical composites. There has been a long history of using metallic biomaterials for human body tissue replacement, especially for hard tissues of bone and teeth. For example, gold has been used for dental devices since its use by Etruscans around 3,000 years ago. At present, despite many recognized issues, metal prostheses have dominated in orthopedics and dentistry. Typical metallic biomaterials include 316L stainless steel, Co-Cr alloy, and Ti-alloy for orthopedic implants and an amalgam for dental filling. With their high strength and stiffness, metal prostheses provide structural and mechanical support in hard tissue repair. However, the main problem for metal prostheses is the mismatch of stiffness between the metal and hard tissue, which will lead to pathological tissue resorption or remodeling according to "Wolff's Law." Reducing the stiffness at least at the interface with biological tissue to achieve or improve mechanical compatibility is an important task in metal–matrix composite development.

Bioceramics have now been widely used in orthopedics and dentistry due to their excellent biocompatibility, high stiffness, and wear/erosion resistance. Among them, hydroxyapatite (HAp), a prominent member of the bioactive calcium phosphate (Ca-P) family, is similar in composition and crystal structure to the inorganic component of bone and has the attractive "osteoconductive" property, which promotes the adhesion, proliferation, and differentiation of osteoblastic cells on HAp implants [4], as well as facilitating the "osteoinductive" activity to mediate genetic expression of mesenchymal stem cells (MSCs) and directing MSC differentiation toward osteogenic phenotypes [25]. β-tricalcium phosphate (β-TCP), another member of the Ca-P family, is biodegradable and can be absorbed once bone tissue repair is completed. Apart from Ca-Ps, bioactive glasses and glass-ceramics represented by Bioglass® (which contains high amounts of calcium and phosphorous with a molar ratio of 5:1) and A-W glass-ceramics are also widely used in orthopedics and dentistry. They show excellent interfacial affinity even with soft tissues, facilitating long-term reliable bio-integration. Certainly, bioceramics are brittle and normally have high stiffness, which requires modulation in ceramic–matrix composite development.

8.2.2 Reinforcements for Composites

In biomedical composites, reinforcements play critical roles in improving mechanical properties (and biological functions for some composites as well). For composites having a ductile matrix with insufficient stiffness (e.g., polymers and hydrogels), much stiffer and stronger reinforcements are usually used for reinforcing the matrix. In this context, bioceramic particles are popular reinforcements. For example, bioactive bioceramic particles, such as Ca-P, Bioglass®, and A-W glass-ceramic particles have been used for making composites for orthopedic and/or dental applications. Such reinforcements not only improve mechanical properties but also bring to the composites desired osteoconductive/osteoinductive properties. Ca-P particles can be synthesized in the lab via a precipitation reaction, resulting in amorphous spherical nanoparticles with sizes ranging from 10 to 30 nm or acicular-shaped nanoparticles. For spherical Ca-P particles, the mechanical properties of resulting composites are determined by the volume fraction and dispersion status of Ca-P nanoparticles in composites. Dispersing treatments are usually required for small-diameter particle reinforcement as they tend to form aggregates within the matrix. For acicular-shaped particles, the aspect ratio (i.e., the length-to-width ratio) and orientation of these particles within the matrix are important factors in mediating composite properties and functions. Compared to the smooth surface of spherical particles used in theoretical analysis, commercial or lab-produced Ca-P particles with rough surfaces and irregular shapes have been found to form an enhanced stable interface with the matrix via mechanical interlocking. However, particles of irregular shapes but with sharp corners/edges such as some glass or glass-ceramic particles made by the conventional melting and quenching techniques can lead to stress concentrations at the reinforcement–matrix interface and subsequent failure of the composite under high mechanical load owing to interfacial debonding.

Fibrous reinforcements are normally used to improve the mechanical performance of biomedical composites. They can be either long (continuous) or short (discontinuous), aligned or randomly oriented, which will result in tunable mechanical properties for the composites. Examples of ceramic short-fiber (whiskers or chopped fibers) include single-crystalline alumina, SiC, and SiN whiskers, which have very high stiffness and can be used for reinforcing metal or ceramic matrices. Chopped metal wires (e.g., 316L stainless steel) have also been used to toughen bioceramics matrices. Long-fiber reinforcements range from polymer fibers (e.g., aramid fibers, UHMWPE fibers, cellulose fibers, and biodegradable polyester fibers) and carbon-based fibers (e.g., carbon fibers formed via graphitization of PAN fibers) to ceramic fibers (e.g., glass fibers and Ca-P fibers). Composites with fibrous reinforcements usually exhibit high axial modulus and strength.

For composites with stiff but low-ductility matrices (i.e., metals or ceramics), reinforcements in another form or, rather, modulus-buffering materials can be employed to improve the mechanical compatibility at the tissue–implant interface. An example is to form a "hydrogel skin" on stiff metal- or ceramic-based implants/devices. Through surface functionalization of the matrix material and *in situ* polymerization [26], a thin layer of hydrogel with a similar modulus (at the magnitude of dozens of kPa) to soft tissues could be formed on the surface, which would significantly improve the mechanical compatibility, thereby lowering the risk of damage to the tissue and even further offering the sensing function of the resulting composite [27].

One other role of the reinforcement is to add or expand the functions for the resulting biomedical composites. In addition to being used to provide or enhance osteoconductivity or osteoinductivity as mentioned earlier, conductive materials have also been used for biomedical composites for the repair of human body tissues having electrophysiological responses such as cardiac tissues, neural tissues, and skeletal muscles [28, 29]. Conductive reinforcements include carbon-based materials (e.g., graphite, carbon black, single-wall/multi-wall carbon nanotubes, graphene, graphene oxide, and nano-diamond [30]), conductive polymers (e.g., polyaniline (PANI), polypyrrole (PPy), and polythiophene (PTH)) [31]), and MXenes [32]. Many of them show bi- or multi-functions in biomedical composites.

8.2.3 *Interfacial Bonds and Bonding Mechanisms*

The reinforcement–matrix interface is also a critical factor in determining the properties of biomedical composites. It is formed through different physical or chemical bonding mechanisms. Generally, the interface formed by chemical bonding is several orders of magnitude stronger than that by physical bonding, leading to high strength but low toughness. A majority of interfaces in biomedical composites are formed via physical interactions between the reinforcement and matrix, e.g., molecular entanglement following interdiffusion, electrostatic interaction (including cation–anionic interactions in layer-by-layer assembly), and mechanical interlocking. Therefore, the interfacial strength of the biomedical composite is highly dependent on surface chemistry, surface charge, and surface geometry/roughness of the reinforcement and matrix. The design and modulation of surface features of each phase can offer effective ways to control the interface and tune the mechanical properties of resulting biomedical composites.

8.2.4 *Control of the Interface*

Based on the bonding mechanisms and characteristics of interfaces in biomedical composites, the properties of biomedical composites can be modulated through the control of the interface. As interfaces formed via chemical bonding are generally significantly stronger than those formed via physical bonding, an effective way to strengthen the interface is to introduce chemical bonding between the reinforcement and matrix, which may be realized by the use of silane coupling agents to generate strong interfacial chemical bonding via a local hydrolysis reaction [33]. However, high interfacial strengths may bring down the toughness of resulting biomedical composites. For biomedical composites to be used in applications that require high toughness such as tendon/ligament repair, the enhancement of toughness could be achieved by controlling the interface. For example, coating the reinforcement (SiC fibers in this case) with a duplex $C/TiB2$ reaction layer led to reinforcing the interface with the metallic matrix by enhancing physical interactions [34].

8.3   Design and Manufacture of Biomedical Composites

8.3.1   *Design Rationale*

When designing a biomedical composite for the repair of a specific human body tissue, comprehensive considerations on constituent materials, macro- and microstructure of the composite, and manufacturing technique should be taken according to the characteristics of the target tissue and its biological environment. A process shown in Fig. 8.3 is normally adopted. The rationale involved in each step of this process will be introduced in the following sections. Materials selected for the composite are generally, and with high preference, US FDA-approved biomedical materials. The design considerations are shown in the following section.

8.3.2   *Architecture, Properties, and Biological Performance*

When using a biomedical composite for body tissue repair, its properties will heavily affect the clinical outcome. The major factors

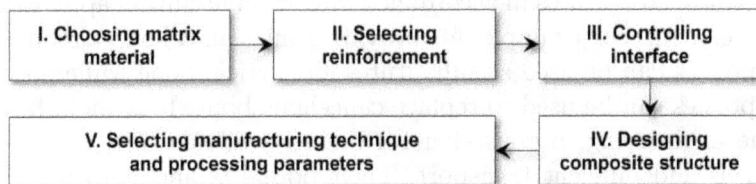

Figure 8.3.   A typical process for designing and manufacturing a biomedical composite.

influencing the performance of biomedical composites include the following:

1. structural features

   (a) overall structure (bulk or thin film, non-porous or porous, pore size, porosity, etc.);
   (b) surface structure (surface roughness, topography, surface pattern, etc.);
   (c) matrix structure (average molecular weight for polymer, average grain size of metal or ceramic, etc.);
   (d) shape, size, size distribution, and volume percentage of the reinforcement;
   (e) distribution (and orientation) of reinforcement in the matrix.

2. physical and mechanical properties

   (a) properties of constituent materials;
   (b) surface wettability of the reinforcement;
   (c) overall mechanical properties (Young's modulus, shear modulus, elongation at fracture, ultimate tensile strength, etc.);
   (d) electroactive properties (conductivity, piezoelectric, pyroelectric, or triboelectric properties).

3. reinforcement–matrix interface and its control.

4. composite–tissue interface and composite biological properties

   (a) biocompatibility (compatible with cells and biological tissues, including biodegradation product(s));
   (b) biodegradability and degradation rate;
   (c) bioactivity or bioinertness;
   (d) tissue–composite interface mechanics (mechanical compatibility, interfacial strength, etc.).

These factors should be carefully considered when designing biomedical composites in accordance with specific clinical application requirements. For example, for providing mechanical support, dense composites can be used as substitutes for cortical bone while porous composites can be used to replace cancellous bone. In scaffold-based tissue engineering, porous structures (i.e., scaffolds) are important for cells and nutrient transport. Their pore size and porosity need to be controlled for the application in the target tissue. Materials for the matrix or reinforcement should be selected according to the mechanical and functional requirements of the specific body tissue to be repaired. For example, stiff and osteoconductive materials such as bioactive Ca-P and glass particles are frequently used as reinforcement in biomedical composites for orthopedic applications. Electroactive materials such as carbon-based materials, conductive polymers, and ferroelectric materials can be used to make biomedical composites for the repair of human body tissues containing electrically excitable cells such as cardiac tissues, neural tissues, and skeletal muscles. Surface features such as surface wettability and electrical charge that can mediate protein adsorption [35] and surface chemistry that can affect interfacial adhesion with the biological tissue [36] are also important factors. They will affect biological responses and implant/device stability after composite implantation in the body.

8.3.3 Manufacture of Particulate Biomedical Composites

In addition to the factors mentioned previously, another major factor that affects the properties and functions of biomedical composites is composite manufacture (including the manufacturing technique and process parameters), which should also be carefully considered prior to composite development. In fact, in most situations, choosing materials for a new composite and selecting a manufacturing technique for the composite are considered together. For different categories of composites, the fabrication of particle-reinforced polymer–matrix biomedical composites appears to be the easiest, although it is not easy, among manufacture of all types of composites. These composites can be processed through extrusion, compression molding, and injection molding, which are common techniques for biomedical polymers. Extrusion and injection molding are often used for fabricating biomedical composites with a thermoplastic polymer matrix, while compression molding can be employed for composites based on thermoplastics or thermosets. Laboratory techniques such as solvent casting can be used for small-quantity production of polymer–matrix composites at the early stage of composite development.

The manufacture of particle-reinforced metal–matrix composites includes liquid-phase processing, solid-state processing, and solid-liquid processing. Liquid-phase processing refers to dispersing particulate reinforcements (usually bioactive ceramic particles) directly in molten metals. Composites are thus formed via, for example, stir casting after solidification of the metal matrix. An example of solid-state processing is powder metallurgy (PM), where solid-state particulate reinforcement and solid-state metal powers for the matrix are thoroughly mixed and then compressed by high pressure and under high temperature, yielding dense and compact composites. (If a sacrificial material is put in the powder mixture during preparation and then removed from the PM-formed dense structure after composite fabrication, porous composite structures, i.e., composite scaffolds, are obtained, which are needed for tissue engineering.) Solid–liquid processing refers to mixing the particulate reinforcement within a metal matrix in a region of the phase diagram where liquid and solid states of the matrix coexist. High temperatures are involved in all the above-mentioned manufacturing routes for particle-reinforced metal–matrix composites. These high temperatures must be carefully chosen as too high a temperature could induce unwanted chemical reactions between the two phases.

As for the manufacture of particle-reinforced ceramic–matrix composites which generally use ceramic particles as the reinforcement, techniques such as pressureless sintering, hot pressing, and hot isostatic pressing (HIPing) are frequently used. The particulate reinforcement must be thoroughly mixed with the ceramic matrix powders prior to form greenbodies. Decomposition of phases during sintering, which may cause problems during composite application, should be avoided. All these manufacturing techniques face the common challenge of forming fully or highly dense ceramic–matrix composites after sintering.

8.3.4   Manufacture of Fibrous Biomedical Composites

Fiber-reinforced polymer–matrix composites have been investigated for implants for human body tissue replacement for human body tissue replacement. Extrusion, compression molding, and injection molding that are used for making particle-reinforced polymer–matrix composites can be extended to manufacturing polymer–matrix composites with short/chopped fiber reinforcements. However, short/chopped brittle fibers are often broken down to shorter lengths during extrusion or injection molding, reducing their reinforcing effect. Besides, fibrous reinforcements in composites made by these two techniques are mostly aligned in the extrusion or injection direction, resulting in anisotropic materials. By contrast, compression molding may avoid these two issues, leading to composites with randomly oriented short/chopped fibers. Nevertheless, the low production rate is a disadvantage for compression molding.

Long/continuous-fiber composites are produced using specialized manufacturing techniques, such as filament winding and pultrusion. Filament winding involves multiple steps: (1) polymer impregnation by pulling long fibers through a low-viscosity resin bath, (2) drawing the long fibers onto a rotating mandrel as successive layers, (3) curing the long fibrous composite on the mandrel, and (4) removal of the mandrel [37]. The alignment and contents of the fibrous reinforcement in the composite can be controlled in the filament winding process. Therefore, filament winding has been widely used for making long/continuous-fiber composites with a directional orientation of the fibrous reinforcement to attain axial high tensile strength. Pultrusion also involves multiple steps [38], with the first step still being polymer impregnation by pulling long fibers through a polymer precursor bath. The fibers are then pulled through a heated die with a microchannel cavity, heated to a temperature near or above their phase transition temperature, and stretched. The composite is finally cooled down and solidified. By controlling the shape/geometry of the microchannel cavity, fibrous composites of different sizes and shapes (e.g., rods, pipes, beams, sheets, or tubes) can be made. Pultrusion has the major advantage of a high production rate, making it attractive for industrial fabrication.

In recent decades, electrospinning has also been investigated for producing biomedical composites with nanofibrous architectures. Electrospinning is a simple and versatile technology. The reinforcement can be simply suspended in a polymer solution which is to be directly electrospun into fibrous composites under a high-voltage electrostatic field [39]. Notably, the composites made by electrospinning show ECM-mimicking nanofibrous structures, making them highly promising as ECM analogues that offer biomimetic structural cues for human body tissue regeneration. Furthermore, the orientation of electrospun fibers can be controlled, leading to the formation of biomedical composites with randomly oriented or aligned fibers for human body tissues.

8.3.5   Manufacture of Laminated Biomedical Composites

Laminated biomedical composites are not often encountered in the biomedical field. They consist of stacked multiple layers, which are normally produced by firstly forming each sheet/panel with unidirectional fiber reinforcement and then compressing the sheets/panels into laminated structures under high pressure and temperature. A vacuum bag/autoclave process is commonly used for fabricating laminated composites. In brief, composite sheets, sometimes partially cured, are first produced, which are stacked one by one in a predetermined order and direction according to the composite design. The stacked sheets are processed into a laminate in a shaped tool, which is then treated in a vacuum bag to remove the air trapped in the laminated structure and cured in an autoclave, finally forming the laminated composite. The mechanical properties of laminated composites can be controlled by using different stacking layers and by changing layer directions (and hence fiber directions).

8.3.6   Manufacture of Porous Composite Scaffolds

In tissue engineering and regenerative medicine, porous scaffolds provide the structural framework and microenvironment of cells [40]. The composite approach gives the possibility of forming porous scaffolds with superior mechanical properties and multiple functions, holding the promise for cell regulation and tissue formation. The techniques commonly used for fabricating porous composite scaffolds include thermally induced phase separation (TIPS), gas foaming, solvent casting and porogen leaching, microsphere sintering, post-fabrication coating (deposition or *in situ* growth of particulate reinforcements on the pore surface of a scaffold), electrospinning, and solid freeform fabrication (known currently and popularly as "additive manufacturing" or "3D printing"). [41] All these techniques can produce composites with interconnected pores (which are essential for cell migration, growth, and perfusion of oxygen and nutrients for cells) and controlled pore size and porosity (by varying process parameters).

Emerging manufacturing technologies such as 3D printing and new materials/structures, such as bicontinuous interfacially jammed emulsion gels ("bijels"), have also been used for fabricating porous nanocomposite scaffolds for tissue engineering. Selective laser sintering (SLS) is a commonly used additive manufacturing technology and shows several advantages for forming porous nanocomposite scaffolds with customized shapes and architectures [42]. The manufacture of porous composite scaffolds under mild fabrication conditions (no toxic solvent, no high temperature, and no high pressure) can be realized by using bijels as templates [43]. The bijel-templating approach also enables the incorporation of drugs, biomolecules, and even live cells into bi-continuous structures, aiming to achieve the best clinical outcome in body tissue regeneration.

8.4 Medical Applications

8.4.1 *Non-Porous Composites for Human Tissue Replacement*

8.4.1.1 *Applications in orthopedics*

Bone is a natural nanocomposite. By using bone as a template, biomedical composites mimicking the bone microstructure structure have been designed and investigated for bone replacement since Bonfield *et al.* introduced the concept of analogue biomaterials in the 1980s [44]. An important motivation for developing biomedical composites for bone substitution is to address the issue of large mismatch in stiffness between natural bone and conventional prostheses made of metals or ceramics, which can result in pathological remodeling or resorption of neighboring bone following "Wolff's law." When under an applied load, the bone adjacent to the implanted much stiffer metal or ceramic prosthesis bears a lower stress according to the load sharing principle, resulting in the phenomena known as "stress shielding," which causes the bone to remodel to lowered mass and hence become weaker.

Biomedical composites may solve the stress shielding problem as their mechanical properties, including stiffness, can be tailored by design and by combining suitable materials. One good example is hydroxyapatite (HAp)-reinforced high-density polyethylene (HDPE) [45], which is termed HAPEXTM commercially and is the first biomedical composite as a bone analogue to be approved for clinical use (used as middle ear implants and orbital floor implants). Many other biomedical composites with different types of reinforcements (HAp particles, Bioglass® particles, A-W glass-ceramic particles, glass fibers, carbon fibers, etc.) and matrix materials (PSU, PEEK, PU, epoxy resins, gelatin, collagen, etc.) have subsequently been made and assessed for bone replacement in orthopedics and other medical fields [46]. As can be seen, the role of reinforcements is not limited to improving mechanical properties; they are also employed to bring in osteoconductivity to composites that can promote the establishment of a biological bond between composite implants and bone, stabilizing the implant–bone interface. As stated in the previous section, high productivity can be achieved using injection molding. Our research has shown that bone analogue biomedical composites such as Hap-reinforced PP could be successfully injection molded [47]. A large content of HAp particles (up to 25 wt%) could be homogeneously dispersed within the PP matrix through injection molding (Figure 8.4). Fully bioabsorbable composites, which consist of bioabsorbable reinforcements (e.g., β-TCP) and biodegradable polymers (e.g., PLGA, PCL and PHBV), have attracted much attention. With their controlled *in vivo* biodegradation, their clinical use can not only avoid second surgery for graft removal but also facilitate bone tissue healing/remodeling [48]. In some high-load-bearing

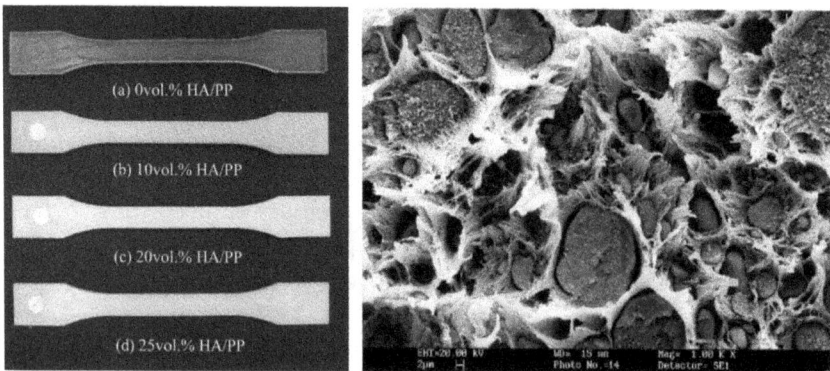

Figure 8.4. HAp-reinforced PP composites as bone analogue for bone replacement. Left: HAp/PP composites with different HAp contents. Right: Good dispersion of HAp particles within the PP matrix for a composite with the HAp content of 25 wt%. Reprinted with permission [47] Copyright 2007 John Wiley & Sons.

situations, biomedical composites of metal or ceramic matrices, rather than polymer matrices, have been investigated. Biodegradable HAp-reinforced Mg [49], HAp-reinforced Ti-6Al-4V [50], and HAp-reinforced zirconia/alumina [51] provide a few examples. Mechanical and biological properties of biomedical composites can be varied by selecting different combinations of materials to form composite bone analogues so as to meet application requirements.

8.4.1.2 *Applications in dentistry*

Biomedical composites have also found applications in dentistry due to the similar nanocomposite nature of teeth and bone. Biomaterial applications in dentistry are usually encountered in cavity filling or tooth replacement. For cavity filling, Amalgam, gold, alumina, zirconia, acrylic resins, silicate cement, etc., are normally used. However, these materials still cannot meet the comprehensive requirements for the ideal dental restorative material, which include the following: (1) low viscosity for easy handling and cavity filling; (2) appropriate thermal expansion coefficient similar to that of teeth; (3) excellent mechanical properties and structural stability, resistance to fatigue, wear, creep, and water absorption; and (4) desirable biocompatibility and reliable integration with teeth. To meet these requirements, biomedical composites, such as barium, aluminum, and silicate glass–resin composites with synergistically high mechanical properties and biocompatibility, have been studied for cavity filling. They have shown high reliability and effectiveness (acceptable ratings in 70% of the fillings and 88% of the inlays) in an 11-year clinical evaluation (88 premolars and 52 molars in 28 adults) [52]. When teeth are severely damaged with limited preserved structures that are insufficient for retaining filling materials, a dental post is usually required, which is inserted in the root canal for mechanical reinforcement. Conventionally, dental posts are made of metallic materials such as Co-Cr and Ti alloy, which do not possess the desirable mechanical properties of varying stiffness along their length (gradually increasing stiffness from the apical end to the coronal end) to accommodate the stress distribution in teeth. Kevlar/carbon/glass-fiber-reinforced epoxy composites were thus investigated for dental posts, whose stiffness could be tuned according to the requirements of gradient mechanics [53]. In situations of complete loss of teeth, tooth analogues will be required for permanent replacement. Conventional materials for artificial teeth include common metal alloys (Au, Co-Cr-Mo alloys, stainless steel, and Ti alloys) and ceramic materials (zirconia, alumina, etc.). To mimic the hierarchical and composite structures of natural teeth, a strong and tough composite tooth analogue — where 250-μm-thick and 10-μm-diameter alumina platelets were dispersed within metallic, polymeric, and ceramic matrices to form a twisted plywood structure — was made via magnetically assisted slip casting [54]. This tooth-mimicking heterogeneous composite showed tunable local microstructure and composition (Fig. 8.5), which could fulfill functional demands for analogues in tooth replacement. Recently, an induced epitaxial crystal growth method for depositing enamel apatite by using calcium phosphate ion clusters as the precursors, which mimicked the natural biomineralization process of crystalline-amorphous frontier formation, was investigated, offering the possibility of repairing tooth enamel with complicated hierarchical composite structures in a mild way [55].

8.4.1.3   *Hybrids in the cardiovascular area*

Cardiovascular diseases are now the leading causes of death worldwide. In clinics, coronary-artery bypass grafting (CABG) is regarded as the gold standard for treating patients with severe cardiovascular diseases such as coronary heart diseases whose coronary arteries are partially or completely obstructed by atherosclerotic plaque [56]. However, relatively high costs and complication risks are associated with CABG in surgery. Therefore, there have been continuous efforts

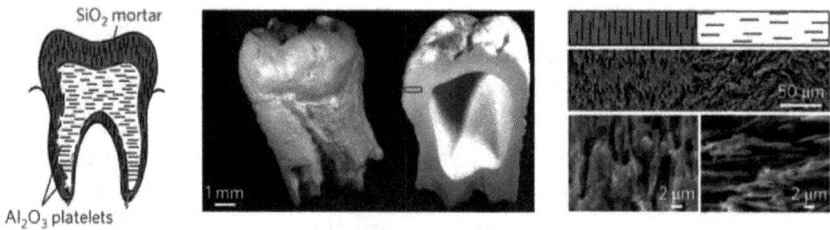

Figure 8.5. Heterogenous composites with a twisted plywood structure as tooth analogues. Reprinted with permission [54] Copyright 2015 Springer Nature.

to develop vascular analogues to substitute the use of native vessels [57]. Early products of bioengineered blood vessels were artificial conduits based on bioinert polymers such as silicone rubber and expanded polytetrafluoroethylene (ePTFE). However, due to difficult remodeling by the host, such artificial conduits tended to induce scar tissue formation and subsequently thrombosis/aneurysm over time after implantation. To avoid the occurrences of complications and to enhance long-term patency, new bioengineered blood vessels should meet the requirements not only in mechanical properties (sufficient resistance to tensile force, burst pressure, rupture, and suturing) but also in biocompatibility (biocompatible with blood and vascular cells and keeping a low level of foreign body responses/immune rejection).

The composite or hybridization approach has offered promising toolkits for constructing bioengineered blood vessels with enhanced and combined functions [58]. For example, a biodegradable polymer–hydrogel composite vascular graft was constructed and studied [59], which consisted of a PLCL nanofibrous lumen layer and a heparin/silk hydrogel shell, which contributed, respectively, to appropriate mechanical support for endothelial remodeling and enhanced biocompatibility. The composite vascular grafts showed feasibility for long-term patency (at least eight months) in a rabbit model. Considering the hierarchical arrangements of different cell types within native blood vessels, composite vascular grafts, whose structures were hierarchical as well for mimicking the vascular anatomies, were also made and investigated [60]. The inner and outer layers of the composite vascular grafts were, respectively, a randomly oriented dense fibrous mesh and a mesh of assembled microfibers with directional orientation. Thanks to the hierarchical composite structure, the composite vascular grafts supported the vessel-mimicking organizations/phenotypes of endothelial cells and smooth muscle cells in the respective tissue layers, potentially facilitating remodeling by the host. The composite approach can also endow other functions in bioengineered blood vessels. Based on liquid metal–polymer composites, an electronic bioengineered blood vessel was designed and made (Fig. 8.6). The integrated circuit made of the conducting composite gave rise to additional functions (electrical stimulation for promoting endothelial proliferation and electroporation for therapeutic gene delivery) of the electronic bioengineered blood vessel [61].

Electronic blood vessel
made from metal-polymer composites

Natural-inspired structure

In situ electroporation/electrical stimulation

Excellent patency in a rabbit model

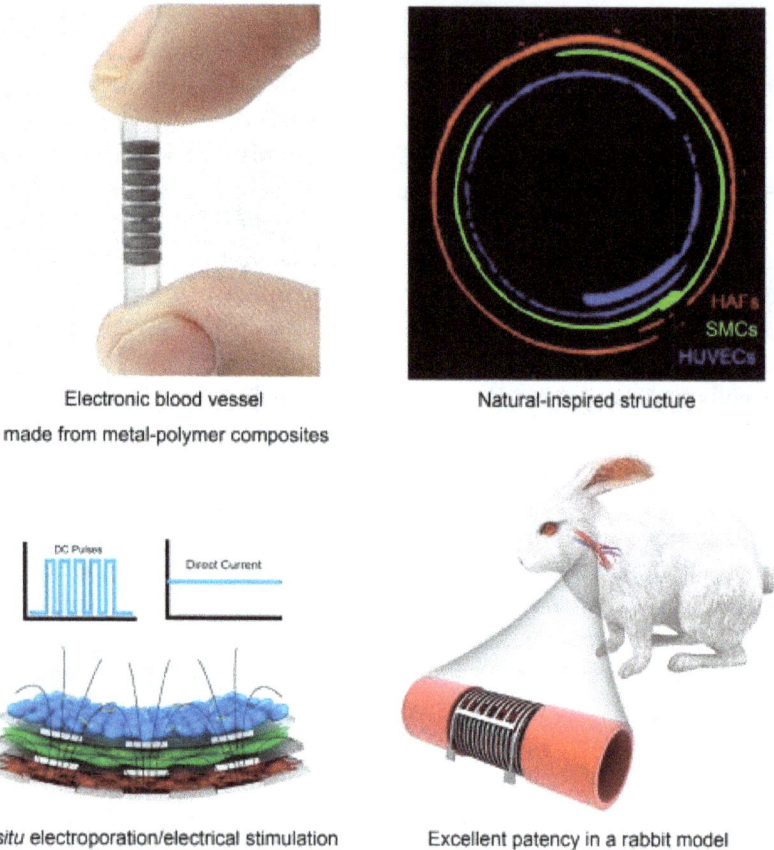

Figure 8.6. A conducting liquid metal–polymer composite-based electronic bio-engineered blood vessel. Reprinted with permission [61] Copyright 2020 Elsevier.

8.4.2 *Porous Composite Scaffolds for Body Tissue Regeneration*

In addition to developing biomaterials (mainly non-porous biomaterials, with occasional use of porous biomaterials) for human body tissue replacement, the design and development of new biomaterials (mainly porous and biodegradable biomaterials) for aiding self-renewal or *in situ* regeneration of body tissues have been increasingly and vigorously pursued, aiming to provide better treatments/therapies for body tissues with diseases, dysfunctions, or injuries, ever since the word/concept of "tissue engineering" was introduced in the late 1980s [62]. The conventional and dominant tissue engineering approach, i.e., scaffold-based tissue engineering, combines live cells, porous scaffolds, and biological signals into constructs that are implanted in the body for directing/promoting new tissue formation at the original diseased or injured sites [63]. As the scaffolds are typically made of biodegradable biomaterials (mainly polymers and their composites even up to present time), inside the body, the constructs biodegrade and are completely integrated with host tissues after completing their repairing and regenerating task. Materials play vital roles in tissue engineering, particularly for scaffolds. Scaffolds and scaffold materials should have these desirable structure and properties: (1) highly porous structure with interconnecting pores for supporting cell development, (2) good biocompatibility for the long-term reliable integration with living tissues, (3) appropriate biodegradation properties for full absorption or elimination after tissue regeneration, and (4) whenever required, good bioactivity to direct cellular behaviors and functions. For biomedical composites, porous composite (or hybrid) scaffolds have provided desired biological performances in the tissue engineering of bone, osteochondral tissue, vasculature, nerve, and many other body tissues.

8.4.2.1   Bone

One major application area for porous composite scaffolds is bone tissue engineering. Osteoconductive biomaterials such as bioactive Ca-P, glasses, and glass-ceramics are usually used as reinforcements in the composite scaffolds for regenerating bone. They serve as both mechanical reinforcement for improving the stiffness and strength of composites and bioactive components for promoting new bone formation and implant integration with the host tissue. So far, a variety of porous composite scaffolds have been made and investigated, which are formed by using different manufacturing techniques and exhibit different mechanical/biological properties [41]. Early research led to composite scaffold manufacture through surface coating of bioactive ceramics onto pre-formed porous polymer scaffolds via biomimetic biomineralization. For example, a layer of bone-like apatite or bone-like apatite/collagen composite could be formed on the pore surface of a PGA scaffold in a high-concentration simulated body fluid

(SBF) [64]. The porous composite scaffolds with a biodegradable polymer strut the matrix and a bone-like apatite coating could support good attachment and proliferation of osteoblast-like cells [65], as well as directing mesenchymal stem cells (MSCs) toward the osteoblast phenotype [66]. Porous composite scaffolds could also be formed via an emulsion freezing/freeze-drying process [67], where the reinforcement (e.g., HAp particles) could be homogenously distributed within the polymer matrix. Electrospinning is a popular method for producing porous composite scaffolds for bone tissue engineering [68]. Even though their stiffness is usually significantly lower than that of natural bone tissue, electrospun composite scaffolds, which possess biomimetic nanofibrous architectures that facilitate cell attachment and 3D organization, offer desirable biointerfaces with bone as bone ECM analogues for promoting *in situ* tissue neoformation and remodeling [69]. In addition, bioactive molecules such as growth factors can be incorporated within composite scaffolds by using suitable electrospinning techniques to achieve the effects on cell regulation and stem cell fate determination, where the release profiles (either burst or sustained release) of the incorporated growth factors may be controlled on demand for stage-specific inducements on tissue regeneration [70–72]. By incorporating and controlling the release of vascular endothelial growth factor (VEGF) in an electrospun composite scaffold, bone formation and vascularization could be synergistically enhanced, accelerating the repair of bone tissue [73].

Additive manufacturing (AM, i.e., "3D printing") is increasingly seen for fabricating porous composite scaffolds for bone tissue engineering. It has multiple advantages such as the ease of forming bone-like hierarchical structures and the production of customized shapes/geometries adaptable to bone defects [74]. In AM processes, "inks" are formulated for specific 3D printing techniques. For example, Ca-P/PHBV nanocomposite microspheres with an average diameter of $\sim 48\,\mu m$ were made via a solid-in-oil-in-water (S/O/W) emulsion solvent evaporation process by dispersing Ca-P nanoparticles uniformly in a PHBV polymer solution [75], which would be suitable "inks" for the SLS process to form porous Ca-P/PHBV nanocomposite scaffolds. The 3D nanocomposite scaffolds thus formed via SLS had hierarchical porous structures, supporting high cell viability and desired attachment of osteoblast-like cells on scaffolds [76]. By using a water-in-oil emulsion as the "ink," which was prepared by dispersing a water phase (Ca-P nanoparticle-suspended and bioactive molecule-supplemented saline) within an oil phase (a PLA polymer solution), hierarchically porous nanocomposite scaffolds for bone tissue engineering could also be formed via a cryogenic 3D printing process [77]. Since the bioactive molecules, i.e., bone morphogenetic protein-2 (BMP-2) in this study, were dispersed in the water phase and were not in direct contact with the cytotoxic organic solvent, which was used to dissolve the polymer to make polymer solutions, and the whole manufacturing process did not involve high temperatures, the bioactivity of the incorporated BMP-2 in the ink and in the 3D nanocomposite scaffolds was well preserved, significantly enhancing the osteoinductive property of the scaffolds. Using similar cryogenic 3D printing processes, a variety of bioactive materials or molecules such as 2D black phosphorus nanosheets, doxorubicin hydrochloride, and osteogenic peptide could be incorporated with well-preserved bioactivity, resulting in multifunctional bone tissue engineering scaffolds capable of simultaneously promoting *in situ* bone tissue regeneration and killing cancer cells, which could be used to treat bone defects after resection of bone tumors [78]. Recently, the digital laser processing (DLP) 3D printing technique was investigated for forming hierarchically porous nanocomposite scaffolds for bone tissue engineering [79]. DLP 3D printing has shown its superiority in printing, yielding scaffolds with Haversian canals, Volkmann canals, and cancellous bone structures mimicking the complex hierarchical structure of native Haversian bone. In another study, by using a nanocomposite "ink" formulated by dispersing β-TCP nanoparticles within a stimulus-responsive polymer solution (i.e., the shape-memory poly(lactic acid-co-trimethylene carbonate) (PLA-co-TMC)), porous nanocomposite scaffolds with changeable stiffness and reconfigurable shapes were made via 4D printing [80]. The 4D printed hierarchically porous nanocomposite scaffolds could be shaped into a temporary, soft-folded geometry for minimally invasive implantation and when at the implantation site, could recover to its permanent stiff, expanded shape, which is triggered by temperature increase, for filling the bone defects (Fig. 8.7). This approach has offered a simple and effective way to treat critical-size bone defects of irregular shapes.

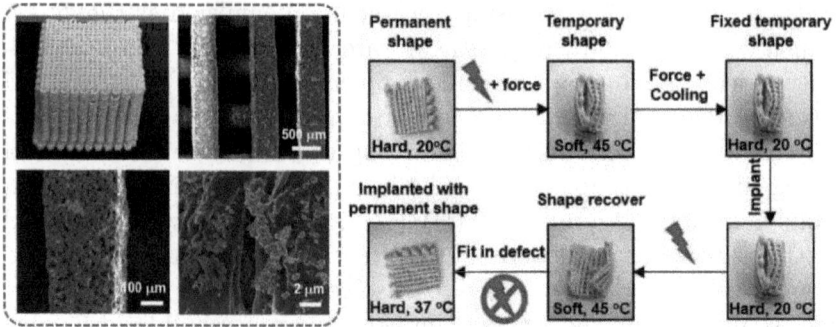

Figure 8.7. 4D printed porous nanocomposite scaffolds (left) for bone tissue engineering with programmable shapes (right). Reprinted with permission [80] Copyright 2020 IOP Publishing.

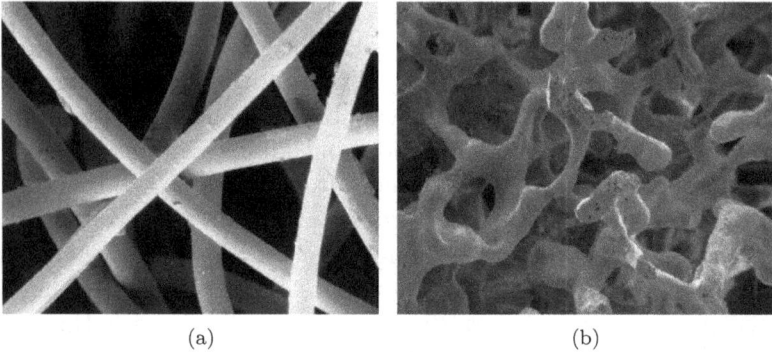

(a)   (b)

Figure 8.8. Microstructures of bilayers in an osteochondral composite scaffold: (a) cartilaginous layer, (b) osteogenic layer. Reprinted with permission [82] 2000 Elsevier.

8.4.2.2 *Osteochondral tissue*

The osteochondral tissue refers to the cartilage–bone interface having a biphasic structure. Composite scaffolds, particularly those with bilayer/biphasic architectures mimicking the native gradient structures of osteochondral tissues and offering varying microenvironments for chondrocytes and osteocytes, are promising for osteochondral tissue engineering [81]. In one study, a bilayer osteochondral composite scaffold consisting of one layer of PGA meshes (Fig. 8.8(a)) and one layer of porous PLGA/PEG blend (Fig. 8.8(b)) was formed and investigated [82]. The bilayer composite scaffold could support *in vitro* formation of well-defined cartilaginous and bone-like tissues by separately culturing chondrocytes and periosteal cells within respective layers, leading to glycosaminoglycan deposition and biomineralization, respectively, in the cartilaginous and bone-like regions. The biological properties of such bilayer/biphasic composite scaffolds in promoting bone-like tissue formation could be optimized by incorporating osteoconductive biomaterials such as HAp nanoparticles to form a nanocomposite layer [83]. To further enhance the tissue-inductive performance of specific layers, chondrogenic/osteogenic factors such as transforming growth factor-$\beta 3$ (TGF-$\beta 3$) and BMP-2 may be incorporated within the respective layers, resulting in bilayer composite scaffolds with improved bioactivity to induce distinct differentiations of MSCs toward a chondrolike or osteo-like phenotype and thereby exhibiting the potential for osteochondral tissue regeneration [84]. Recently, biphasic cell-laden constructs having GelMA hydrogel as the matrix, with osteogenic β-TCP and chondrogenic methacrylated HyAc (HAMA, derived from Streptococcus zooepidemicus) being incorporated in individual phases, were made and studied, which exhibited preserved viability of MSCs and upregulation on osteochondral phenotype [85]. Despite these advances and successes, there is still a long way to go for translational applications of osteochondral composite scaffolds, which have been limited by the spatiotemporally sophisticated biomechanics of the osteochondral tissue. The future direction of developing osteochondral composite scaffolds could involve producing/gaining precisely controlled hierarchical structures and even dynamically tunable mechanical properties [86].

8.4.2.3 *Cardiac Tissue*

The heart plays a vital role in human life. But it lacks sufficient self-renewal/self-repair capabilities after injuries or lesions. Myocardial infarction is a common disease caused by inadequate blood flow to the myocardium, which can cause various types of irreversible damage to the heart, including loss of cardiomyocytes, scar formation, cardiac tissue remodeling, and arrhythmias. Developing scaffolds/constructs to repair cardiac tissue with myocardial infarction is therefore of great importance and an urgent demand. Both scaffolds for cardiac tissue engineering and engineered cardiac constructs must be biocompatible (allowing attachment/growth of cells such as myocytes), mechanically stable (anti-fatigue, resistance to continuous contraction/relaxation), and electrically conductive (supporting the propagation of electrical impulses to maintain the synchronized contraction of myocardium) [28]. Composite scaffolds are desirable candidates as they can integrate multiple properties/functions to meet the comprehensive requirements of cardiac tissue engineering. Through reinforcement with an electrically conductive filler, graphene oxide (GO), a soft GO–hydrogel composite was made and assessed [87]. The composite scaffold for cardiac repair showed high conductivity ($2.84 \times 104\,\text{S/cm}$) and excellent resistance to fatigue, resulting in significant improvements in heart functions with myocardial infarction such as a distinct increase of ejection fraction and vessel density and reduced infarction and fibrosis areas. The underlying mechanism for the mediating effects of conductive constituents in composites on cardiomyocytes was studied via immunochemical staining and western blotting in a CNT-reinforced GelMA hydrogel composite [88]. The study showed that β1-integrin-mediated FAK and RhoA signaling pathways were responsible for mechano-electric transduction, contributing to cardiomyocyte adhesion and maturation. Based on the insights, different types of composites, e.g., collagen-hyaluronic acid-PAN composite hydrogels [89] and MXene-PEG composite scaffolds [32], that possessed tunable mechanical (slightly higher mechanical properties than the native myocardium) and electrical (comparable electrical conductivity to the native myocardium) properties have been investigated for cardiac tissue engineering, which showed excellent performance for treating hearts with myocardial infarction. Given the poor renewal ability of native cardiomyocytes and risky immune responses arising from allogeneic cells, the incorporation of human induced pluripotent stem cells (iPSCs) in composite scaffolds for directional induction of iPSCs and engineering cardiac-mimicking tissues *in vitro* to aid in the regeneration of cardiac tissues can be explored in the future [90].

8.4.2.4 *Neural tissue*

Composite scaffolds, particularly electroactive scaffolds formed by incorporating conductive constituents, have also shown promise in nerve tissue engineering due to the essential role of electrical signal propagation in the development of neural circuitry [91]. For example, a conductive nerve conduit was prepared based on compositing conductive poly N-vinylpyrrole (PNVPY) or poly(3-hexylthiophene) (P3HT) with a nanofibrous electrospun cellulose matrix through *in situ* polymerization [92]. The conductive PNVPY/P3HT coating layers were found to effectively promote the proliferation and neurite growth of neuronal cells, showing promise in neural tissue engineering. By combining a conductive neural conduit (i.e., polypyrrole/silk fibroin conductive composite scaffold) with electrical stimulation, the viability, proliferation, migration, and expression of neurotrophic factors of Schwann cells could be all upregulated via activating the MAPK signal transduction pathway [93]. The results suggest good potential for the conductive composite nerve conduits to repair and regenerate peripheral nerves. However, great challenges remain in developing and employing appropriate composite scaffolds for the repair and regeneration of the central nervous system.

8.4.2.5 *Other body tissues*

In addition to the aforementioned tissue engineering applications, porous composite scaffolds have also been used for the regeneration of many other body tissues. For example, composite scaffolds with conductive reinforcements have been studied and used for muscle tissue engineering in accordance with the electrically excitable nature of skeleton muscle cells [94]. Notably, the composite approach leads to multicomponent and multifunctional scaffolds. For example, nanofibrous and nanocomposite scaffolds have been produced via concurrent electrospinning (to obtain nanofibers) and electrospraying (for obtaining microspheres) [95]. In these scaffolds, highly branched theranostic nanoparticles were encapsulated in electrosprayed core-shell structured microspheres (Figure 8.9). The nanocomposite scaffold could support desirable cellular attachment and growth owing to its ECM-mimicking nanofibrous matrix architecture, thereby promoting *in situ* tissue regeneration by offering an appropriate structural platform. Meanwhile, through local delivery of the theranostic nanoparticles with well-preserved highly branched structures after the breakup of the encapsulating electrosprayed microspheres, the nanocomposite scaffolds could offer additional functions of targeting, detecting, and selective killing of cancer cells

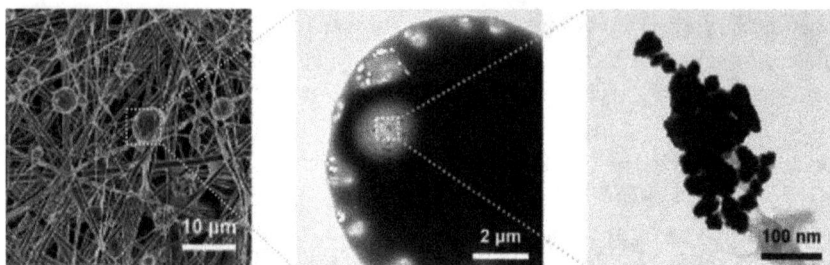

Figure 8.9. Multicomponent and multifunctional nanocomposite scaffolds with encapsulated theranostic nanoparticles. Reprinted with permission [95] 2023 John Wiley & Sons.

based on the folic acid-mediated ligand-receptor binding, surface-enhanced Raman scattering (SERS) activity, and near-infrared-responsive photothermal effect of the theranostic nanoparticles. The multiple functions make these nanocomposite scaffolds highly promising for post-operative cancer management that requires both tissue regeneration and cancer recurrence inhibition.

8.5   Concluding Remarks

Compared to mono-component biomaterials (polymers, metals, or ceramics), a biomaterial formed through the composite/hybridization approach by either combining multiple materials into one material or modifying one material with the use of other materials can offer enhanced performance or unique properties for human body tissue replacement or regeneration. Inspired by biological composites, a great number of biomedical composites with outstanding properties (physiochemical, mechanical, electrical, etc.) or multiple functions have been fabricated and studied. Many of these biomedical composites have a high potential for tissue replacement as substitutes/prostheses or for tissue regeneration as scaffolds. Nowadays, not constrained by conventional concepts for materials development, living organisms ranging from microorganisms to mammalian cells have been employed as elements for constructing living biomedical composites [96–98], opening new avenues for self-adaptive sensing and actuating biomedical composites for autonomous tasks in the physiological environments. There are still clear and sometimes large gaps in properties and functions between current biomedical composites and biological composites such as bone and teeth. Reconstituting or replicating the complex hierarchical architectures of biological composites is a formidable task that challenges the whole materials community and shapes perhaps the ultimate goal for developing biomedical composites of superior clinical performance. It should be noted that biological composites are formed or "grow" at ambient temperature and under atmospheric pressure. We should learn well from nature when developing new manufacturing techniques to produce high-performance biomedical composites in mild conditions or even in the human body environment. Owing to the complexities in structure and composition of new biomedical composites, more comprehensive and careful considerations should be taken for their biological performances prior to their clinical applications, ranging from cellular responses *in vitro* to long-term foreign body responses *in vivo*. On such a solid foundation, we can envision that biomedical composites will benefit patients and society greatly by addressing grand challenges in human body tissue replacement and regeneration.

Acknowledgments

Min Wang thanks the University of Hong Kong (HKU), Hong Kong's Research Grants Council (RGC), and China's National Natural Science Foundation of China (NSFC) for supporting his research in the biomaterials and tissue engineering field through various research grants. Qilong Zhao thanks the NSFC, the Youth Innovation Promotion Association of the Chinese Academy of Sciences (CAS), and the Natural Science Foundation of Guangdong Province for funding his research on biomaterials and tissue engineering.

References

[1] C. F. Guimarães, L. Gasperini, A. P. Marques, and R. L. Reis, The stiffness of living tissues and its implications for tissue engineering, *Nature Reviews Materials*, 2020, 5(5):351–370.

[2] T. S. Jay, Wolff's law (bone functional adaptation), in *The International Encyclopedia of Biological Anthropology*, eds. W. Trevathan, (Wiley, Berlin, 2018), ieba0521.

[3]   L. S. Nair and C. T. Laurencin, Biodegradable polymers as biomate-
      rials, *Progress in Polymer Science*, 2007, 32(8–9):762–798.
[4]   J. M. Bouler, P. Pilet, O. Gauthier, *et al.*, Biphasic calcium phosphate
      ceramics for bone reconstruction: A review of biological response,
      Acta Biomaterialia, 2017, 53:1–12.
[5]   P. Cai, B. Hu, W. R. Leow, *et al.*, Biomechano-interactive materials
      and interfaces, *Advanced Materials*, 2018, 30(31):1800572.
[6]   Y. Liu, D. Luo, and T. Wang, Hierarchical structures of bone and
      bioinspired bone tissue engineering, *Small*, 2016, 12(34):4611–4632.
[7]   G. L. Koons, M. Diba, and A. G. Mikos, Materials design for bone-
      tissue engineering, *Nature Reviews Materials*, 2020, 5(8):584–603.
[8]   L. J. Gibson, The hierarchical structure and mechanics of plant mate-
      rials, *Journal of the Royal Society Interface*, 2012, 9(76):2749–2766.
[9]   C. Chen, Y. Kuang, S. Zhu, et al., Structure–property–function rela-
      tionships of natural and engineered wood, *Nature Reviews Materials*,
      2020, 5(9):642–666.
[10] T. Li, C. Chen, A. H. Brozena, *et al.*, Developing fibrillated cellu-
      lose as a sustainable technological material, *Nature*, 2021, 590(7844):
      47–56.
[11] J. Song, C. Chen, S. Zhu, *et al.*, Processing bulk natural wood
      into a high-performance structural material, *Nature*, 2018, 554(7691):
      224–228.
[12] L. B. Mao, H. L. Gao, H. B. Yao, *et al.*, Synthetic nacre by pre-
      designed matrix-directed mineralization, *Science*, 2016, 354(6308):
      107–110.
[13] X. S. Meng, L. C. Zhou, L. Liu, *et al.*, Deformable hard tissue with
      high fatigue resistance in the hinge of bivalve Cristaria plicata, *Sci-
      ence*, 2023, 380(6651):1252–1257.
[14] M. Eder, S. Amini, and P. Fratzl, Biological composites-complex
      structures for functional diversity, *Science*, 2018, 362(6414):543–547.
[15] M. Wang and Q. Zhao, Biomedical composites. *Encyclopedia of
      Biomedical Engineering*. eds. R. Narayan (Elsevier, Amsterdam,
      2018), pp. 34–52.
[16] H. Zhang, L. Zhang, Z. Zhang, *et al.*, Unique bi-continuous phase
      structure can facilitate the development of fire-resistant surface,
      Chemical Engineering Journal, 2024, 479:147547.
[17] J. Steck, J. Kim, Y. Kutsovsky, *et al.*, Multiscale stress decon-
      centration amplifies fatigue resistance of rubber, *Nature*, 2023,
      624(7991):303–308.
[18] E. S. Place, J. H. George, C. K. Williams, *et al.*, Synthetic poly-
      mer scaffolds for tissue engineering, *Chemical Society Reviews*, 2009,
      38(4):1139–1151.

[19] W. Wang, J. Li, H. Liu, *et al.*, Advancing versatile ferroelectric materials toward biomedical applications, *Advanced Science*, 2020, 8(1):2003074.

[20] M. P. Lutolf and J. A. Hubbell, Synthetic biomaterials as instructive extracellular microenvironments for morphogenesis in tissue engineering, *Nature Biotechnology*, 2005, 23(1):47–55.

[21] Y. S. Zhang and A. Khademhosseini, Advances in engineering hydrogels, *Science*, 2017, 356(6337):eaaf3627.

[22] S. Correa, A. K. Grosskopf, H. Lopez Hernandez, *et al.*, Translational applications of hydrogels, *Chemical Reviews*, 2021, 121(18): 11385–11457.

[23] H. Yuk, J. Wu, X. and Zhao, Hydrogel interfaces for merging humans and machines, *Nature Reviews Materials*, 2022, 7(12):935–952.

[24] K. Yue, G. Trujillo-De Santiago, M. M. Alvarez, *et al.*, Synthesis, properties, and biomedical applications of gelatin methacryloyl (GelMA) hydrogels, *Biomaterials*, 2015, 73:254–271.

[25] A. M. Barradas, H. Yuan, J. Van Der Stok, *et al.*, The influence of genetic factors on the osteoinductive potential of calcium phosphate ceramics in mice, *Biomaterials*, 2012, 33(23):5696–5705.

[26] H. Yuk, T. Zhang, G. A. Parada, *et al.*, Skin-inspired hydrogel-elastomer hybrids with robust interfaces and functional microstructures. *Nature Communications*, 2016, 7:12028.

[27] S. Park, H. Yuk, R. Zhao, *et al.*. Adaptive and multifunctional hydrogel hybrid probes for long-term sensing and modulation of neural activity, *Nature Communications*, 2021, 12(1):3435.

[28] K. Ashtari, H. Nazari, H. Ko, *et al.*, Electrically conductive nanomaterials for cardiac tissue engineering, *Advanced Drug Delivery Reviews*, 2019, 144:162–179.

[29] B. Guo, and P. X. Ma., Conducting polymers for tissue engineering, *Biomacromolecules*, 2018, 19(6):1764–1782.

[30] W. Zhang, A. A. Dehghani-Sanij, R. S. Blackburn, Carbon based conductive polymer composites, *Journal of Materials Science*, 2007, 42(10):3408–3418.

[31] T. Nezakati, A. Seifalian, A. Tan, *et al.*, Conductive polymers: Opportunities and challenges in biomedical applications, *Chemical Reviews*, 2018, 118(14):6766–6843.

[32] G. Basara, M. Saeidi-Javash, X. Ren, *et al.*, Electrically conductive 3D printed Ti3C2T MXene-PEG composite constructs for cardiac tissue engineering, *Acta Biomaterialia*, 2022, 139:179–189.

[33] Y. J. Xie, C. A. S. Hill, Z. F. Xiao, *et al.*, Silane coupling agents used for natural fiber/polymer composites: A review, *Composites Part A-Applied Science and Manufacturing*, 2010, 41(7):806–819.

[34] M. C. Watson and T. W. Clyne, Reaction-induced changes in interfacial and macroscopic mechanical-properties of SiC monofilament-reinforced titanium, *Composites*, 1993, 24(3):222–228.

[35] Y. Arima and H. Iwata, Effect of wettability and surface functional groups on protein adsorption and cell adhesion using well-defined mixed self-assembled monolayers, *Biomaterials*, 2007, 28(20): 3074–3082.

[36] S. Nam, and D. Mooney, Polymeric tissue adhesives, *Chemical Reviews*, 2021, 121(18):11336–11384.

[37] M. Munro, Review of manufacturing of fiber composite components by filament winding, *Polymer Composites*, 2004, 9(5):352–359.

[38] A. M. Fairuz S. M. Sapuan, E. S. Zainudin, *et al.*, Polymer composite manufacturing using a pultrusion process: A review, *American Journal of Applied Sciences*, 2014, 11(10):1798–1810.

[39] X. Lu, C. Wang, and Y. Wei, One-dimensional composite nanomaterials: Synthesis by electrospinning and their applications, *Small*, 2009, 5(21):2349–2370.

[40] S. J. Hollister, Porous scaffold design for tissue engineering, *Nature Materials*, 2005, 4(7):518–524.

[41] K. Rezwan, Q. Z. Chen, J. J. Blaker, *et al.*, Biodegradable and bioactive porous polymer/inorganic composite scaffolds for bone tissue engineering. Biomaterials, 2006, 27(18):3413–3431.

[42] J. H. Lai, C. Wang, M. Wang, 3D printing in biomedical engineering: Processes, materials, and applications, *Applied Physics Reviews*, 2021, 8(2):021322.

[43] J. Li, M. Wang, Fabrication and evaluation of multiwalled carbon nanotube-containing bijels and bijels-derived porous nanocomposites, Langmuir, 2023, 39(4):1434–1443.

[44] W. Bonfield, Composites for bone replacement, *Journal of Biomedical Engineering*, 1988, 10(6):522–526.

[45] M. Wang, P. Porter, W. Bonfield, Processing, characterisation, and evaluation of hydroxyapatite reinforced polyethylene composites, *British Ceramic Transactions*, 1994, 93:91–95.

[46] M. Wang, Developing bioactive composite materials for tissue replacement, *Biomaterials*, 2003, 24(13):2133–2151.

[47] Y. Liu, M. Wang, Fabrication and characteristics of hydroxyapatite reinforced polypropylene as a bone analogue biomaterial, *Journal of Applied Polymer Science*, 2007, 106(4):2780–2790.

[48] L. J. Chen, M. Wang, Production and evaluation of biodegradable composites based on PHB-PHV copolymer, *Biomaterials*, 2002, 23(13):2631–2639.

[49] F. Witte, F. Feyerabend, P. Maier, *et al.* Biodegradable magnesium-hydroxyapatite metal matrix composites, *Biomaterials*, 2007, 28(13):2163–2174.

[50] Y. W. Gu, K. A. Khor, and P. Cheang. *In vitro* studies of plasma-sprayed hydroxyapatite/Ti-6Al-4V composite coatings in simulated body fluid (SBF). *Biomaterials*, 2003, 24(9):1603–1611.

[51] Y. M. Kong, C. J. Bae, S. H. Lee, *et al.* Improvement in biocompatibility of ZrO2-Al2O3 nano-composite by addition of HA, *Biomaterials*, 2005, 26(5):509–517.

[52] U. Pallesen and V. Qvist. Composite resin fillings and inlays, An 11-year evaluation, *Clinical Oral Investigations*, 2003, 7(2):71–79.

[53] H. Fouad, A. I. Mourad, A. L. Ba, *et al.* Fracture toughness, vibration modal analysis and viscoelastic behavior of Kevlar, glass, and carbon fiber/epoxy composites for dental-post applications, *Journal of the Mechanical Behavior of Biomedical Materials*, 2020, 101:103456.

[54] H. Le Ferrand, F. Bouville, T. P. Niebel, *et al.*, Magnetically assisted slip casting of bioinspired heterogeneous composites, *Nature Materials*, 2015, 14(11):1172–1179.

[55] C. Shao, B. Jin, Z. Mu, *et al.* Repair of tooth enamel by a biomimetic mineralization frontier ensuring epitaxial growth, *Science Advances*, 2019, 5(8):eaaw9569.

[56] J. H. Alexander and P. K. Smith. Coronary-artery bypass grafting, *The New England Journal of Medicine*, 2016, 374(20):1954–1964.

[57] L. E. Niklason and J. H. Lawson. Bioengineered human blood vessels, *Science*, 2020, 370(6513):eaaw8682.

[58] A. W. Zia, R. Liu, X. Wu. Structural design and mechanical performance of composite vascular grafts, *Bio-Design and Manufacturing*, 2022, 5(4):757–785.

[59] H. Kuang, Y. Wang, Y. Shi, *et al.*, Construction and performance evaluation of Hep/silk-PLCL composite nanofiber small-caliber artificial blood vessel graft, *Biomaterials*, 2020, 259:120288.

[60] T. Jungst, I. Pennings, M. Schmitz, *et al.*, Heterotypic scaffold design orchestrates primary cell organization and phenotypes in cocultured small diameter vascular grafts, *Advanced Functional Materials*, 2019, 29(24):1905987.

[61] S. Cheng, C. Hang, L. Ding, *et al.* Electronic blood vessel, *Matter*, 2020, 3(5):1664–1684.

[62] R. Langer and J. P. Vacanti, Tissue engineering, *Science*, 1993, 260(5110):920–926.

[63] L. G. Griffith and G. Naughton. Tissue engineering — current challenges and expanding opportunities, *Science*, 2002, 295(5557): 1009–1014.

[64]   Y. Chen, A. F. Mak, J. Li, *et al.,* Formation of apatite on poly(alpha-hydroxy acid) in an accelerated biomimetic process, *Journal of Biomedical Materials Research Part B: Applied Biomaterials,* 2005, 73(1):68–76.

[65]   Y. Chen, A. F. T. Mak, M. Wang, *et al.,* PLLA scaffolds with biomimetic apatite coating and biomimetic apatite/collagen composite coating to enhance osteoblast-like cells attachment and activity, *Surface and Coatings Technology,* 2006, 201(3–4):575–580.

[66]   Y. Chen, M. R. Cho, A. F. Mak, *et al.,* Morphology and adhesion of mesenchymal stem cells on PLLA, apatite and apatite/collagen surfaces, *Journal of Materials Science: Materials in Medicine,* 2008, 19(7):2563–2567.

[67]   N. Sultana and M. Wang, Fabrication of HA/PHBV composite scaffolds through the emulsion freezing/freeze-drying process and characterisation of the scaffolds, *Journal of Materials Science: Materials in Medicine,* 2008, 19(7):2555–2561.

[68]   H. W. Tong, M. Wang, Z. Y. Li, *et al.* Electrospinning, characterization and *in vitro* biological evaluation of nanocomposite fibers containing carbonated hydroxyapatite nanoparticles, *Biomedical Materials,* 2010, 5(5):054111.

[69]   C. Wang and M. Wang. Electrospun multicomponent and multifunctional nanofibrous bone tissue engineering scaffolds, *Journal of Materials Chemistry B,* 2017, 5(7):1388–1399.

[70]   Y. Zhou, Q. Zhao, and M. Wang. Dual release of VEGF and PDGF from emulsion electrospun bilayer scaffolds consisting of orthogonally aligned nanofibers for gastrointestinal tract regeneration, *MRS Communications,* 2019, 9(03):1098–1104.

[71]   Q. Zhao and M. Wang. Manipulating the release of growth factors from biodegradable microspheres for potentially different therapeutic effects by using two different electrospray techniques for microsphere fabrication, *Polymer Degradation And Stability,* 2019, 162: 169–179.

[72]   Q. Zhao, W. W. Lu and M. Wang. Modulating the release of vascular endothelial growth factor by negative-voltage emulsion electrospinning for improved vascular regeneration, Materials Letters, 2017, 193:1–4.

[73]   C. Wang, W. W. Lu, and M. Wang. Multifunctional fibrous scaffolds for bone regeneration with enhanced vascularization, *Journal of Materials Chemistry B,* 2020, 8(4):636–647.

[74]   C. Wang, W. Huang, Y. Zhou, *et al.,* 3D printing of bone tissue engineering scaffolds, *Bioactive Materials,* 2020, 5(1): 82–91.

[75]   B. Duan, M. Wang, W. Y. Zhou, *et al.,* Synthesis of Ca-P nanoparticles and fabrication of Ca–P/PHBV nanocomposite microspheres for

bone tissue engineering applications, *Applied Surface Science*, 2008, 255(2):529–533.

[76] B. Duan, M. Wang, W. Y. Zhou, *et al.*, Three-dimensional nanocomposite scaffolds fabricated via selective laser sintering for bone tissue engineering, *Acta Biomaterialia*, 2010, 6(12):4495–4505.

[77] C. Wang, Q. Zhao and M. Wang. Cryogenic 3D printing for producing hierarchical porous and rhBMP-2-loaded Ca-P/PLLA nanocomposite scaffolds for bone tissue engineering, *Biofabrication*, 2017, 9(2):025031.

[78] C. Wang, X. Ye, Y. Zhao, *et al.*, Cryogenic 3D printing of porous scaffolds for *in situ* delivery of 2D black phosphorus nanosheets, doxorubicin hydrochloride and osteogenic peptide for treating tumor resection-induced bone defects, *Biofabrication*, 2020, 12(3):035004.

[79] M. Zhang, R. Lin, X. Wang, *et al.*, 3D printing of Haversian bone-mimicking scaffolds for multicellular delivery in bone regeneration, *Science Advances*, 2020, 6(12):eaaz6725.

[80] C. Wang, H. Yue, J. Liu, *et al.*, Advanced reconfigurable scaffolds fabricated by 4D printing for treating critical-size bone defects of irregular shapes, Biofabrication, 2020, 12(4):045025.

[81] Y. Liu, G. Zhou, and Y. Cao, Recent progress in cartilage tissue engineering—our experience and future directions, *Engineering*, 2017, 3(1):28–35.

[82] D. Schaefer, I. Martin, P. Shastri, *et al.*, *In vitro* generation of osteochondral composites, *Biomaterials*, 2000, 21(24):2599–2606.

[83] X. Liang, P. Duan, J. Gao, *et al.*, Bilayered PLGA/PLGA-HAp composite scaffold for osteochondral tissue engineering and tissue regeneration, *ACS Biomaterials Science & Engineering*, 2018, 4(10): 3506–3521.

[84] J. Lee, S. Lee, S. J. Huh, *et al.* Directed regeneration of osteochondral tissue by hierarchical assembly of spatially organized composite spheroids, *Advanced Science*, 2021, 9(3):2103525.

[85] M. L. Bedell, A. L. Torres, K. J. Hogan, *et al.*, Human gelatin-based composite hydrogels for osteochondral tissue engineering and their adaptation into bioinks for extrusion, inkjet, and digital light processing bioprinting, *Biofabrication*, 2022, 14(4):045012.

[86] W. Wei and H. Dai, Articular cartilage and osteochondral tissue engineering techniques: Recent advances and challenges, *Bioactive Materials*, 2021, 6(12):4830–4855.

[87] R. Bao, B. Tan, S. Liang, *et al.* A π-π conjugation-containing soft and conductive injectable polymer hydrogel highly efficiently rebuilds cardiac function after myocardial infarction, *Biomaterials*, 2017, 122: 63–71.

[88] H. Sun, J. Tang, Y. Mou, *et al.*, Carbon nanotube-composite hydrogels promote intercalated disc assembly in engineered cardiac tissues through β1-integrin mediated FAK and RhoA pathway, *Acta Biomaterialia*, 2017, 48:88–99.

[89] K. Roshanbinfar, L. Vogt, F. Ruther, *et al.*, Nanofibrous composite with tailorable electrical and mechanical properties for cardiac tissue engineering, *Advanced Functional Materials*, 2019, 30(7):1908612.

[90] S. Cho, D. E. Discher, K. W. Leong, *et al.* Challenges and opportunities for the next generation of cardiovascular tissue engineering, *Nature Methods*, 2022, 19(9):1064–1071.

[91] L. I. Zhang, M. M. Poo. Electrical activity and development of neural circuits. *Nature Neuroscience*, 2001, 4 Suppl: 1207–1214.

[92] F. Zha, W. Chen, L. Hao, *et al.*, Electrospun cellulose-based conductive polymer nanofibrous mats: Composite scaffolds and their influence on cell behavior with electrical stimulation for nerve tissue engineering, *Soft Matter*, 2020, 16(28):6591–6598.

[93] Y. Zhao, Y. Liang, S. Ding, *et al.*, Application of conductive PPy/SF composite scaffold and electrical stimulation for neural tissue engineering, *Biomaterials*, 2020, 255:120164.

[94] R. Dong, P. X. Ma and B. Guo. Conductive biomaterials for muscle tissue engineering, *Biomaterials*, 2020, 229:119584.

[95] L. Guo, Q. Zhao, L. W. Zheng, *et al.*, Multifunctional nanofibrous scaffolds capable of localized delivery of theranostic nanoparticles for postoperative cancer management, *Advanced Healthcare Materials*, 2023, 12(32):2302484.

[96] L. K. Rivera-Tarazona, V. D. Bhat, H. Kim, *et al.* Shape-morphing living composites, *Science Advances*, 2020, 6(3):eaax8582.

[97] M. Y. Rotenberg, N. Yamamoto, E. N. Schaumann, *et al.*, Living myofibroblast-silicon composites for probing electrical coupling in cardiac systems, *Proceedings of the National Academy of Sciences of the United States of America*, 2019, 116(45):22531–22539.

[98] R. M. Mcbee, M. Lucht, N. Mukhitov, *et al.*, Engineering living and regenerative fungal-bacterial biocomposite structures, *Nature Materials*, 2022, 21(4):471–478.

Chapter 9

Composites in Biomedical Applications

Zheng-Ming Huang[*,‡] **and S. Ramakrishna**[†,§]

*School of Aerospace Engineering & Applied Mechanics, Tongji University,
1239 Siping Road, Shanghai 200092, P. R. China
†Department of Mechanical Engineering, National University of Singapore,
10 Kent Ridge Crescent, Singapore 119260, Singapore
‡huangzm@tongji.edu.cn
§seeram@nus.edu.sg*

Composites are materials that contain two or more distinct constituent phases on a scale larger than that of atomic. Compared with traditional homogeneous materials such as metals, ceramics, and polymers, the main advantage of composites is that their mechanical, biological, and other physical properties can be tailored to the requirements of specific applications. This chapter focuses on composites that are suitable for biomedical applications. Various application practices documented in the literature have been summarized in this chapter. Some of the commonly used methods for composite fabrications are introduced. Attention has been given to the mechanics of composites: a study which aims at estimating the mechanical properties of different composites using only the material parameters and geometric information of their constituents. Some future trends are also given at the end of this chapter.

Abbreviations

Acronym	Meaning
BIS–GMA	bis-phenol A glycidyl methacrylate
C	Carbon
CF	Carbon fibers
GF	Glass fibers
HA	Hydroxyapatite
HDPE	High-density polyethylene
KF	Kevlar fiber
LCP	Liquid crystalline polymer
LDPE	Low-density polyethylene
MMA	Methylmethacrylate
PA	Polyacetal
PBT	Polybutylene terephthalate
PC	Polycarbonate
PCL	Polycaprolactone
PE	Polyethylene
PEA	Polyethylacrylate
PEEK	Polyetheretherketone
PEG	Polyethylene glycol
PELA	Block copolymer of lactic acid and polyethylene glycol
PET	Polyethylene terephthalate
PGA	Polyglycolic acid
PHB	Polyhydroxybutyrate
PHEMA	Poly(HEMA) or Poly(2–hydroxyethyl methacrylate)
PLA	Polylactic acid
PLDLA	Poly L–DL–lactide
PLLA	Poly(L–lactic acid)
PMA	Polymethylacrylate
PMMA	Polymethylmethacrylate
Polyglactin	Copolymer of PLA and PGA
PP	Polypropylene
PS	Polysulfone
PTFE	Polytetrafluroethylene

Acronym	Meaning
PU	Polyurethane
PVC	Polyvinylchloride
SR	Silicone rubber
THFM	Tetrahydrofurfuryl methacrylate
UHMWPE	Ultra-high molecular weight polyethylene

9.1　Introduction

A composite material considered in this chapter is a physical mixture of two or more distinct constituents. It has radically different properties from those of each constituent. Except for some interfacial reactions to ensure good bonding, no chemical reactions or any alloying exists between the constituents in a composite. Though a composite can be made of two or more constituents, in most cases, the composite comprises only two constituents: the matrix phase and the reinforcing one. The matrix phase is continuous and provides the overall form. A reinforcing phase, such as fibers or particulates, is generally stronger than the matrix. Biocomposites are a special form of composites which can be used in biomedical applications, either inside or in contact with the human body. A key advantage of composites over monolithic materials is that the material properties of the composites can be tailored according to different requirements in the mechanical, chemical, biological, and other physical aspects. This is achieved by altering the composition, interfacial bonding, and physical arrangement of the constituent phases in the composites.

The composites in common use can be classified based on either the reinforcing or the matrix phase. For the classification based on the reinforcing phase, there are mainly three kinds of reinforcements: continuous fibers, short or chopped fibers, and particulates, which are roughly classified as follows:

- A continuous fiber has an aspect ratio (the ratio of its length over its diameter) generally greater than 10^5 — the resulting composites are called continuous fiber reinforced composites.

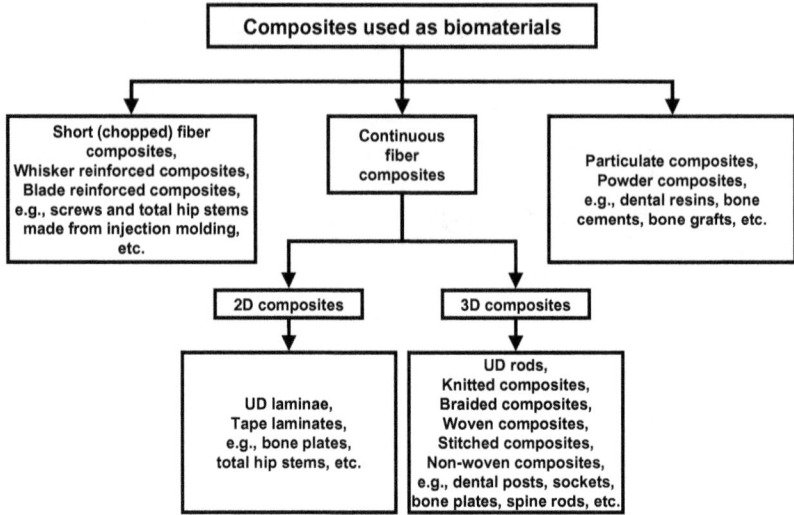

Figure 9.1.   Classification of composites based on reinforcing phase.

- Short or chopped fibers have an aspect ratio of between 5 and 200 (included in this category are whiskers and blades also) — the resulting composites are called short (chopped) fiber reinforced composites.
- Particulates or powders have an aspect ratio from less than 1 to about 2 — the resulting composites are called particulate-reinforced composites.

Rigorous definitions for the three kinds of composites are given later, see Figure 9.13.

These three kinds of composites together with their biomedical application examples are summarized in Figure 9.1. Note that among various kinds of continuous fiber composites, a unidirectional (UD) fiber-reinforced composite is fundamental. This composite, which is abbreviated as UD composite, is fabricated by arranging all the fibers in the same direction.

Besides the classification by the reinforcing phase, composites can also be classified according to the matrix materials used. For example, monolithic metals, ceramics, and polymers can be used as matrix materials. The resulting composites are then named as metal matrix composites, ceramic matrix composites, and polymer matrix composites. As most composites in biomedical applications are polymer matrix composites, this chapter focuses only on this type of composite.

Polymers can be either thermoset or thermoplastic, according to their thermal behaviors. A thermoplastic polymer can be molten at high temperatures and solidified at low temperatures many times. Hence, a thermoplastic composite can be reshaped to some extent after its fabrication. On the other hand, a thermoset polymer cannot be molten at high temperatures. Hence, a thermoset composite, once it is made, cannot be reshaped without destroying its structure.

Apart from categorization by thermal behaviors, polymer matrix composites can also be grouped by their biodegradable property. A biodegradable material is one that can be absorbed by the human body once it is implanted within the body. If both the polymer matrix phase and the reinforcing phase (such as fiber) are biodegradable, the resulting composite is called a fully resorbable composite. If only the polymer matrix is biodegradable but the reinforcing phase is not, the resulting composite is partially resorbable. A non-resorbable composite is one where all of its constituent substances are not biodegradable.

To date, the majority of biomedical devices used either as implants in the human body or as external prostheses are made of biocompatible homogeneous materials, such as metals, ceramics, or polymers. However, there are recognized limitations in these monolithic material devices. For example, though most implants in orthopedic surgery are made of metals, their drawbacks include the following:

(1) They are too stiff such that stress protection of the fractured bone can occur during healing [1].
(2) Considerable artifacts are produced under X-ray, which makes the interpretation of radiographs difficult [2].
(3) Metal sensitization can occur and the implants may cause mutagenicity.

In contrast, these drawbacks can be overcome if implants were made of polymer matrix composites. Moreover, biodegradable implants can be developed based on composite technology, which no longer needs a second operation to remove the implants once they are fixed into host tissues [3]. This unique feature is not presented in any metal implant.

Composite materials can offer numerous advantages over the traditional homogeneous materials in biomedical applications. As such, a fundamental knowledge of composite materials is necessary for the development of biomaterials as well as for the design of medical devices. The purpose of this chapter is to provide an introductory description on composite theory, fabrication, characterization, the potential in biomedical applications, as well as an outlook on future advances.

9.2   Biomedical Applications

As aforementioned, a biomedical device can be an external prosthesis or an implant used within the human body. An implant then needs to be in contact with host tissues. The human tissues can be categorized as hard and soft tissues. Only bones, teeth, and cartilages are hard tissues [4]. All other tissues are of the soft category. In this respect, the biomedical applications of composites can be grouped into those for hard tissues and some others for soft tissues. A schematic show of various possible composite biomaterials in the human body is given in Figure 9.2. Following this, some medical devices (such as bone plates, dental materials, and vascular grafts) are discussed in more detail.

9.2.1   *Bone Plates*

The majority of composites used in biomedical applications are targeted for bone-repairing purposes. Bone constitutes the skeleton of a human being and sustains all kinds of loads including gravity applied to the human body. Therefore, bone can be easily injured under an external load. There are many types of bone fractures depending on the crack size, orientation, morphology, and location, which have to be treated in different ways. In general, medical devices are necessary to fix the fractured bone for proper healing. The most commonly used such devices are the bone plates.

Bone plates, also known as osteosynthesis plates, are conventionally made of stainless steel, Cr–Co, and Ti alloys. The rigid fixation is designed to provide high axial pressures (also known as dynamic compression) in the fragments of the bone, in order to facilitate primary bone healing without the formation of external callus. A secondary operation is generally required to remove the plate once the bone

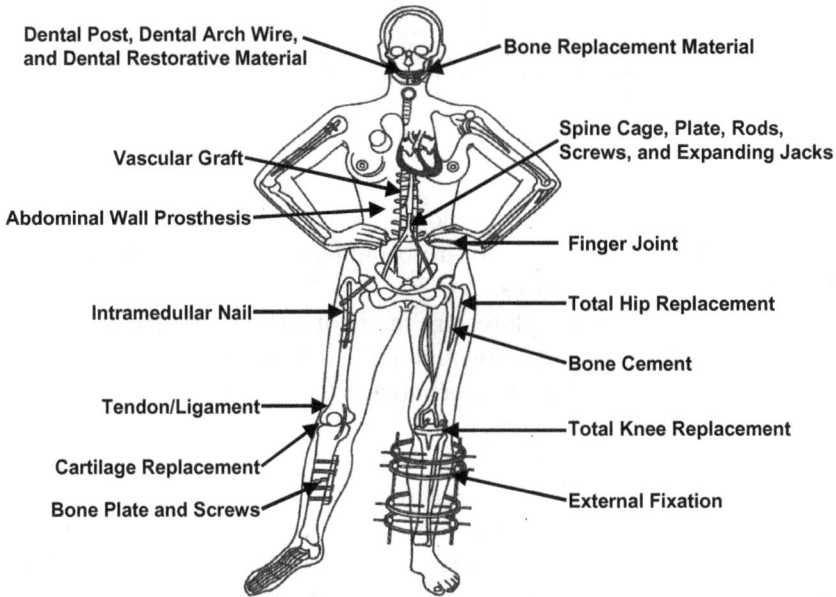

Figure 9.2. Medical devices which can be fabricated using composites.

healing is completed, which may take one to two years. However, the high rigidity of the metal plate fixation can result in bone atrophy. The bone underneath the plate adapts to the low stress and becomes less dense and weak. Due to bone atrophy, there is a possibility of bone refractures after the plate is removed. This is recognized as the "stress shielding" effect. It may be noted that the modulus of stainless steel $(210-230\,\mathrm{GPa})$ is much higher than the 10–$18\,\mathrm{GPa}$ modulus of the bone. In the plate and the fractured bone system, the amount of stress carried by each of them is directly related to its stiffness. Thus, bone is insufficiently loaded compared to the implanted plate, resulting in "stress-shielding" or stress protection. Many investigators [5–7] have shown that the degree of stress protection is proportional to the degree of stiffness mismatch. This suggests that 'less rigid fixation plates' diminish the stress-shielding problem and that it is desirable to use plates whose stiffness is close to that of the bone. However, low stiffness should not be accompanied with low fatigue strength, since the plate/bone system will have to sustain severe cyclic loading while the bone is healing. Polymer composite materials offer the desired high strength and bone-like elastic properties and

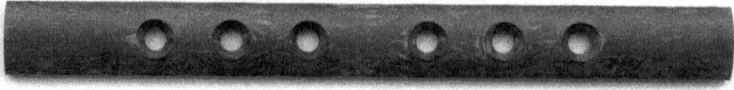

Figure 9.3.   A composite bone plate.

hence have been proposed for bone plate applications (Figure 9.3). They may be grouped into non-resorbable, partially resorbable, and fully resorbable bone plates.

Non-resorbable bone plates are made of either thermoset or thermoplastic polymer composite materials. CF/epoxy and GF/epoxy are a few examples of non-resorbable thermoset composites [8–10]. However, there is a concern over the toxic effects of monomers in partially cured epoxy composite materials [11, 12]. Thermoplastic composite bone plates using carbon fibers and various polymer matrix materials have been made available, including CF/PMMA, CF/PP, CF/PS, CF/PE, CF/nylon, CF/PBT, and CF/PEEK [13]. Among them, the CF/PEEK material system has shown promising characteristics [14]. Unlike thermoset composites, thermoplastic composites are considered free from the complications associated with unused monomers. Moreover, like a metal alloy plate, a thermoplastic composite plate can be bent or contoured to the shape of the bone at the time of surgery.

As the bone healing progresses, it is desirable that the bone be subjected to gradual increase of stress, thus reducing the stress-shielding effect. In other words, the stress on the plate should decrease with time, whereas the stress on the bone should increase. This is possible only if the plate loses rigidity gradually in the body environment. The non-resorbable polymer composites do not display this desired characteristic. To meet this need, resorbable polymer composites have been introduced for bone plate applications. Polymers such as poly(lactic acid) (PLA) and poly(glycolic acid) (PGA) resorb or degrade upon implantation into the human body. Many bioresorbable polymers are found to loose most of their mechanical properties in a few weeks. Tormala *et al.* [3] and Choueka *et al.* [15] proposed fully resorbable composites by reinforcing resorbable matrices with resorbable fibers, such as poly(L–lactic acid) (PLLA) fibers. One of the advantages often cited for resorbable composite prostheses is that they need not be removed with a second operative procedure, as is recommended with metallic or non-resorbable composite implants. However, the low mechanical property of resorbable materials remains a drawback, and hence they are only limited to applications where the loads are moderate.

To improve the mechanical properties, resorbable polymers are reinforced with a variety of non-resorbable materials, including carbon fibers [16–18] and polyamide fibers. Due to the non-resorbable nature of reinforcements used, these composites are called partially resorbable composites. According to Zimmerman *et al.* [16], CF/PLA composites possessed superior mechanical properties before implantation. However, they lost mechanical properties too rapidly in the human body because of delamination.

9.2.2 *Intramedullary Nails*

Intramedullary nails or rods are mainly used to fix long bone fractures. It is inserted into the intramedullary cavity of the bone and fixed in position using screws or friction fit method (Figure 9.2). The insertion often requires reaming of the medullary canal and can affect intramedullary blood vessels and nutrient arteries. The nail must have sufficient strength to carry the weight of the patient without bending in either flexure or torsion and should not completely disrupt the blood supply. Stainless steel is one of the widely used materials in intramedullary nails. Researchers have attempted to make composite nails. Lin *et al.* [19] developed short GF/PEEK composite material for intramedullary applications, whereas Kettunen *et al.* [20] made an intramedullary rod from a unidirectional carbon fiber-reinforced liquid crystalline (Vectra, A950) polymer composite. It was reported that the non-resorbable composite nails were biologically inert with good flexural strength and elastic modulus close to the bone.

To date, the most successful applications of fully bioresorbable implants are in the form of pins, rods, and screws [21]. Most implants are manufactured from hydroxy fatty acids, such as PGA (polyglycolic acid), PLA (polylactic acid), and copolymers, with a self-reinforcing technique in which oriented filaments are used as a scaffold for the matrix of the same chemical structure to produce strong implants [22,23]. Due to their modest mechanical properties, these implants were restricted to low-stress applications in cancellous bone, mainly in the small fracture regions of the ankle and foot, knee, elbow, wrist, and hand [24]. These biodegradable devices have a key advantage in that they dissolve during implantation. Hence, this advantage obviates the need for a second operation to remove the biodegradable implants. However, a new type of infectious complication, the sterile sinus formation, has been observed. Santavirta *et al.* [25] reported an incidence of this aseptic inflammatory response that varies from 3% in Chevron osteotomies to 22% in distal radius fractures. Bostman *et al.* [26] conducted another survey and found that out of 216 patients with malleolar fractures, 24 developed a transient local inflammatory reaction with a painful erythematous fluctuant swelling. The average postoperative period in these studies was three months.

9.2.3 *Spine Instrumentation*

Spine is a linked structure consisting of 33 vertebrae superimposed one on another. The vertebrae are separated by fibrocartilaginous intervertebral discs (IVD) and are united by articular capsules and ligaments. Spine disorders commonly include metastasis of the vertebral body and disc, disc herniation, facet degeneration, stenosis, and structural abnormalities, such as kyphosis, scoliosis, and spondylolistheses. These disorders are caused by various reasons, such as birth deformities, aging, tumorous lesions (metastasis), and mechanical loads induced by work and sports.

When the spine defect is limited to some vertebrae, alternative treatments such as spinal fusion and disc replacement are used. Ignatius *et al.* [27] and Claes *et al.* [28] developed Bioglass/PU composite material for vertebral body replacement, whereas Marcolongo *et al.* [29] proposed Bioglass/PS composite material for bone grafting purposes. Preliminary experiments indicated that these materials are bioactive and that they facilitate direct bone bonding (osseous integration). Brantigan *et al.* [30] and Ciappetta *et al.* [31] developed CF/PEEK and CF/PS composite cages for lumbar interbody fusion. The composite cage has an elastic modulus close to that of the bone, thus eliciting maximum bone growth into the cage. The composite cages are radiolucent and hence do not hinder radiographic evaluation of bone fusion. Moreover, they produce fewer artifacts on CT images than other implants constructed of metal alloys. Researchers also developed CF/PEEK and CF/PS [7] composite plates and screws for stabilizing the replacement body and spine. Flexural and fatigue properties of CF/PEEK composites are comparable to those of stainless steel, which is normally used for spine plates and screws.

Problems related to intervertebral discs are treated by replacing the affected nucleus with a substitute material or by replacing the total disc (nucleus and annulus) with an artificial disc [32]. A variety of materials such as stainless steel, Co–Cr alloy, PE, SR, PU, PET/SR [33,34], and PET/hydrogel [35] composites have been proposed for disc prostheses — either being utilized alone or in combinations. However, their performance has not yet been acceptable for long-term applications. To date, no artificial disc is able to reproduce the unique mechanical and transport behaviors of natural disc satisfactorily.

Structural abnormalities or curvatures (lordosis, kyphosis, and spondylolistheses) of the spine are corrected using either external or internal fixations. Splints and casts form the external fixation devices. The internal fixations require surgery, and many types of instrumentation (screws, plates, rods, and expanding jacks) are available [36]. In some cases, an adjustable stainless steel rod — also known as the Harrington spinal distraction rod — is used to stabilize or straighten the curvature. Schmitt-Thomas *et al.* [37] made initial attempts to develop a polymer composite rod using unidirectional and braided carbon fibers and biocompatible epoxy resin. The main motivation for this work was to overcome the problems of metal alloys such as corrosion and interference with the diagnostic techniques. To date, specific mechanical and physical properties required for ideal spine instrumentation have not yet been attained.

9.2.4 *Total Hip Replacement (THR)*

Joints enable the movement of the body and its parts. THR is the most common artificial joint in human beings. For example, over 150,000 THRs are conducted each year in the USA alone. A typical THR consists of a cup-type acetabular component and a femoral component (also called the femoral stem). The latter's head is designed to fit into the acetabular cup and enables joint articulations. Conventional THRs use stainless steel, Co–Cr, and Ti alloys for the femoral stem. Acetabular cups are often made of

UHMWPE. Although the short-term function of UHMWPE acetabular cups is satisfactory, their long-term performance has been a concern for many years. To improve creep resistance, stiffness, and strength, researchers proposed reinforcing UHMWPE with carbon fibers [38] or UHMWPE fibers [39]. Deng and Shalaby [39] found no appreciable difference in wear properties of reinforced and unreinforced UHMWPE. However, the effect of carbon fibers on the wear characteristics of UHMWPE is a controversial subject because of the negatively opposite results reported in the literature.

Although metal THRs are used widely, one of the major unsolved problems is the mismatch between the stiffness of the femur bone and that of the prosthesis. It has been acknowledged that metallic stems, due to stiffness mismatch, induce unphysiological stresses in the bone and hence lead to bone resorption and eventual aseptic loosening of the prosthesis. This may cause severe pain and clinical failure, thus necessitating a repeat surgery. Gese *et al.* [40] demonstrated that Ti alloy stems result in a 50% reduction in the femur peak stress compared to the Co–Cr alloy stem. This suggests that implant loosening and eventual failure could be reduced through improvement in the prosthesis design and the use of a less stiff material with mechanical properties close to those of bone. Researchers introduced CF/PS [41] and CF/C [42] composite stems. They reported faster bone bonding in the case of composite implants as compared to high-stiffness conventional implants. The composite stems were found to be stable with no release of soluble compounds and also favorably possessing high static and fatigue strengths. Chang *et al.* [43] proposed CF/epoxy stems by laminating 120 layers of unidirectional plies in a predetermined orientation and stacking sequence. Simoes *et al.* [44] made composite stems using braided hybrid carbon–glass fiber preforms and epoxy resin. Some researchers [45–47] also designed CF/PEEK composite stems (Figure 9.4) through injection molding, which exhibit a mechanical behavior similar to that of the femur. Animal studies indicated that CF/PEEK composite elicits minimal response from muscular tissue.

9.2.5   *Bone Grafts*

Synthetic bone grafts are necessary to fill bone defects or replace fractured bones. The bone graft material must be sufficiently strong and

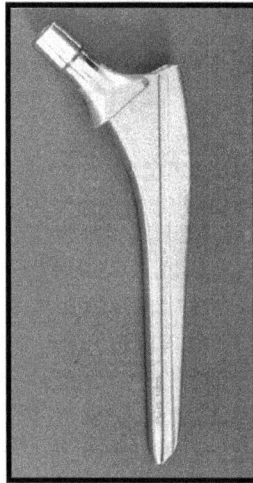

Figure 9.4. A total hip replacement stem made of CF/PEEK composite.

stiff and also capable of bonding to the residual bones. PE is considered biocompatible from its satisfactory utilization in hip and knee joint replacements for many years. However, its stiffness and strength are much lower than those of the bone. To improve the mechanical properties, bioactive HA particulates have been used to reinforce PE. The resulting composite has an elastic modulus of 1–8 GPa and a strain-to-failure value from over 90% to 3% as the volume fraction of HA increases from 0% to 50%. It was reported that when the HA particulate volume fraction is above 40%, the composite becomes brittle. Moreover, the bioactivity of the composite is less than optimal because the surface area of HA available is low and the bonding rate between bone and HA is slow. To increase the interface between HA particles and the bone tissues, some researchers developed partially resorbable composites. They reinforced resorbable polymers such as PEG, PBT [48], PLLA [49], PHB [50], alginate, and gelatin [51] with bioactive particles. Upon implantation, as the matrix polymer resorbs, more and more bioactive particles come in contact with the growing tissues — thus resulting in good integration of the biomaterial into the bone. The wide range of material combinations offers the possibility of making composites with various desired properties, such as stiffness, strength, biodegradation, and bioactivity.

9.2.6   *Dental Materials*

Dental treatment is one of the most frequent medical treatments for human beings, which ranges from filling cavities to replacing fractured or decayed teeth. Dental restorative materials — as the name suggests — are used to fill tooth cavities (caries) and sometimes to mask discoloration (veneering) or correct contour and alignment deficiencies. Amalgam, gold, alumina, zirconia, acrylic resins, and silicate cements have been traditionally used for restoring decayed teeth. Dental composite resins — which are translucent with a refractive index matching that of the enamel — have virtually replaced some of these traditional materials; presently, they are very commonly used to restore posterior teeth as well as anterior teeth. The dental composite resin comprises BIS–GMA as the matrix polymer and quartz, barium glass, and colloidal silica as fillers. Polymerization can be started by a thermochemical initiator or by a photochemical initiator that generates free radicals when subjected to ultraviolet light from a lamp used by the dentist. In other types of composites, a urethane dimethacrylate resin is used rather than BIS–GMA. The filler particle concentration varies from 33% to 78% by weight, and the size varies from $0.05\,\mu$m to $50\,\mu$m. The glass fillers reduce the shrinkage during resin polymerization as well as the coefficient of thermal expansion mismatch between the resin and the teeth. Strong bonding between the fillers and resin is achieved using silane-coupling agents [52]. Active research is still being carried out to develop dental composite resins with improved performance.

When a severely damaged tooth lacks the structure to adequately retain a filling or restoration, a dental post or cast dowel is used to reinforce the remaining tooth structure. The post is normally inserted in the root canal and fixed in position using dental cement. Traditional posts made of stainless steel, Ni–Cr, Au–Pt, or Ti alloys are attributed to the hypothesis that the post should be rigid. In recent years, this old basic tenet has been strongly challenged. As a result, it has been suggested to reduce the modulus mismatch between the post and the dentine so as to minimize the occurrence of root fractures (where root fracture frequency is between 2% and 4%) and restoration failures. Newer posts made of zirconia, short glass fiber reinforced polyester, and unidirectional carbon fiber reinforced epoxy composite [53] are introduced. These new posts are adequately rigid and resistant to corrosion and fatigue. In addition to providing support to the core, the dental post also helps direct occlusal and excursive forces more apically along the length of the root. Recent findings have suggested that an ideal post should have varying stiffness along its length. Specifically, the coronal end of the post should have higher stiffness for better retention and rigidity of the core, while the apical end of the post should have lower stiffness matching that of the dentine to overcome root fractures (that arise due to stress concentration). A post with varying stiffness but no change in the cross-sectional geometry along its length is only possible by using functionally graded composite materials. Ramakrishna *et al.* [54] proposed a functionally graded dental post using braided CF/epoxy composite technology. It has a high stiffness in the coronal region, and this stiffness gradually reduces to a value comparable to the stiffness of dentine at the apical end.

Orthodontic arch wires (approximately 0.5 mm in diameter) are used to correct teeth alignment. An arch wire is placed through orthodontic brackets and retained in position using ligature — a small plastic piece. By changing the tension in the arch wire, the alignment of the teeth is adjusted. Traditionally, arch wires are made of stainless steel and Ni–Ti (beta titanium) alloys. To date, composite arch wires based on glass fiber reinforcement have been developed [55, 56]. The advantages of using composite arch wires include improved aesthetics, easy forming in the clinic, and the possibility of varying stiffness without changing component dimensions [57].

9.2.7 *Prosthetic Sockets*

Artificial legs are designed primarily to restore walking of the amputees and were previously made of wood or metallic materials. These materials are limited by their weight and poor durability due to corrosion and moisture-induced swelling. A typical artificial leg system consists of three parts: socket, shaft, and foot (Figure 9.5). The most highly customized and important part of the prosthesis is the socket, which has to be fabricated individually to the satisfaction of each amputee. Sockets can be divided into two categories: direct and indirect sockets. A widely used indirect socket is fabricated by wrapping several layers of knitted or woven fabrics [58] on a customized plastic mold, vacuuming the fabrics enclosed in a plastic bag, and impregnating the vacuumed fabrics with polyester resin. The socket

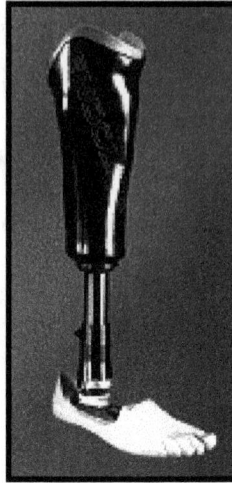

Figure 9.5. An artificial leg consisting of a socket, shank, and foot [59].

is formed after the resin is cured under vacuum pressuring condition. It is reported that the performance of an indirect socket depends on the quality of the mold, especially on the prosthetist skills. A direct socket — as the name suggests — is fabricated directly on the stump of a patient, without using any mold. Compared with indirect sockets, the benefit of direct socket fabrication is that it helps reduce reliance on socket molding/creation skills, hence leading to reduction of fitting errors between the stump and the socket. In addition, direct socket fabrication also reduces the number of patient visits, hence improving the quality of service to the physically disabled people. The direct sockets appeared in the market only in recent years. They are made using a combination of knitted or braided carbon or glass fiber fabrics and water-curable (water-activated) resins. As expected, braided fabric-reinforced sockets are stiff and strong, whereas knitted fabric-reinforced sockets are flexible and more conformable to the patient's stump [59].

9.2.8   *Tendons and Ligaments*

Tendons and ligaments hold the bones of a joint, thus facilitating their stability and movement. They are essentially composite materials comprising undulated collagen fiber bundles aligned along the length and immersed in a ground substance, which is a complex made of elastine and mucopolysaccharide hydrogel [60]. Synthetic biomaterials used thus far in repairing tendons/ligaments include UHMWPE, PP, PET, PTFE, PU, Kevlar 49, carbon, and reconstituted collagen fibers in a multi-filament or braided form. Clinical experience with synthetic prostheses has been disappointing thus far. Problems with synthetic prostheses include difficulty anchoring to the bone, and abrasion and wear of prostheses, whose strength deteriorates in the long term and leads to mechanical failure (such as fatigue). Furthermore, particulate matter generated by abrasion against rough bony surfaces may cause synovitis, as well as inflammation of the lymph nodes should the size of the particulate matter produced allow its migration to the nodes [61]. To reduce particle migration and improve handling properties, prostheses are coated with polymers, such as SR, poly(2–hydroxyethyl methacrylate) (PHEMA), and PLA. Pradas and Calleja [60] reported that by combining a flexible polymer such as PMA or PEA with crimped Kevlar–49 fibers, the stress–strain behavior of natural ligaments can be reproduced to a certain extent. Iannace *et al.* [62] and Ambrosio *et al.* [63] developed a ligament prosthesis by reinforcing a hydrogel matrix (PHEMA) with helically wound rigid PET fibers and demonstrated that both static and dynamic mechanical behavior of natural ligaments can be reproduced. Note that PET maybe sensitive to hydrolytic, stress-induced degradation. Surgeons are still looking for suitable synthetic materials to adequately reproduce the mechanical behavior of natural tissue for long-term applications. To many researchers, a combination of autogenous tissue and synthetic materials maybe an ideal choice for tendon/ligament prostheses.

9.2.9 *Vascular Grafts*

Arterial blood vessels are complex, multi-layered structures comprising collagen and elastin fibers, smooth muscle, ground substance, and endothelium. The blood vessel is anisotropic because of the orientation of inherent fibrous components. Vascular grafts are used to replace displaced or blocked segments of the natural cardiovascular system, such as in atherosclerosis, where deposits on the inner surface of blood vessels restrict the flow of blood and increase blood pressure. However, the use of vascular grafts is mainly successful in the case of blood vessels with the lumen diameter exceeding 5 mm. The most widely used vascular grafts are woven or knitted fabric tubes of PET

material or extruded porous wall tubes of PTFE and PU materials.
The most important property of a graft is its porosity. An appropriate degree of porosity is desirable as it promotes tissue growth
and acceptance of the graft by the host tissues. However, excessive porosity leads to blood leakage. In addition to porosity, other
key requirements of vascular graft include good handling and suturing characteristics, satisfactory healing (i.e., rapid tissue growth),
and mechanical and chemical stability (i.e., good tensile strength
and resistance to deterioration). Since vascular grafts are subjected
to static pressure and repeated stress of pulsation in application,
they should have good dilation and creep resistance. Therefore, fabric tubes are crimped to make them bulky, resilient, and soft. This
is because crimping facilitates extensibility and enables bending of
fabric tubes without kinks and stress concentrations, which are very
important considerations in blood-transporting vascular grafts.

Conventional vascular prostheses are predominantly rigid structures that lack anisotropy and nonlinear compliance. Gershon
et al. [64, 65] and Klein *et al.* [66] developed composite grafts
which comprised Lycra-type polyurethane fibers and Pellethane-type
polyurethane matrix with PELA (block copolymer of lactic acid and
polyethylene glycol) mixture. The nonlinear stress–strain behavior
of the composite graft was obtained by controlling the fiber orientation. The composite graft is anisotropic and isocompliant with the
natural artery. The matrix material is designed to resorb in animal
testing conditions. At the time of implantation, the impervious graft
prevents any blood loss. The resorption of matrix material during
healing process will result in pores. The ingrowth of granulation tissue into the pores provides a stable anchorage for the development
of a viable cellular lining. The optimum pore size of the outer and
inner layers of the graft can be designed to meet the exact needs of
ingrowth and anchorage. Presently, the composite grafts are still in
the clinical research phase and yet to be used clinically.

9.3   Composite Fabrication

A number of methods on how to fabricate polymer matrix composites have been proposed in numerous literature works. Most methods
are applicable to specific kinds of composites: some may be suitable

for thermoplastic composites and others for thermoset composites but only a few for both composite types. In terms of fabrication techniques, some are limited to particulate and short fiber reinforcements, whereas others are best suited for handling continuous fiber reinforcements. In terms of fabrication processes, some make use of dry reinforcement, whereas others use prepregs — in which fibers are already combined with the polymer matrix — as raw materials. Brief descriptions of some of the most widely used fabrication methods are given in the following sections. Before making his own composites, the reader may refer to other references such as Agarwal and Broutman [67], Astrom [68], and Chawla [69] for more detailed information.

9.3.1 *Filament Winding*

Filament winding (Figure 9.6) is a process in which continuous fiber yarns are passed through a low-viscosity resin bath for impregnation and then precisely wound over a rotating or stationary mandrel. Successive layers are laid on at a constant or varying angle until the desired thickness is obtained. After the wound part is cured, the mandrel will be removed if necessary. Sometimes (such as for thermoplastic polymers), a hot-melt or solvent-dip process is used to

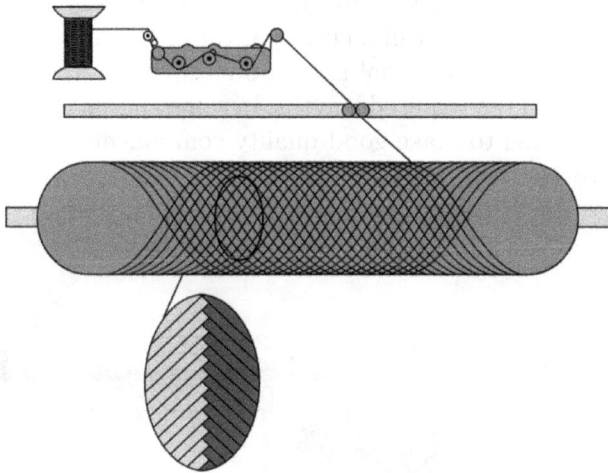

Figure 9.6. Illustration of filament winding for composite fabrication.

impregnate the fibers. In another approach (called tow winding), thermoplastic prepreg tape is heated to the melting point of the polymer just before it is wound onto the mandrel. To avoid uneven cooling across the laminate's thickness, which may generate residual stresses, the mandrel is normally heated to a temperature which is above the glass transition temperature of the polymer.

Filament winding is best suited for making parts with rotational symmetry (e.g., tubes and cylinders). Due to good control of fiber orientation, this process can generate higher fiber contents by up to 65% by volume. Care should be taken to avoid void formation at yarn crossover and at regions between layers of different fiber orientations. As the process uses only one-sided tooling, some cases may lead to poor surface finishing (depending on the process control).

9.3.2 *Pultrusion*

Many composite biomedical devices can be made through pultrusion (Figure 9.7). It is a process that involves pulling the reinforcement through a bath of liquid thermosetting resin and then directly and continuously through a heated die to produce a continuous section. While passing through the bath, the reinforcement is properly impregnated with the resin. The die has a constant cross-sectional cavity almost along its entire length, except at the tapered entrance, which is designed to squeeze out any excess resin from the reinforcement. The heated die permits curing of the thermosetting resin and determines the cross-sectional shape. Subsequently, the hot solid is cooled and cut to the required lengths. In some special cases, prepregs are also pultruded to make good quality components.

This process can also be applied to produce thermoplastic composites. In such a case, the feedstock possesses both the

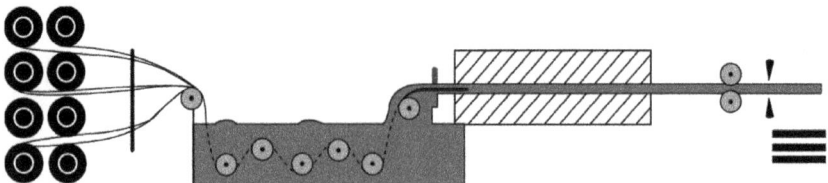

Figure 9.7.   Schematic diagram of pultrusion in composite fabrication.

reinforcement fibers and matrix (prepreg) a pre-consolidated or non-preconsolidated form (e.g., a commingled yarn containing both reinforcement and thermoplastic polymer matrix fibers). A preheating system is used to heat the feedstock to a temperature near to or in excess of the softening point of the matrix. The feedstock then enters a heated die, which melts the matrix polymer and determines the cross-sectional shape of the composite. Subsequently, the composite is consolidated in a cooling die, pulled out, and cut according to the desired lengths.

Pultrusion is best suited for making parts with constant cross-section (e.g., rods, tubes, pipes, beams, angles, and sheets) in large quantities. Very good fiber alignment and fiber volume fractions (as high as 60%) can be obtained. However, there are some limitations to which this process can achieve fiber orientations. Reinforcements in different forms — such as unidirectional fibers (rovings), continuous strand mats, and braided, woven, and stitched fabrics — can be used as feedstock.

9.3.3 *Extrusion*

An extrusion machine (Figure 9.8) consists mainly of rotating screws in a heated barrel. At one end of the barrel, a die is attached — the design of the die cavity is based on the desired cross-sectional geometry of the component. The feedstock is a combined form of polymer matrix and reinforcement fibers. It is fed in the form of pellets from a hopper at the other end of the barrel. The feedstock is mixed and

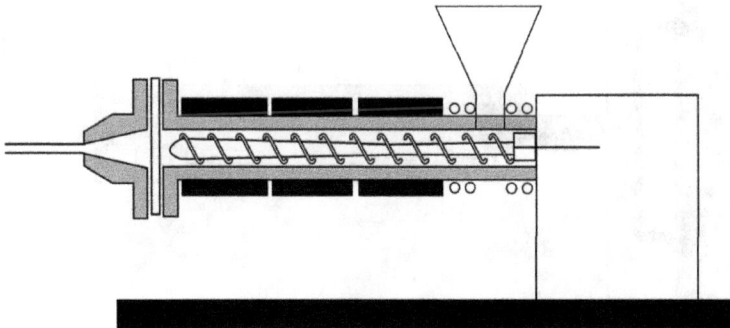

Figure 9.8. Schematic diagram of an extrusion process.

heated to plasticity and then passed through the die. The extruded product is cooled and cut according to the desired dimensions.

This process is limited to particulate and short fiber reinforcements with sections of uniform cross-section. The capital cost is high. Typical reinforcement contents are in the range of 10–30% by volume.

9.3.4 *Injection Molding*

In injection molding (IM) (Figure 9.9), the feedstock containing polymer matrix and reinforcement in a combined form is heated to plasticity in a cylindrical barrel at a controlled temperature. By means of a rotating screw inside the barrel, the material is forced through a nozzle into spruces, runners, gates, and cavities of the mold. Upon solidification or cross-linking of the polymer, the mold is opened and the part ejected. This process is widely used for making thermoplastic composites and to a lesser extent, thermoset composites.

The fierce rotating action of the screw inside the barrel aids in reducing the reinforcement's length. As such, this process is limited to particulate or short fiber reinforcement, where typical reinforcement contents are in the range of 10–30% by volume. Moreover, this process is capable of mass-producing complicated parts with very accurately controlled dimensions, which is another contributing factor to the high capital cost of the injection molding equipment.

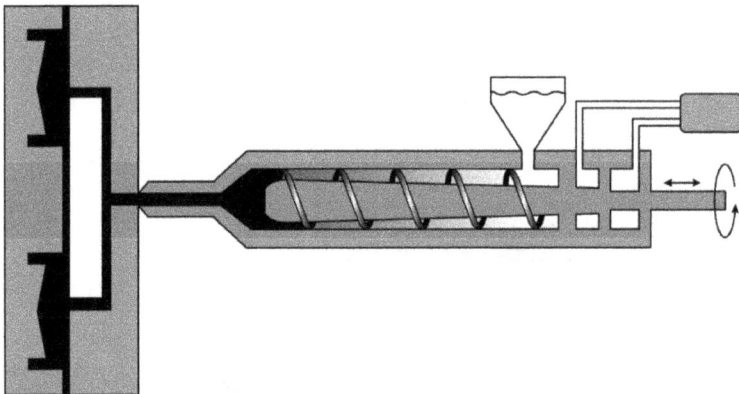

Figure 9.9. Schematic show of injection molding.

9.3.5 *Thermoforming*

Thermoforming (Figure 9.10) is a technique that transforms a flat sheet of composite into a three-dimensional shape. 'Press forming' or 'sheet forming' is the simplest of such method. The composite sheet, heated to a temperature above the softening point of the polymer, is squeezed into shape between two tools. Both tools may be made of metal (as in the case of compression molding) or one tool made of metal and the other made of rubber (the latter is called rubber-block molding). The rubber tool generates an even pressure and reduces the risk of wrinkles on the part. A related method called 'hydroforming' uses hydraulic fluid pressure and membrane to force the composite sheet into shape.

A variant is the 'diaphragm forming' method, in which stacked composite sheets are sandwiched between two diaphragms (superplastic aluminum sheets or polyamide films). The edges of the diaphragms (not the composite sheets) are clamped to a frame and heated to a temperature above the melting point of the polymer. Pressure is applied to one side, which conforms the diaphragms to the shape of a one-sided tool. To aid the forming process, air is evacuated from between the assembly and the tool. The component is

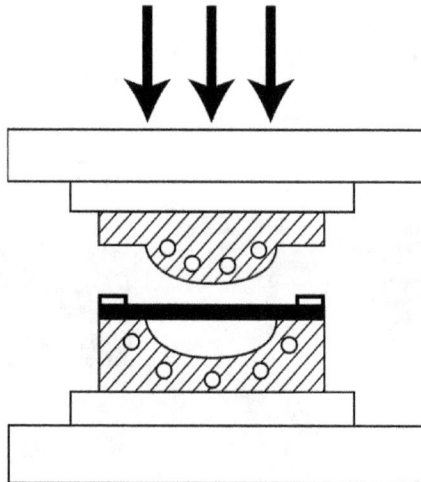

Figure 9.10. A thermoforming process.

formed after the assembly is cooled and the diaphragms removed. This process is also carried out in purpose-built autoclaves.

9.3.6   *A Fabrication Example*

Besides the aforesaid fabrication techniques, many composites in laboratory-development level are fabricated through some simple methods by hand. Such an example is given here. The composite was developed for bone plate application (Figure 9.3) using carbon fiber and a PEEK matrix material system. The PEEK matrix, also in a fiber form, was combined with the reinforcing carbon fibers through a micro-braiding technique [14] to form a commingled yarn (Figure 9.11(a)). In the next step, the micro-braiding yarns were made into braided fabrics using a flat braiding machine, as seen in Figure 9.11(b). Then, the fabrics were placed in a stainless steel mold to make the composite bone plate. As screws are necessary to fix the plate to human bone, the bone plate must be fabricated with the screw holes. It is recognized that drilling a hole on a fabricated composite can drastically reduce its load-carrying capacity due to breakage of fiber continuity. Conversely, if the hole is formed before matrix impregnation and without causing significant fiber damage, good fracture resistance around the hole can be expected [70]. In this

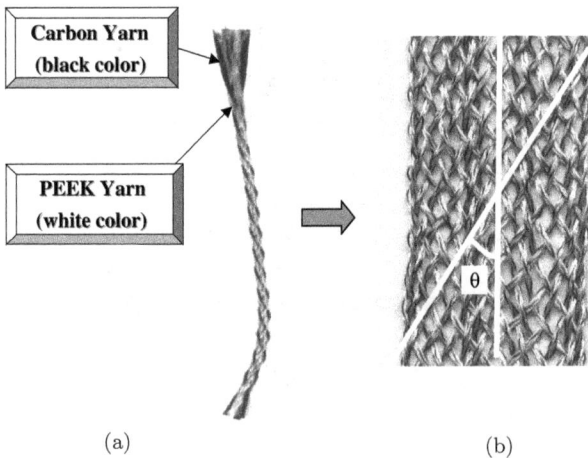

(a)   (b)

Figure 9.11.   (a) A micro-braiding CF/PEEK yarn; (b) a flat braided fabric using such yarns.

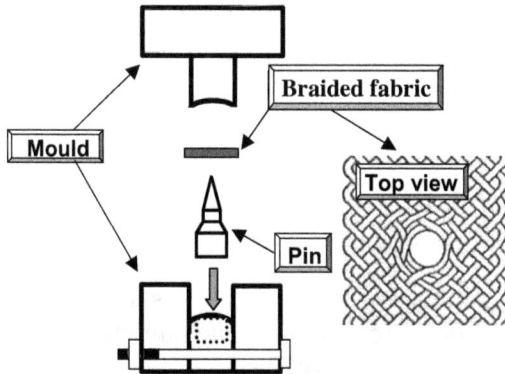

Figure 9.12. Schematic show for braided composite bone plate.

regard, a fabrication mold with six inserted pins was prepared. The diameter of each pin was equal to that of the screws (Figure 9.12). The female mold consisted of three parts — all connected through screw bolts. The central part had a convex curvature, giving a curve form for the bone plate. Flat braided fabrics — of nine layers — were placed in between the mold. The pins were carefully penetrated through the fabrics, without breaking the continuity of yarns. The mold was then put into a vacuumed hot press machine for a further melt-and-press treatment, with an average holding pressure of 5.6MPa and a heating temperature of 400°C for 60 minutes. The bone plate (Figure 9.3) was achieved when the mold was cooled down to room temperature and removed, with an average fiber volume fraction of 48.1% (measured through a burning method). Good impregnation of PEEK matrix into carbon fiber braided fabrics was recognized.

9.4 Mechanics of Composites

A key advantage for composites to be used in biomedical applications is that their mechanical properties can be customized to meet the specific requirements of each application. To achieve this, the composite's structure–property relationship must be clearly understood. The study of the mechanics of composites aims to explore this relationship based on the knowledge of the behaviors and geometries of the composites' constituents.

9.4.1   RVE and Effective Property

From fundamental mechanics of materials textbook, a stress of a solid is defined as an averaged value of those on an infinitesimally small unit element through

$$\sigma_i = \frac{1}{V'} \int_{V'} \tilde{\sigma}_i dV, \quad V' \to 0 (i = 11, 22, 33, 23, 13, 12) \qquad (9.1)$$

where $\tilde{\sigma}_i$ is a point-wise stress and V' is the volume of the unit element. For a composite, however, such an element (called a representative volume element or RVE) cannot be infinitesimal, since both the fiber and matrix must be contained in it. The resulting stress of the composite on the left-hand side is a homogenized value, which is obtained from Equation (9.1) as

$$\sigma_i = \frac{1}{V'} \int_{V'} \tilde{\sigma}_i dV = \left(\frac{V_f'}{V'}\right)\left(\frac{1}{V_f'} \int_{V_f'} \tilde{\sigma}_i dV\right)$$

$$+ \left(\frac{V_m'}{V'}\right)\left(\frac{1}{V_m'} \int_{V_m'} \tilde{\sigma}_i dV\right)$$

$$= V_f \sigma_i^f + V_m \sigma_i^m \qquad (9.2)$$

where $V' = V_m' + V_f'$, V_f' and V_m' are fiber and matrix volumes in the RVE. $V_f = V_f'/V'$ and $V_m = V_m'/V'$ are volume fractions of the fiber and matrix with $V_f + V_m = 1$. σ_i^f and σ_i^m are the homogenized internal stresses in the fiber and matrix, respectively. Similarly, a homogenized strain of the composite is given by

$$\varepsilon_i = V_f \varepsilon_i^f + V_m \varepsilon_i^m \qquad (9.3)$$

From the very fundamental definition, the RVE should be as small as possible. One of the smallest RVEs for continuous and short fiber/particulate composites is shown in Figures 9.13(a) and 9.13(b), respectively. The difference between the latter from the former is that the lengths of the fiber and matrix cylinders are not the same. Both the RVEs are transversely isotropic, resembling a unidirectional

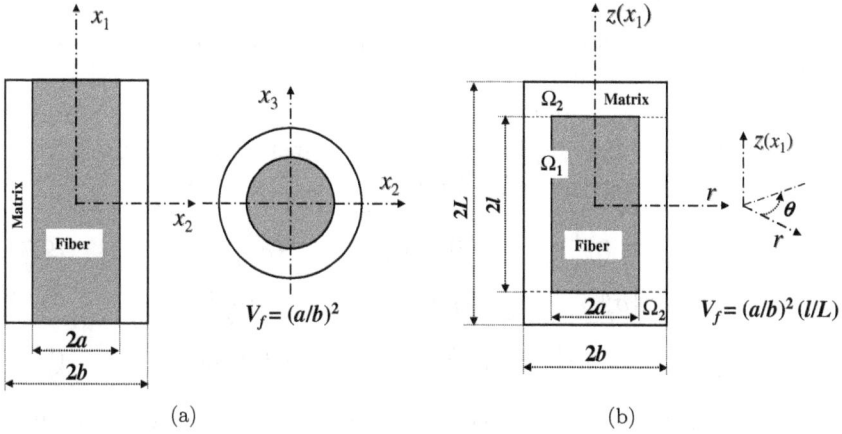

Figure 9.13. RVE of (a) continuous fiber composite and (b) short fiber composite, in which $l/a \approx 1$ corresponds to a particle composite.

(UD) and a uniaxially aligned short fiber composites in mechanical behaviors, respectively. It is noticed that when a fiber aspect ratio (Figure 9.13(b)) $l/a = 1$, the short fiber composite becomes a particulate one.

In all of the above and following Equations, the suffixes (either superscripts or subscripts) "f" and "m" stand for fiber and matrix phases, respectively. A quantity without any suffix denotes a composite or, sometimes, a special kind of material. Equations (9.2) and (9.3) are valid for every $i = 1, 2,\ldots, 6$. Thus, the following two relationships are written instead:

$$\{\sigma_i\} = V_f\{\sigma_i^f\} + V_m\{\sigma_i^m\} \qquad (9.4a)$$

$$\{\varepsilon_i\} = V_f\{\varepsilon_i^f\} + V_m\{\varepsilon_i^m\} \qquad (9.4b)$$

Further, Let $[S_{ij}^f]$ and $[S_{ij}^m]$ be the compliance matrices of the fiber and matrix materials, respectively. These two matrices are invariant with respect to homogenization. Thus,

$$\{\varepsilon_i^f\} = [S_{ij}^f]\{\sigma_j^f\} \qquad (9.5a)$$

$$\{\varepsilon_i^m\} = [S_{ij}^m]\{\sigma_j^m\} \qquad (9.5b)$$

$$\{\varepsilon_i\} = [S_{ij}]\{\sigma_j\} \qquad (9.6)$$

where $[S_{ij}]$ denotes the compliance matrix of the composite. Note that any fiber-reinforced composite can be subdivided into a series of UD or uniaxially aligned short fiber composites.

Using a bridging equation, $\{\sigma_i^m\} = [a_{ij}]\{\sigma_j^f\}$ where $[a_{ij}]$ is a bridging matrix, the following basic equations can be easily derived from Equations (9.4) together with Equations (9.5) and (9.6):

$$\{\sigma_i^f\} = (V_f[I] + V_m[a_{ij}])^{-1}\{\sigma_j\} \tag{9.7}$$

$$\{\sigma_i^m\} = [a_{ij}](V_f[I] + V_m[a_{ij}])^{-1}\{\sigma_j\} \tag{9.8}$$

$$[S_{ij}] = (V_f[S_{ij}^f] + V_m[S_{ij}^m][a_{ij}])(V_f[I] + V_m[a_{ij}])^{-1} \tag{9.9}$$

Thus, determination of the composite compliance matrix is equivalent to that of the bridging matrix. Since the basic equations of the composite are derived based on the homogenized stresses and strains, a resulting composite property is called an averaged or effective quantity.

A composite in reality is usually subjected to a 2D (two-dimensional) stress state, $\{\sigma_i\}_{2D} = \{\sigma_{11}, \sigma_{22}, \sigma_{12}\}^T$. The resulting internal stresses in the fiber and matrix can be calculated upon either a 2D bridging matrix $[a_{ij}]_{2D}$, corresponding to the 2D constitutive relation, or the 3D one $[a_{ij}]_{3D}$ for which the external load is denoted as $\{\sigma_i\}_{3D} = \{\sigma_{11}, \sigma_{22}, 0, 0, 0, \sigma_{12}\}^T$. A necessary condition for the resulting two sets of the internal stresses to be consistent or equal to each other is that the bridging matrix $[a_{ij}] = [a_{ij}]_{3D}$ is of an upper triangular form. In fact, e.g., when $a_{32} \neq 0$, it follows from Equations (9.7) and (9.8) that $\sigma_{33}^f = b_{32}\sigma_{22} \neq 0$ and $\sigma_{33}^m = a_{32}\sigma_{22}^f + a_{33}\sigma_{33}^f \neq 0$, where $[b_{ij}] = (V_f[I] + V_m[a_{ij}])^{-1}$.

9.4.2 *Bridging Matrix*

As aforementioned, a micromechanics model is characterized by its bridging matrix. A different model corresponds to a different bridging matrix. Although a number of such models are available to calculate the composite effective elastic properties and the homogenized internal stresses in the fiber and matrix, almost all of the well-known micromechanics models are non-consistent except for the bridging model [80]. This means that the use of the other models should be in 3D equations to achieve a higher accuracy. In addition, very complicated explicit expressions for the internal stresses would be obtained, since the inversion to their 3D bridging matrices required in Equations (9.7) and (9.8) would be very complicated in explicit forms. Finally, most models are not directly applicable to the analysis of a short fiber composite. Compact and very simple expressions for the elastic moduli and homogenized internal stresses of either a UD or a uniaxially aligned short fiber composite can be obtained in terms of the bridging model. Moreover, many assessments have shown that the bridging model is overall more accurate than most other micromechanics models [71–76]. As such, we only summarize the bridging matrix elements by the bridging model in an elastic region as follows. More details can be found in, e.g., [77]:

$$
a_{11} = \begin{cases} E^m/E_{11}^f, \text{ for continuous fiber composite} \\ \dfrac{V_f E^m}{V_m E_{11}^f} \dfrac{\sigma_{11}L - E_{11}^f[\varepsilon_L^1 l + \varepsilon_L^2(L-l)]}{E^m[\varepsilon_L^1 l + \varepsilon_L^2(L-l)] - \sigma_{11}L}, \text{ for short fiber composite} \end{cases} \quad (9.10)
$$

$$
a_{22} = a_{33} = a_{44} = 0.3 + 0.7\frac{E^m}{E_{22}^f} \quad (9.11)
$$

$$
a_{55} = a_{66} = 0.3 + 0.7\frac{G^m}{G_{12}^f} \quad (9.12)
$$

$$
a_{12} = a_{13} = \frac{S_{12}^f - S_{12}^m}{S_{11}^f - S_{11}^m}(a_{11} - a_{22}) \quad (9.13)
$$

All of the other bridging matrix elements not given in Equations (9.10)–(9.13) are zero. In Equation (9.13), $S_{11}^f = 1/E_{11}^f$, $S_{12}^f = -\nu_{12}^f/E_{11}^f$, $S_{11}^m = 1/E^m$, and $S_{12}^m = -\nu^m/E^m$. In Equation (9.10), ε_L^1 and ε_L^2 are the homogenized longitudinal strains of Ω_1 and Ω_2 in Figure 9.13(b), which are determined from the following simultaneous equations [78]:

$$
\begin{bmatrix} 0 & 0 & \frac{l}{L}[gE_{11}^f + (1-g)E^m] & (1-l/L)E^m \\ \frac{2\nu^m E^m}{(1+\nu^m)(1-2\nu^m)} & \frac{2g\nu^m E^m}{(1+\nu^m)(1-2\nu^m)} & 0 & \frac{(1-\nu^m)E^m}{(1+\nu^m)(1-2\nu^m)} \\ \frac{E^m[g\nu_{12}^f+\nu^m(1-g)]}{0.5(1+\nu^m)(1-2\nu^m)} & -\frac{2g\nu_{12}^f E^m}{1+\nu^m} & k_1 & 0 \\ k_2 & k_3 & k_4 & 0 \end{bmatrix}
$$

$$
\times \begin{Bmatrix} C_1 \\ \frac{C_2}{a^2} \\ \varepsilon_L^1 \\ \varepsilon_L^2 \end{Bmatrix} = \begin{Bmatrix} \sigma_{11} \\ \sigma_{11} \\ \sigma_{11} \\ 0 \end{Bmatrix} \quad (9.14)
$$

$$k_1 = \frac{2g\nu^m\nu_{12}^f + (1-\nu^m)(1-g)}{(1+\nu^m)(1-2\nu^m)}E^m + gE_{11}^f, g = (a/b)^2 \quad (9.15)$$

$$k_2 = E_{11}^f \frac{E^m\nu_{12}^f(1+\nu_{23}^f) + \nu_{12}^f E_{22}^f - (1+2\nu^m)\nu^m\nu_{12}^f E_{22}^f}{(1+\nu^m)(1-2\nu^m)[E_{11}^f - E_{22}^f(\nu_{12}^f)^2]}$$

$$-\frac{2E^m\nu_{12}^f}{(1+\nu^m)(1-2\nu^m)} \quad (9.16)$$

$$k_3 = E_{11}^f \frac{\nu_{12}^f(1+\nu^m)E_{22}^f - (1+\nu_{23}^f)E^m\nu_{12}^f}{(1+\nu^m)[E_{11}^f - E_{22}^f(\nu_{12}^f)^2]} + \frac{2E^m\nu_{12}^f}{1+\nu^m} \quad (9.17)$$

$$k_4 = E_{11}^f \frac{E_{22}^f(\nu_{12}^f)^2(1+\nu^m)(1-2\nu^m) + E^m\nu^m\nu_{12}^f(1+\nu_{23}^f)}{(1+\nu^m)(1-2\nu^m)[E_{11}^f - E_{22}^f(\nu_{12}^f)^2]}$$

$$-\frac{2\nu^m E^m\nu_{12}^f}{(1+\nu^m)(1-2\nu^m)} \quad (9.18)$$

where E_{11}^f, ν_{12}^f, and G_{12}^f are longitudinal Young's modulus, Poisson's ratio, and shear modulus of the fiber material, whereas E_{22}^f, G_{23}^f, and ν_{23}^f are transverse Young's modulus, shear modulus, and Poisson's ratio of the fiber with $G_{23}^f = 0.5E_{22}^f/(1+\nu_{23}^f)$. E^m, ν^m, and G^m are the elastic modulus, Poisson's ratio, and shear modulus of the matrix with $G^m = 0.5E^m/(1+\nu^m)$.

With no loss of generality, one can set the axial stress in Equations (9.10) and (9.14) to be $\sigma_{11} = 1$. It can be verified that the A_{11} in Equation (9.10) for a discontinuous fiber composite approaches that for a continuous one when $l \to L$ or $l/a \to \infty$.

For the RVE of a continuous fiber composite shown in Figure 9.13(a), only the fiber volume fraction V_f is required, while for that in Figure 9.13(b), except for the V_f, there are two other geometric parameters, i.e., the fiber aspect ratio l/a and the fiber length ratio l/L, must be provided as well. Only the V_f and l/a are measurable, but the length ratio l/L can hardly be measured directly. Reference [79] proposed an empirical formula for the length ratio, reading as

$$\frac{l}{L} = \left[\sqrt{V_f} \frac{l}{a} \tan\left\{ \arctan(a/l) \right. \right.$$

$$\left. \left. -c(l-a)\frac{\arctan(a/l) - \arctan(a/(l\sqrt{V_f}))}{c(l-a)+a} \right\} \right]^{2/3} \quad (9.19)$$

where $c = 0.03$ is an empirical parameter [79]. For the definition of the other parameters, refer to Figure 9.13(b).

9.4.3 *Elastic Moduli*

The five elastic moduli of a UD or uniaxially aligned short fiber composite are expressed as follows [77]:

$$E_{11} = \frac{(V_f + V_m a_{11})E_{11}^f E^m}{V_f E^m + V_m a_{11} E_{11}^f} \quad (9.20)$$

$$\nu_{12} = \frac{E_{11}(V_f \nu_{12}^f E^m + V_m a_{11} \nu^m E_{11}^f)}{E_{11}^f E^m (V_f + V_m a_{11})} \quad (9.21)$$

$$E_{22} = \frac{(V_f + V_m a_{11})(V_f + V_m a_{22})}{(V_f + V_m a_{11})(V_f S_{22}^f + a_{22} V_m S_{22}^m) + V_f V_m (S_{21}^m - S_{21}^f)a_{12}} \quad (9.22)$$

$$G_{12} = \frac{G_{12}^f G^m (V_f + V_m a_{66})}{V_f G^m + V_m G_{12}^f a_{66}} \quad (9.23)$$

$$G_{23} = \frac{G_{23}^f G^m (V_f + V_m a_{22})}{V_f G^m + V_m G^f {}_{23} a_{22}} \quad (9.24)$$

9.4.4 *Homogenized Internal Stresses*

Explicit formulae for the homogenized internal stresses of the fiber and matrix in the UD or uniaxially short fiber composite subjected to any arbitrary load are given as follows [77]:

$$\sigma_{11}^f = \frac{\sigma_{11}}{V_f + V_m a_{11}} - \frac{V_m a_{12}(\sigma_{22} + \sigma_{33})}{(V_f + V_m a_{11})(V_f + V_m a_{22})} \tag{9.25}$$

$$\sigma_{22}^f = \frac{\sigma_{22}}{V_f + V_m a_{22}} \tag{9.26}$$

$$\sigma_{33}^f = \frac{\sigma_{33}}{V_f + V_m a_{22}} \tag{9.27}$$

$$\sigma_{23}^f = \frac{\sigma_{23}}{V_f + V_m a_{22}} \tag{9.28}$$

$$\sigma_{13}^f = \frac{\sigma_{13}}{V_f + V_m a_{66}} \tag{9.29}$$

$$\sigma_{12}^f = \frac{\sigma_{12}}{V_f + V_m a_{66}} \tag{9.30}$$

$$\sigma_{11}^m = \frac{a_{11}\sigma_{11}}{V_f + V_m a_{11}} + \frac{V_f a_{12}(\sigma_{22} + \sigma_{33})}{(V_f + V_m a_{11})(V_f + V_m a_{22})} \tag{9.31}$$

$$\sigma_{22}^m = \frac{a_{22}\sigma_{22}}{V_f + V_m a_{22}} \tag{9.32}$$

$$\sigma_{33}^m = \frac{a_{22}\sigma_{33}}{V_f + V_m a_{22}} \tag{9.33}$$

$$\sigma_{23}^m = \frac{a_{22}\sigma_{23}}{V_f + V_m a_{22}} \tag{9.34}$$

$$\sigma_{13}^m = \frac{a_{66}\sigma_{13}}{V_f + V_m a_{66}} \tag{9.35}$$

$$\sigma_{12}^m = \frac{a_{66}\sigma_{12}}{V_f + V_m a_{66}} \tag{9.36}$$

in which $\{\sigma_{11}, \sigma_{22}, \sigma_{33}, \sigma_{23}, \sigma_{13}, \sigma_{12}\}$ are arbitrary external loads applied on the RVE (Figures 9.13(a) or 9.13(b)), i.e., on the UD or the uniaxially aligned short fiber composite. These formulae show that the upper triangularity of the bridging tensor is also a sufficient condition for a constitutive relation to be consistent in internal stress calculation at least in an elastic range.

9.4.5 *Strengths of UD Composite — Bridging Model Formulae*

It is difficult to calculate the strength of a composite by using only the properties of its constituent materials. The key reason is that the introduction of a reinforcement (stood by a fiber throughout the following) into the matrix causes stress concentrations in the matrix around the fiber. One cannot compare a homogenized stress of the matrix obtained from Equation (9.8) with its strengths to assess a matrix and further composite failure. A true stress of the matrix must be obtained first, which equals the homogenized stress of the matrix multiplied by its stress concentration factor (SCF) caused by the fiber reinforcement. This SCF is no longer obtainable by a classical method. Otherwise, the resulting SCF would be infinite if an interface between the fiber and matrix is debonded. Almost all of the possible matrix SCFs have been explicitly derived [77], and only some of them are summarized in the following. The others are complicated or very complicated in expressions. The authors can refer to [77] to find the other expressions and, more importantly, to download the Excel data-based program to calculate the required SCF.

Different from a matrix-caused composite failure which must be detected on the matrix true stresses, a fiber-induced composite failure can be assessed from the fiber-homogenized stresses. This is because a stress field of the fiber in a composite is always uniform no matter whichever external load is applied to the composite as demonstrated by Eshelby [80].

9.4.5.1 *True stresses of matrix*

Let $\{d\sigma_i^m\} = \{d\sigma_{11}^m, d\sigma_{22}^m, d\sigma_{33}^m, d\sigma_{23}^m, d\sigma_{13}^m, d\sigma_{12}^m\}$ be the matrix homogenized stress increments obtained from Equation (9.8) by replacing an overall applied stress vector $\{\sigma_j\}$ on its right-hand side using an incremental one $\{d\sigma_j\}$. The overall true stresses of the matrix, $\{\bar{\sigma}_i^m\}_n$, at the current load step are updated through the following formulae:

$$\{\bar{\sigma}_i^m\}_n = \{\bar{\sigma}_{11}^m, \bar{\sigma}_{22}^m, \bar{\sigma}_{33}^m, \bar{\sigma}_{23}^m, \bar{\sigma}_{13}^m, \bar{\sigma}_{12}^m\}_n$$

$$= \{\bar{\sigma}_i^m\}_{n-1} + \{d\bar{\sigma}_i^m\}, n = 1, 2, \ldots \quad (9.37)$$

$$\{d\bar{\sigma}_i^m\} = \{K_{11}d\sigma_{11}^m, K_{22}d\sigma_{22}^m, K_{33}d\sigma_{33}^m,$$

$$K_{23}d\sigma_{23}^m, \bar{K}_{12}d\sigma_{13}^m, \bar{K}_{12}d\sigma_{12}^m\} \quad (9.38)$$

$$\text{where } K_{11} = \begin{cases} 1, \text{ for continuous fiber composite} \\ K_{11}^t, \text{ forshort fiber or particlecomposite} \\ \quad \text{with } d\sigma_{11}^m \geq 0 \\ K_{11}^c, \text{ for short fiber or particlecomposite} \\ \quad \text{with } d\sigma_{11}^m < 0 \end{cases} \quad (9.39)$$

$$K_{22} = \begin{cases} K_{22}^t, \text{ if } d\sigma_{22}^m > 0 \text{ with perfect interface bonding} \\ \hat{K}_{22}^t, \text{ if } d\sigma_{22}^m > 0 \text{ with debonded interface} \\ K_{22}^c, \text{ if } d\sigma_{22}^m < 0 \end{cases} \quad (9.40)$$

$$K_{33} = \begin{cases} K_{22}^t, \text{ if } d\sigma_{33}^m > 0 \text{ with perfect interface bonding} \\ \hat{K}_{22}^t, \text{ if } d\sigma_{33}^m > 0 \text{ with debonded interface} \\ K_{22}^c, \text{ if } d\sigma_{33}^m < 0 \end{cases} \quad (9.41)$$

$$\bar{K}_{12} = \begin{cases} K_{12}, \text{ for perfect interface bonding} \\ \hat{K}_{12}, \text{ for debonded interface} \end{cases} \quad (9.42)$$

$$K_{22}^t = \left[1 + \frac{\sqrt{V_f}}{2} A + \frac{\sqrt{V_f}}{2} (3 - V_f - \sqrt{V_f}) B \right]$$
$$\times \frac{(V_f + 0.3V_m) E_{22}^f + 0.7 V_m E^m}{0.3 E_{22}^f + 0.7 E^m} \quad (9.43)$$

$$K_{22}^c = \left\{ 1 - \frac{\sqrt{V_f}}{2} A \frac{\sigma_{u,c}^m - \sigma_{u,t}^m}{2\sigma_{u,c}^m} \right.$$
$$+ \frac{B}{2(1 - \sqrt{V_f})} \left[-V_f^2 \left(1 - 2 \left(\frac{\sigma_{u,c}^m - \sigma_{u,t}^m}{2\sigma_{u,c}^m} \right)^2 \right) \right.$$
$$+ \frac{(\sigma_{u,c}^m + \sigma_{u,t}^m) V_f}{\sigma_{u,c}^m} \left(1 + \frac{\sigma_{u,c}^m - \sigma_{u,t}^m}{\sigma_{u,c}^m} \right)$$
$$\left. \left. - \sqrt{V_f} \left(\frac{\sigma_{u,c}^m - \sigma_{u,t}^m}{\sigma_{u,c}^m} + 1 - 2 \left(\frac{\sigma_{u,c}^m - \sigma_{u,t}^m}{2\sigma_{u,c}^m} \right)^2 \right) \right] \right\}$$
$$\times \frac{(V_f + 0.3V_m) E^f{}_{22} + 0.7 V_m E^m}{0.3 E^f{}_{22} + 0.7 E^m} \quad (9.44)$$

$$K_{23} = 2\sigma_{u,s}^m \sqrt{\frac{K_{22}^t K_{22}^c}{\sigma_{u,t}^m \sigma_{u,c}^m}} \tag{9.45}$$

$$K_{12} = \left[1 - V_f \frac{G_{12}^f - G^m}{G^f_{12} + G^m} \left\{ W(V_f) - \frac{1}{3} \right\} \right]$$

$$\times \frac{(V_f + 0.3V_m)G^f_{12} + 0.7V_m G^m}{0.3G^f_{12} + 0.7G^m} \tag{9.46}$$

$$A = \frac{\begin{array}{c} 2E_{22}^f E^m (\nu_{12}^f)^2 + E_{11}^f \{ E^m (\nu_{23}^f - 1) \\ -E_{22}^f [2(\nu^m)^2 + \nu^m - 1] \} \end{array}}{\begin{array}{c} E_{11}^f [E_{22}^f + E^m (1 - \nu_{23}^f) + E_{22}^f \nu^m] \\ -2E_{22}^f E^m (\nu_{12}^f)^2 \end{array}} \tag{9.47}$$

$$B = \frac{E^m (1 + \nu_{23}^f) - E_{22}^f (1 + \nu^m)}{E_{22}^f [\nu^m + 4(\nu^m)^2 - 3] - E^m (1 + \nu_{23}^f)} \tag{9.48}$$

$$W(V_f) = \pi \sqrt{V_f} \left[\frac{1}{4V_f} - \frac{1}{32} - \frac{1}{256} V_f - \frac{5}{4096} V_f^2 \right] \tag{9.49}$$

$\sigma_{u,t}^m, \sigma_{u,c}^m$, and $\sigma_{u,s}^m$ are the tensile, compressive, and shear strengths of the matrix, respectively. $\hat{K}_{22}^t$ and $\hat{K}_{12}$ are the transverse tensile and in-plane shear SCFs of the matrix after interface debonding. K_{11}^t and K_{11}^c are, respectively, the longitudinal tensile and compressive SCFs of the matrix in a short fiber/particle composite. Analytical formulae for all of the SCFs not listed above can be found in, e.g., [77].

The fiber true stresses are updated through

$$\{\bar{\sigma}_i^f\}_n = \{\bar{\sigma}_i^f\}_{n-1} + \{d\sigma_j^f\}, n = 1, 2, \cdots \tag{9.50}$$

$\{\bar{\sigma}_i^m\}_0$ and $\{\bar{\sigma}_i^f\}_0$ are the initial true stresses of the matrix and fiber, which are generally induced from thermal residual stresses or simply set to zero.

9.4.5.2 *Longitudinal tensile strength*

If a UD or uniaxially aligned short fiber composite with perfect inter-face bonding up to failure is subjected only to a longitudinal tensile load (σ_{11}), its strength is given as follows [77, 81]:

$$\sigma_{11}^u = \min \left\{ \frac{\sigma_{u,t}^f - (\alpha_{e1}^f - \alpha_{p1}^f)\sigma_{11}^0}{\alpha_{p1}^f}, \right.$$

$$\left. \times \frac{\sigma_{u,t}^m - K_{11}^t(\alpha_{e1}^m - \alpha_{p1}^m)\sigma_{11}^0}{K_{11}^t \alpha_{p1}^m} \right\} \qquad (9.51\text{a})$$

$$\sigma_{11}^0 = \min \left\{ \frac{\sigma_Y^m}{K_{11}^t \alpha_{e1}^m}, \frac{\sigma_{u,t}^f}{\alpha_{e1}^f} \right\} \qquad (9.51\text{b})$$

$$\alpha_{e1}^f = \frac{E_{11}^f}{V_f E_{11}^f + (1 - V_f)E^m} \qquad (9.51\text{c})$$

$$\alpha_{e1}^m = \frac{E^m}{V_f E_{11}^f + (1 - V_f)E^m} \qquad (9.51\text{d})$$

$$\alpha_{p1}^f = \frac{E_{11}^f}{V_f E_{11}^f + (1 - V_f)E_T^m} \qquad (9.51\text{e})$$

$$\alpha_{p1}^m = \frac{E_T^m}{V_f E_{11}^f + (1 - V_f)E^m_T} \qquad (9.51\text{f})$$

In the above, $\sigma_{u,t}^f$ is the fiber tensile strength (in axial direction). σ_Y^m and E_T^m are the yield strength and hardening modulus of the matrix (Figure 9.14). Note that a bilinear elastic–plastic behavior

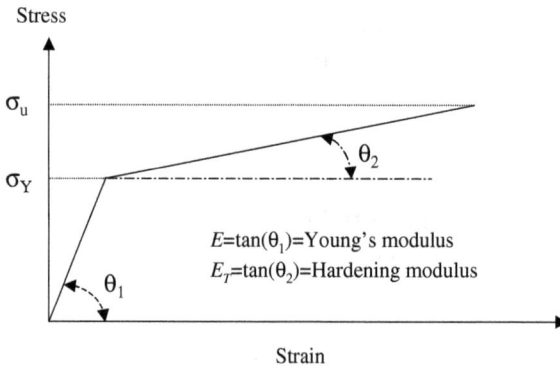

Figure 9.14. Schematic bilinear stress–strain curve of a matrix material.

has been assumed for the matrix and that the fiber material has been assumed to be linearly elastic until rupture.

9.4.5.3 *Transverse tensile strength*

If the composite is subjected only to a transverse tensile load (σ_{22}), its strength is determined from

$$\sigma_{22}^u = \min \left\{ \frac{\sigma_{u,t}^f - (\alpha_{e2}^f - \alpha_{p2}^f)\sigma_{22}^0}{\alpha_{p2}^f}, \right.$$

$$\left. \times \frac{\sigma_u^m - K_{22}^t(\alpha_{e2}^m - \alpha_{p2}^m)\sigma_{22}^0}{K_{22}^t \alpha_{p2}^m} \right\} \qquad (9.52a)$$

$$\text{Where} \quad \sigma_{22}^0 = \min \left\{ \frac{\sigma_Y^m}{K_{22}^t \alpha_{e2}^m}, \frac{\sigma_u^f}{\alpha_{e2}^f} \right\} \qquad (9.52b)$$

$$\alpha_{e2}^f = \frac{E_{22}^f}{V_f E_{22}^f + 0.5(1 - V_f)(E^m + E_{22}^f)} \qquad (9.52c)$$

$$\alpha_{e2}^m = \frac{0.5(E_{22}^f + E^m)}{V_f E_{22}^f + 0.5(1 - V_f)(E^m + E_{22}^f)} \qquad (9.52d)$$

$$\alpha_{p2}^f = \frac{E_{22}^f}{V_f E_{22}^f + 0.5(1 - V_f)(E_T^m + E_{22}^f)} \qquad (9.52e)$$

$$\alpha_{p2}^m = \frac{0.5(E_{22}^f + E_T^m)}{V_f E_{22}^f + 0.5(1 - V_f)(E^m{}_T + E_{22}^f)} \qquad (9.52f)$$

9.4.5.4 *In-plane shear strength*

The ultimate strength of the composite due to an in-plane shear load (σ_{12}) alone is calculated through

$$\sigma_{12}^u = \min \left\{ \frac{\sigma_{u,t}^f - (\alpha_{e3}^f - \alpha_{p3}^f)\sigma_{12}^0}{\alpha_{p3}^f}, \right.$$

$$\left. \times \frac{\sigma_{u,s}^m - K_{12}(\alpha_{e3}^m - \alpha_{p3}^m)\sigma_{12}^0}{K_{12}\alpha_{p3}^m} \right\} \qquad (9.53a)$$

$$\text{where} \quad \sigma^0_{12} = \min \left\{ \frac{\sigma^m_Y}{\sqrt{3}K_{12}\alpha^m_{e3}}, \frac{\sigma^f_{u,t}}{\alpha^f_{e3}} \right\} \tag{9.53b}$$

$$\alpha^f_{e3} = \frac{G^f_{12}}{V_f G^f_{12} + 0.5(1 - V_f)(G^m + G^f_{12})} \tag{9.53c}$$

$$\alpha^m_{e3} = \frac{0.5(G^f_{12} + G^m)}{V_f G^f_{12} + 0.5(1 - V_f)(G^m + G^f_{12})} \tag{9.53d}$$

$$\alpha^f_{p3} = \frac{3G^f_{12}}{3V_f G^f_{12} + 0.5(1 - V_f)(E^m{}_T + 3G^f_{12})} \tag{9.53e}$$

$$\alpha^m_{p3} = \frac{0.5(3G^f_{12} + E^m_T)}{3V_f G^f_{12} + 0.5(1 - V_f)(E^m{}_T + 3G^f_{12})} \tag{9.53f}$$

9.4.6 Example

A SiC-fiber reinforced titanium (Ti) matrix UD composite has properties of $E^f = 400\,\text{GPa}$, $\nu^f = 0.25$, $\sigma^f_{u,t} = 3480\,\text{MPa}$, $E^m = 110\,\text{GPa}$, $\nu^m = 0.33$, $E^m_T = 2.16\,\text{GPa}$, $\sigma^m_Y = 850\,\text{MPa}$, and $\sigma^m_{u,s} = \sigma^m_{u,t} = 1000\,\text{Mpa}$ [82]. The fiber volume fraction is 0.15. Calculate the uniaxial strengths of this composite and identify its corresponding failure modes. Suppose the composite is in perfect fiber and matrix interface bonding up to failure.

Solution

(A) *SCFs of Matrix*

From Equations (9.42) and (9.45), it is found that $K^t_{11} = 1$, $K^t_{22} = 1.41$, and $K_{12} = 0.99$.

(B) *Longitudinal Strength*

Substituting the relevant parameters into Equations (9.52a)–(9.52f), we have

$$\alpha^f_{e1} = (400)/[(0.15)(400) + (0.85)(110)] = 2.606$$

$$\alpha^m_{e1} = (110)/[(0.15)(400) + (0.85)(110)] = 0.717$$

$$\alpha^f_{p1} = (400)/[(0.15)(400) + (0.85)(2.16)] = 6.550$$

$$\alpha^m_{p1} = (2.16)/[(0.15)(400) + (0.85)(2.16)] = 0.0349$$

$$\sigma_{11}^0 = \min\{(850)/(1^*0.717), (3480)/(2.606)\}$$

$$= \min\{1185.5, 1335.4\} = 1185.5$$

$$\sigma_{11}^u = \min\{[3480 - (2.606 - 6.55)(1185.5)]/6.55,$$

$$[1000 - (1)(0.717 - 0.0349)(1185.5)]/(1^*0.0349)\}$$

$$= \min\{1245.1, 5483.4\} = 1245.1 (\text{MPa})$$

The last expression indicated that it was fiber fracture that caused the composite failure (since under the longitudinal load the fiber failure corresponded stress is 1245.1 MPa, whereas the matrix failure corresponded stress is 5483.4 MPa).

(C) *Transverse Strength*

According to Equations (9.53a)–(9.53f), we obtain the following:

$$\alpha_{e2}^f = (400)/[(0.15)(400) + (0.5)(0.85)(110 + 400)] = 1.445$$

$$\alpha_{e2}^m = (0.5)(110 + 400)/[(0.15)(400)$$

$$+ (0.5)(0.85)(110 + 400)] = 0.921$$

$$\alpha_{p2}^f = (400)/[(0.15)(400)$$

$$+ (0.5)(0.85)(2.16 + 400)] = 1.732$$

$$\alpha_{p2}^m = (0.5)(400 + 2.16)/[(0.15)(400)$$

$$+ (0.5)(0.85)(402.16)] = 0.871$$

$$\sigma_{22}^0 = \min\{(850)/(1.41^*0.921), (3480)/(1.445)\}$$

$$= \min\{922.9, 2408.3\} = 654.5$$

$$\sigma_{22}^u = \min\{[(3480) - (1.445 - 1.732)(654.5)]/(1.732),$$

$$[1000 - (1.41)(0.921 - 0.871)(654.5)]/(1.41^*0.871)\}$$

$$= \min\{2117.7, 776.7\} = 776.7 (\text{MPa})$$

The last expression indicated that it was matrix fracture that caused the composite failure (since under the transverse load the fiber failure corresponded stress is 2117.7MPa, whereas the matrix failure corresponded stress is 776.7MPa).

(D) *In-plane Shear Strength*

First, we have $G^f = (400)/[(2)(1 + 0.25)] = 160 \, \text{GPa}$ and $G^m = (110)/[(2)(1 + 0.33)] = 41.4 \, \text{GPa}$, as both the fiber and matrix are isotropic. Then, Equations (9.53a)–(9.53f) give the following:

$$\alpha_{e3}^{f} = (160)/[(0.15) + (0.5)(0.85)(160 + 41.4)] = 1.460$$

$$\alpha_{e3}^{m} = (0.5)(201.4)/[(0.15)(160) + (0.5)(0.85)(201.4)] = 0.919$$

$$\alpha_{p3}^{f} = (3)(160)/[(3)(0.15)(160)$$
$$\qquad\qquad + (0.5)(0.85)(2.16 + 480)] = 1.733$$

$$\alpha_{p3}^{m} = (0.5)(480 + 2.16)/[(3)(0.15)(160)$$
$$\qquad\qquad + (0.5)(0.85)(2.16 + 480)] = 0.871$$

$$\sigma_{12}^{0} = \min\{(850)/[(1.732)(0.99)(0.919)], (3480)/(1.46)\}$$
$$\qquad = \min\{539.4, 2383.6\} = 539.4$$

$$\sigma_{12}^{u} = \min\{[3480 - (1.46 - 1.733)(539.4)]/(1.733),$$
$$\qquad\qquad [1000 - (0.99)(0.919 - 0.871)(539.4)]/(0.99^{*}0.871)\}$$

$$= \min\{2093, 1130\} = 1130(\text{MPa})$$

The last expression indicated that it was matrix fracture that caused the composite failure (since under the in-plane shear load the fiber failure corresponded stress is 2093 MPa, whereas the matrix failure corresponded stress is 1130 MPa).

9.4.7 Structure–Property Relationship

The stiffness and strength formulae given in the preceding subsections are applicable only to the simplest cases, i.e., UD composites subjected to uniaxial loads. In most cases, UD composites are used as laminae to construct multidirectional tape laminates in which the UD composites are subjected to a planar load condition. Even for such conditions, the previous micromechanics strength formulae are not applicable nor sufficient. In reality, we often have to deal with problems such as a textile composite laminate (i.e., a laminate consisting of multi-layer textile fabric reinforced composites) which can be much more complicated.

9.4.7.1 Mechanical properties of UD composite

Suppose the UD composite is subjected to an arbitrary planar stress state, $\{\sigma\} = \{\sigma_{11}, \sigma_{22}, \sigma_{12}\}^{T}$ (Figure 9.15(a)). What will be the composite's response to failure? For this purpose, the homogenized stresses in the fiber and matrix are calculated first. This can be

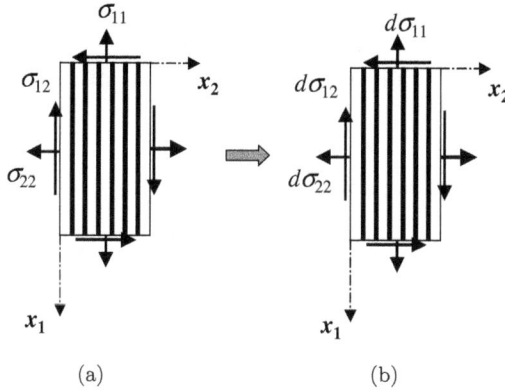

Figure 9.15. (a) UD composite subjected to any planar load; (b) an incremental approach.

accomplished using the bridging model [77, 83], in which an incremental solution strategy (Figure 9.15(b)) is generally applied when the analysis is out of an inelastic deformation range or an interface debonding already occurs. The benefit of applying the incremental solution is that the composite stiffness (compliance) at the current load level can be regarded as unchanged when incremental loads are applied subsequently.

9.4.7.2 *Internal homogenized stress increments*

The homogenized stress increments in the fiber and matrix are given as follows:

$$
\left\{ \begin{array}{c} d\sigma_{11}^f \\ d\sigma_{22}^f \\ d\sigma_{12}^f \end{array} \right\} = \begin{bmatrix} b_{11} & b_{12} & b_{13} \\ 0 & b_{22} & b_{23} \\ 0 & 0 & b_{33} \end{bmatrix} \left\{ \begin{array}{c} d\sigma_{11} \\ d\sigma_{22} \\ d\sigma_{12} \end{array} \right\} = [b_{ij}] \left\{ \begin{array}{c} d\sigma_{11} \\ d\sigma_{22} \\ d\sigma_{12} \end{array} \right\} \quad (9.54\text{a})
$$

$$
\left\{ \begin{array}{c} d\sigma_{11}^m \\ d\sigma_{22}^m \\ d\sigma_{12}^m \end{array} \right\} = \begin{bmatrix} a_{11} & a_{12} & a_{13} \\ 0 & a_{22} & a_{23} \\ 0 & 0 & a_{33} \end{bmatrix} \begin{bmatrix} b_{11} & b_{12} & b_{13} \\ 0 & b_{22} & b_{23} \\ 0 & 0 & b_{33} \end{bmatrix} \left\{ \begin{array}{c} d\sigma_{11} \\ d\sigma_{22} \\ d\sigma_{12} \end{array} \right\}
$$

$$
= [a_{ij}][b_{ij}] \left\{ \begin{array}{c} d\sigma_{11} \\ d\sigma_{22} \\ d\sigma_{12} \end{array} \right\} \quad (9.54\text{b})
$$

where $[a_{ij}]$ is a bridging matrix and $[b_{ij}]$ is closely related to $[a_{ij}]$.

Substituting the stress increments from Equations (9.53a) and (9.53f) into the right-hand sides of Equations (9.60) and (9.37), respectively, the overall true stresses of the matrix and fibers are obtained.

9.4.7.3 *Instantaneous compliance matrix*

Under an incremental load, $\{d\sigma\} = \{d\sigma_{11}, d\sigma_{22}, d\sigma_{12}\}^T$, the composite generates an incremental strain response, $\{d\varepsilon\} = \{d\varepsilon_{11}, d\varepsilon_{22}, 2d\varepsilon_{12}\}^T$, through the following expression:

$$\{d\varepsilon_i\} = [S_{ij}]\{d\sigma_j\} \tag{9.55}$$

where the instantaneous compliance matrix of the composite is determined by Equation (9.9), in which $[S_{ij}^f]$ and $[S_{ij}^m]$ are the instantaneous compliance matrices of the fiber and matrix materials, respectively.

Bridging Matrix Elements

When the matrix is able to undergo plastic deformation, the bridging matrix becomes complicated [77]. In a 2D case and when the composite is a UD, however, the bridging matrix elements are explicitly expressed as follows:

$$a_{11} = E_m/E_{11}^f \tag{9.56a}$$

$$a_{22} = 0.3 + 0.7E_m/E_{22}^f \tag{9.56b}$$

$$a_{33} = 0.3 + 0.7G_m/G_{12}^f \tag{9.56c}$$

$$a_{12} = (S_{12}^f - S_{12}^m)(a_{11} - a_{22})/(S_{11}^f - S_{11}^m) \tag{9.56d}$$

$$a_{13} = \frac{d_2\beta_{11} - d_1\beta_{21}}{\beta_{11}\beta_{22} - \beta_{12}\beta_{21}} \tag{9.56e}$$

$$a_{23} = \frac{d_1\beta_{22} - d_2\beta_{12}}{\beta_{11}\beta_{22} - \beta_{12}\beta_{21}} \tag{9.56f}$$

$$d_1 = S_{13}^m(a_{11} - a_{33})$$

$$d_2 = S_{23}^m(V_f + V_m a_{11})(a_{22} - a_{33}) + S_{13}^m(V_f + V_m a_{33})a_{12}$$

$$\beta_{11} = S_{12}^m - S_{12}^f, \beta_{12} = S_{11}^m - S_{11}^f,$$

$$\beta_{22} = (V_f + V_m a_{22})(S_{12}^m - S_{12}^f)$$

$$\beta_{21} = V_m(S_{12}^f - S_{12}^m)a_{12} - (V_f + V_m a_{11})(S_{22}^f - S_{22}^m)$$

$$E_m = \begin{cases} E^m, & when \ \bar{\sigma}_e^m \leq \sigma_Y^m \\ E_T^m, & when \ \bar{\sigma}_e^m > \sigma_Y^m \end{cases}$$

$$G_m = \begin{cases} 0.5E^m/(1+\nu^m), & when \ \bar{\sigma}_e^m \leq \sigma_Y^m \\ E_T^m/3, & when \ \bar{\sigma}_e^m > \sigma_Y^m \end{cases}$$

$$\bar{\sigma}_e^m = \sqrt{(\bar{\sigma}_{11}^m)^2 + (\bar{\sigma}_{22}^m)^2 - (\bar{\sigma}_{11}^m)(\bar{\sigma}_{22}^m) + 3(\bar{\sigma}_{12}^m)^2}$$

The elements of $[B]$ are then found to be as follows:

$$b_{11} = (V_f + V_m a_{22})(V_f + V_m a_{33})/c,$$

$$b_{12} = -(V_m a_{12})(V_f + V_m a_{33})/c \tag{9.57a}$$

$$b_{13} = [(V_m a_{12})(V_m a_{23}) - (V_f + V_m a_{22})(V_m a_{13})]/c,$$

$$b_{22} = (V_f + V_m a_{11})(V_f + V_m a_{33})/c \tag{9.57b}$$

$$b_{23} = -(V_m a_{23})(V_f + V_m a_{11})/c,$$

$$b_{33} = (V_f + V_m a_{22})(V_f + V_m a_{11})/c \tag{9.57c}$$

$$c = (V_f + V_m a_{11})(V_f + V_m a_{22})(V_f + V_m a_{33})$$

9.4.7.4 *Constituent compliances*

The instantaneous compliance matrices of the constituents are assumed to be known. For example, Hooke's law can be used to define the fiber compliance matrix if it is linearly elastic until rupture and Prandtl–Reuss theory can be used to define the matrix compliance matrix when it is in a plastic deformation range [77].

9.4.7.5 *Ultimate strength*

When a composite fails, the corresponding applied load is defined as an ultimate stress state for the composite and the ultimate strength follows. How to identify composite failure? As there are only two constituents, composite failure occurs as soon as one of the constituents attains a failure stress state. Constituent failure can be detected using, e.g., the maximum normal stress criterion, that is, composite failure is attained if any of the following conditions are fulfilled:

$$\times \frac{\bar{\sigma}_{11}^f + \bar{\sigma}_{22}^f}{2} + \frac{1}{2}\sqrt{(\bar{\sigma}_{11}^f - \bar{\sigma}_{22}^f)^2 + 4(\bar{\sigma}_{12}^f)^2} \geq \sigma_{u,t}^f \qquad (9.58a)$$

$$\times \frac{\bar{\sigma}_{11}^f + \bar{\sigma}_{22}^f}{2} - \frac{1}{2}\sqrt{(\bar{\sigma}_{11}^f - \bar{\sigma}_{22}^f)^2 + 4(\bar{\sigma}_{12}^f)^2} \leq -\sigma_{u,c}^f \qquad (9.58b)$$

$$\times \frac{\bar{\sigma}_{11}^m + \bar{\sigma}_{22}^m}{2} + \frac{1}{2}\sqrt{(\bar{\sigma}_{11}^m - \bar{\sigma}_{22}^m)^2 + 4(\bar{\sigma}_{12}^m)^2} \geq \sigma_{u,t}^m \qquad (9.58c)$$

$$\times \frac{\bar{\sigma}_{11}^m + \bar{\sigma}_{22}^m}{2} - \frac{1}{2}\sqrt{(\bar{\sigma}_{11}^m - \bar{\sigma}_{22}^m)^2 + 4(\bar{\sigma}_{12}^m)^2} \leq -\sigma_{u,c}^m \qquad (9.58d)$$

Other more powerful failure criteria can be found in, e.g., [77]. It is noticed that a constituent failure must be detected on a true stress level.

9.4.7.6   *Mechanical properties of laminated composite*

Suppose a laminated composite consists of N layers of UD laminae stacked in different ply angles (Figure 9.16). A global coordinate system, (x, y, z), is assumed to have its origin on the middle surface of the laminate, with x and y in the laminate plane and z along the thickness direction. Let the fiber direction of the kth lamina

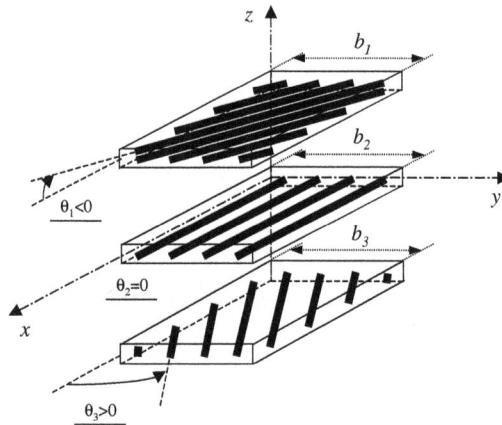

Figure 9.16.   Schematic showing multi-layer laminae to constitute a laminate.

have an inclined ply-angle θ_k with the global x direction, where θ is measured in anticlockwise direction from x to the fiber axis direction of the ply.

The analysis of the laminate is based on the classical lamination theory [84]. A schematic procedure of the analysis is shown in Figure 9.17. For each lamina in the laminate, only in-plane stress and strain increments, i.e., $\{d\sigma\}^G = \{d\sigma_{xx}, d\sigma_{yy}, d\sigma_{xy}\}^T$ and $\{d\varepsilon\}^G = \{d\varepsilon_{xx}, d\varepsilon_{yy}, 2d\varepsilon_{xy}\}^T$ are retained, where "G" refers to the global coordinate system (Figure 9.17(b)). They are correlated by Equation (9.55), but in the global system, as shown in Figure 9.17(b),

$$\{d\sigma\}^G = [C_{ij}^G]\{d\varepsilon\}^G = [T]_c[S]^{-1}[T]_c^T\{d\varepsilon\}^G \tag{9.59}$$

where $[S]$ is the lamina's instantaneous compliance matrix and is determined using Equation (9.9) in which the bridging matrix and the matrix instantaneous compliance matrix must be of instantaneous quantities and $[T]_c$ is a coordinate transformation matrix dependent on the ply-angle and is given by

$$[T]_c = \begin{bmatrix} l_1^2 & l_2^2 & 2l_1l_2 \\ m_1^2 & m_2^2 & 2m_1m_2 \\ l_1m_1 & l_2m_2 & l_1m_2+l_2m_1 \end{bmatrix},$$
$$l_1 = m_2 = \cos\theta, l_2 = -m_1 = \sin\theta \tag{9.60}$$

According to the classical laminate theory, the global strain increments of the kth lamina in the laminate can be expressed as follows:

$$\{d\varepsilon\}_k^G = \left\{ d\varepsilon_{xx}^0 + \frac{z_k+z_{k-1}}{2}d\kappa_{xx}^0, d\varepsilon_{yy}^0 + \frac{z_k+z_{k-1}}{2} \right.$$
$$\left. d\kappa_{yy}^0, 2d\varepsilon_{xy}^0 + (z_k+z_{k-1})d\kappa_{xy}^0 \right\}^T \tag{9.61}$$

where z_{k-1} and z_k are the z-coordinates of the bottom and top surfaces of the kth ply, and $d\varepsilon_{xx}^0$, etc. and $d\kappa_{xx}^0$, etc. are the strain and curvature increments of the middle surface, respectively. They can be determined from the following formulae:

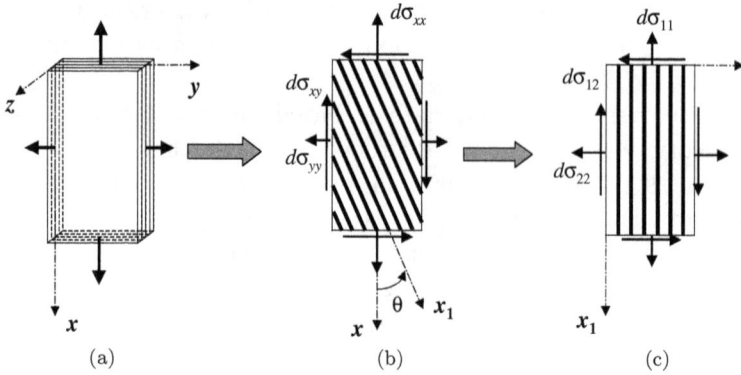

Figure 9.17. Analysis procedure for a tape laminate.

$$
\begin{Bmatrix} dN_{xx} \\ dN_{yy} \\ dN_{xy} \\ dM_{xx} \\ dM_{yy} \\ dM_{xy} \end{Bmatrix} = \begin{bmatrix} Q_{11}^{I} & Q_{12}^{I} & Q_{16}^{I} & Q_{11}^{II} & Q_{12}^{II} & Q_{16}^{II} \\ Q_{12}^{I} & Q_{22}^{I} & Q_{26}^{I} & Q_{12}^{II} & Q_{22}^{II} & Q_{26}^{II} \\ Q_{16}^{I} & Q_{26}^{I} & Q_{66}^{I} & Q_{16}^{II} & Q_{26}^{II} & Q_{66}^{II} \\ Q_{11}^{II} & Q_{12}^{II} & Q_{16}^{II} & Q_{11}^{III} & Q_{12}^{III} & Q_{16}^{III} \\ Q_{12}^{II} & Q_{22}^{II} & Q_{26}^{II} & Q_{12}^{III} & Q_{22}^{III} & Q_{26}^{III} \\ Q_{16}^{II} & Q_{26}^{II} & Q_{66}^{II} & Q_{16}^{III} & Q_{26}^{III} & Q_{66}^{III} \end{bmatrix}
$$

$$
\times \begin{Bmatrix} d\varepsilon_{xx}^{0} \\ d\varepsilon_{yy}^{0} \\ 2d\varepsilon_{xy}^{0} \\ d\kappa_{xx}^{0} \\ d\kappa_{yy}^{0} \\ 2d\kappa_{xy}^{0} \end{Bmatrix} \qquad (9.62a)
$$

$$
Q_{ij}^{I} = \sum_{k=1}^{N} (C_{ij}^{G})_k (z_k - z_{k-1}), \, Q_{ij}^{II} = \frac{1}{2}\sum_{k=1}^{N}(C_{ij}^{G})_k(z_k^2 - z_{k-1}^2),
$$

$$
Q_{ij}^{III} = \frac{1}{3}\sum_{k=1}^{N}(C_{ij}^{G})_k(z_k^3 - z_{k-1}^3) \qquad (9.62b)
$$

In Equation (9.62a), the quantities dN_{xx}, dN_{yy}, dN_{xy}, dM_{xx}, dM_{yy}, and dM_{xy} are the overall incremental in-plane forces and moments per unit length exerted on the laminate, respectively. Once the overall stress increments of the kth lamina are calculated through

Equation (9.59), they should be transformed into the local system (Figure 9.17(c)) before being substituted into the right-hand side of Equations (9.54a) and (9.54b) to determine the internal stress increments. The transformation formula from the global to the local systems is

$$\{d\sigma\} = [T]_s^T \{d\sigma\}^G \tag{9.63}$$

where $[T]_s = \begin{bmatrix} l_1^2 & l_2^2 & l_1 l_2 \\ m_1^2 & m_2^2 & m_1 m_2 \\ 2l_1 m_1 & 2l_2 m_2 & l_1 m_2 + l_2 m_1 \end{bmatrix}$ (9.64)

As with the application of external loads, some laminae must fail before the others. Once a lamina fails, its stiffness must be discounted for the remaining analysis. For simplicity, let a total stiffness discount be applied. Supposing that the k_0^{th} lamina ply has failed, the remaining laminate stiffness elements are defined as follows [?]:

$$Q_{ij}^I = \sum_{\substack{k=1 \\ k \neq k_0}}^{N} (C_{ij}^G)_k (z_k - z_{k-1}), \quad Q_{ij}^{II} = \frac{1}{2} \sum_{\substack{k=1 \\ k \neq k_0}}^{N} (C_{ij}^G)_k (z_k^2 - z_{k-1}^2)$$

$$Q_{ij}^{III} = \frac{1}{3} \sum_{\substack{k=1 \\ k \neq k_0}}^{N} (C_{ij}^G)_k (z_k^3 - z_{k-1}^3) \tag{9.65}$$

In this way, a progressive failure process of the laminate can be identified and accordingly, its ultimate strength can be determined. The scheme represented by Equations (9.65) is called a total stiffness discount scheme can be found in, e.g., [77].

9.4.7.7 *Modeling procedure for a textile composite*

As shown in Figure 9.1, composites reinforced with textile fabrics are widely used in biomedical applications. A textile fabric refers to a fibrous structure made of continuous fiber yarns (bundles) by means of a textile technique. Three basic textile techniques can be employed to develop fibrous preforms (fabric structures) for biocomposite reinforcement. They are weaving, braiding, and knitting.

Subdivision ➡

| Textile composite | ⇄ | Unit cell | ⇄ | RVE | ⇄ | UD composites |

⬅ Assemblage

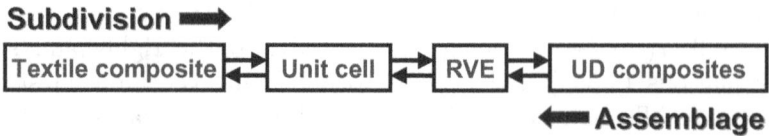

Figure 9.18. Analysis procedure for a textile fabric-reinforced composite.

Correspondingly, the resulting composites are called woven fabric composites, braided fabric composites, and knitted fabric composites.

Although the fibrous structure of a textile composite is much more complicated than that of a tape laminate, the structure–property relationship of the former is analyzed in a manner somewhat similar to that of the latter. A schematic diagram to show the analysis procedure for a textile fabric-reinforced composite is given in Figure 9.18. It essentially consists of three steps — subdivision, analysis, and assemblage — which are similar to those applied to a tape laminate. In the first step, the textile composite is subdivided in an arbitrary way into a number of smallest slides, each of which contains at most one straight yarn segment. Such a slide can be considered as a UD composite (lamina) in its local coordinate system with, possibly, a different fiber volume fraction. Some slides may even contain no fiber. Once the textile composite is subdivided into UD laminae, the second step is the analysis of these laminae using the bridging model micromechanics theory summarized previously. Namely, the internal true stress increments in the fiber and matrix are calculated and the instantaneous compliance matrix of the UD composite is determined through Equation (9.9). The third and final step deals with the assemblage of the contributions of all the UD laminae to obtain the overall response of the textile composite. Roughly speaking, the last step is somewhat a reverse to the first step.

9.4.7.8 *Analysis outline for braided fabric composites*

As can be understood from the aforementioned procedure, the difference in the analyses of different fabric-reinforced composites lies in the first (discretization) and last (assemblage) steps, which are more related to a geometrical rather than mechanical analysis. A schematic diagram to show the discretization of a diamond braided composite into UD laminae is graphed in Figure 9.19. The whole fabric structure

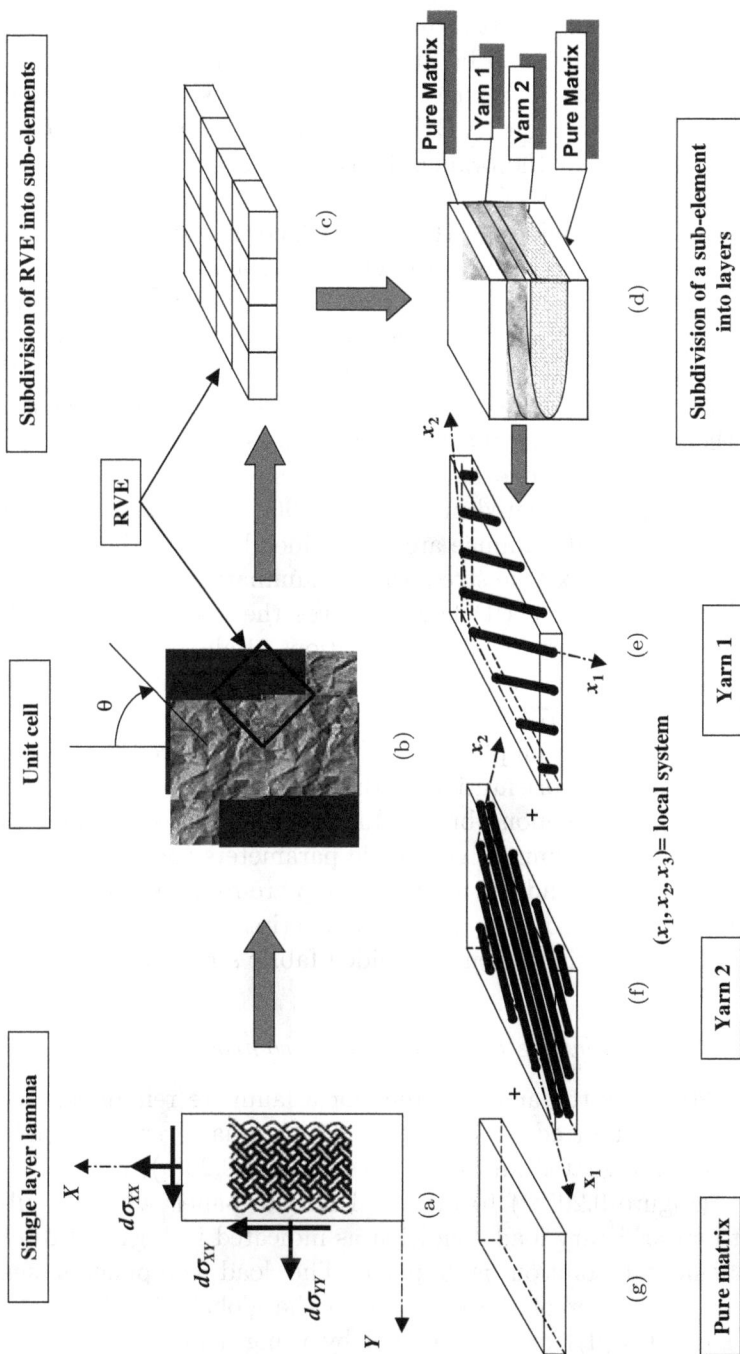

Figure 9.19. Subdivision of a braided fabric composite into UD laminae.

(Figure 9.19(a)) can be constructed by repeating some unit cells
(Figure 9.19(b)), which can be further divided into four identical or
symmetrical sub-cells. One such sub-cell together with the surrounding matrix is taken as an RVE for the composite (Figure 9.19(a)).
Thus, the analysis for the braided fabric composite can be achieved
by the analysis of the RVE.

The RVE is subdivided in the fabric plane into sub-elements, as
shown in Figure 9.19(c). Each sub-element (Figure 9.19(d)) has at
most four material layers: braider yarn 1 (e.g., warp yarn), braider
yarn 2 (e.g., fill yarn), and the top and bottom pure matrix layers.
Note that the warp and fill yarns have already been impregnated with
the polymer matrix. These material layers are considered as UD laminae in their respective local coordinate systems, while both the pure
matrix layers are regarded as a UD composite with zero fiber volume fraction — as indicated in Figures 9.19(e)–(g). The mechanical
responses of these UD laminae are determined by using the bridging
model and the matrix true stress theory summarized previously. An
assemblage of the three UD laminae gives the responses of a sub-
element. An assemblage of the contributions of all the sub-elements
then gives rise to the overall properties of the composite (RVE). For
more details, refer to [77, 86].

To successfully accomplish the subdivision followed by assemblage, the fiber yarn orientation in the RVE must be specified. For
a plain weave or a diamond braid, Huang [86] proposed a geometric
model in which only limited geometric parameters such as the yarn
thickness and width and the inter-yarn gap are required. Huang and
Ramakrishna [87] also gave a general description of the geometric
model for a 2D biaxial woven or braided fabric structure.

9.4.7.9 Analysis outline for knitted fabric composites

Figure 9.20 shows the analysis steps for a laminate reinforced with
multi-layers of knitted fabric composite laminae. Several single-
layer resin-impregnated knitted fabrics (Figure 9.20(a)) are stacked
together (Figure 9.20(b)) to make a laminate panel, which is subjected to an arbitrary load condition as indicated in Figure 9.20(c).
An incremental solution is applied. The load components sustained by each layer of the laminate in the global coordinate system (Figure 9.20(d)) are determined by using a laminate analysis

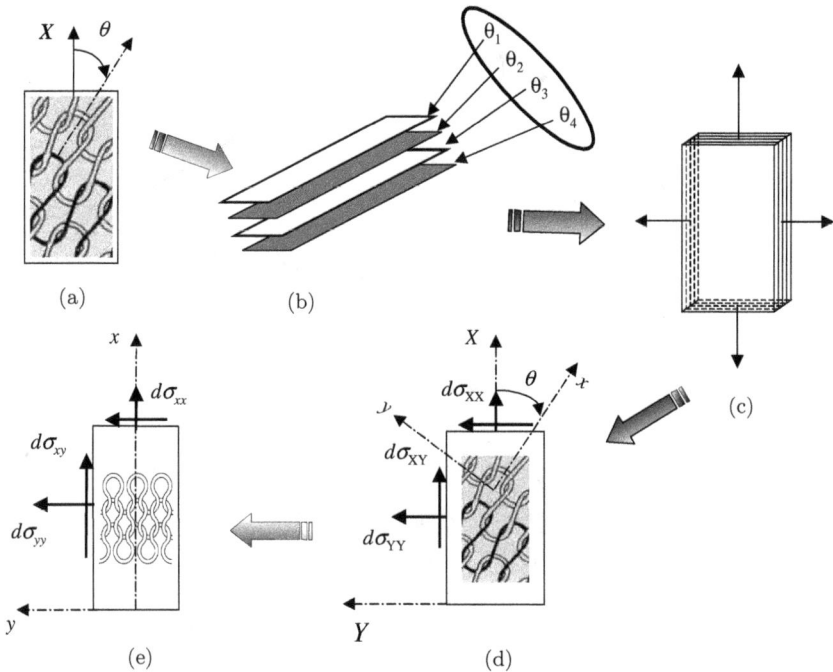

Figure 9.20. Analysis of a knitted fabric-reinforced laminate.

procedure [88]. Before proceeding to the analysis for a single layer of the knitted fabric composite, a coordinate transformation is necessary to transform the stress state in the global coordinate system into the ply system (Figure 9.20(e)).

The analysis steps for a single layer of the knitted fabric composite are schematically shown in Figure 9.21, with respect to the ply coordinate system. Figure 9.21(a) shows that the entire fabric can be constructed using a repeating unit cell (Figure 9.21(b)), which can be further divided into four symmetrical or identical sub-cells. One such sub-cell is taken as the RVE for the knitted fabric composite, as indicated in Figure 9.21(c).

There are two yarns in the RVE, whose geometric positions are critical. Fortunately, for the present plain weft-knitted fabric structure, the Leaf and Glaskin model can be employed to specify its geometry [89]. For the geometrical descriptions of some other fabric structures, please refer to Huang and Ramakrishna [90].

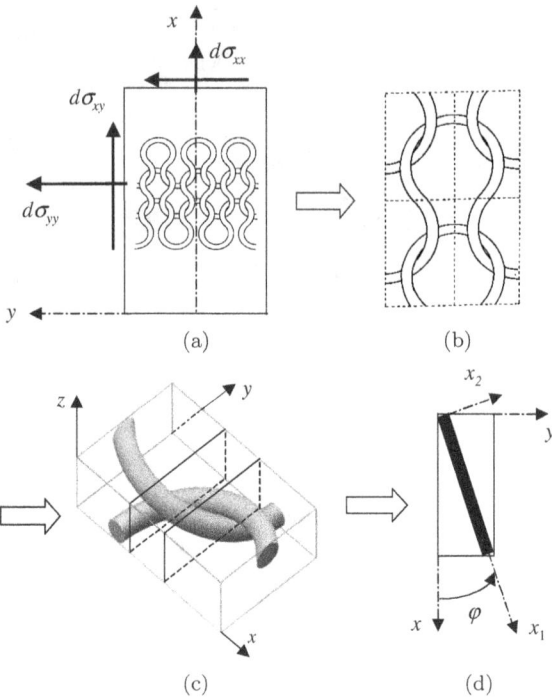

Figure 9.21. Analysis steps for a single layer of knitted fabric-reinforced composite.

The RVE in Figure 9.21(c) is subdivided into even smaller elements along the x-direction. Due to the small element size after subdivision, the yarn segment together with its surrounding matrix can be regarded as a UD composite which has an inclined angle with the x-direction (Figure 9.21(d)). The response of the UD composite in its local coordinate system is determined through the bridging model and the matrix true stress theory. Then, the RVE properties can be obtained by assembling the contributions of all the sub-elements. More details can be found in [77, 88, 90].

9.4.7.10   *Analysis outline for short fiber/particulate composites*

Composite reinforcements by short (chopped or whisker) fibers or particulates are generally in random form, as shown in Figure 9.22.

Loading

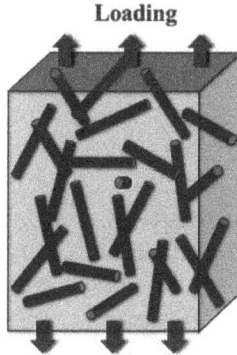

Figure 9.22. A schematic composite with random short fiber reinforcements.

The analysis for such composites follows a similar procedure as for the previous textile composites. Namely, the short fiber/particulate composites are subdivided into arbitrary smallest slides, each with at most one straight fiber yarn segment. As before, such a slide can be considered as a UD composite, if the fiber yarn length is the same as the matrix length in the fiber axial direction (Figure 9.13(a)), or a uniaxially aligned short fiber/particulate composite when the fiber yarn length is shorter than the matrix length (Figure 9.13(b)). The homogenized stress increments in the fiber and matrix of the uniaxially aligned short fiber composite are still calculated using Equations (9.54a) and (9.54b). Only the axial bridging matrix element, a_{11}, needs to be defined differently, as given by Equation (9.10).

It noted that when the matrix undergoes a plastic deformation, Equations (9.14), in which the matrix elastic modulus E^m and Poisson's ratio ν^m must be replaced by their plastic counterparts, E_m^T and 0.5, respectively, are solved simultaneously to determine an instantaneous axial bridging matrix element a_{11}.

Once the fiber and matrix true stress increments of each UD/uniaxially aligned short fiber composite are determined, they are transformed into those in the global coordinate system, and the overall global true stresses of the fiber and matrix are updated step by step. Meanwhile, the instantaneous compliance matrix of the composite is obtained from the contributions of all the slides. Failure detections on the various composite failures can be made upon the overall true stresses of the composite.

9.5   Future Advances

It is a relatively recent clinical practice where composite materials are used in biomedical applications. For implants which have been developed based on composite technology, many are still at the laboratory development stage. One major flaw is the lack of proper design theory with composite materials [91]. Many researchers used directly the design standards which were originally developed for isotropic materials to produce polymer composite implants. However, composite materials are distinctly different from homogenous materials in terms of anisotropy, fracture behavior, and environmental sensitivity. As such, polymer composite implants must be designed using criteria separate from those intended for isotropic material-based implants. Innovations, such as spatially varying fiber contents and reinforcing structures, are adding new types of functionally graded composite materials to implant applications. New design criteria need to be developed to explore the potential of this new class of materials and to design implants with improved performance.

The success of polymer composites as biomaterials also relies substantially on the implants' quality, which is determined by the reproducibility of the fabrication process. Current practices use a trial-and-error approach, resulting in limited success in clinical applications. The composite fabrication methods employed in engineering applications have been directly adopted for producing implants. It is important to realize that the requirements for the two applications are different. Hence, the composite fabrication methods for biomedical applications must be modified to meet the specific needs of each application. For example, in a hip joint replacement application, the composite material surface should be completely covered with a continuous matrix layer to prevent any potential release of fiber particle debris during implantation. Moreover, the fabrication method needs to be optimized such that it enables desired local and global arrangements of reinforcement phase so as to make the composite implant structurally compatible with the host tissues. Thus far, the polymer composite biomaterials are mainly reinforced with particulates, short fibers, and unidirectional fiber prepregs — very few reports on woven fabric composites are available. The many advantages offered by textile composite materials have not been well exploited in the biomedical field. Efforts should be made to harness the potential of textile composite materials in designing implants with improved performance.

It is now clear that for greater success, implants should be surface-compatible as well as structurally compatible with the host tissues. In this regard, polymer composite biomaterials are particularly attractive because of their tailorable structure designability, as well as properties that are comparable to those of the host tissues. In addition, other factors help heighten the appeal of polymer composite biomaterials. Innovations in composite material design, improvements in polymer matrices, and fabrication processes raise the possibility of achieving implants with improved performance. However, for successful application, surgeons must be convinced of the long-term durability and reliability of polymer composite biomaterials. Monolithic materials have long been used and there are considerable experimental and clinical data supporting their continued usage. Such data in terms of polymer composite biomaterials are relatively scarce. Considerable research efforts are required to elucidate the long-term durability of composite biomaterials in human body conditions. Nevertheless, in view of their promising potential for high performance, composite materials are likely to be increasingly utilized as biomaterials in the future.

References

[1] G. O. Hofmann, Biodegradable implants in orthopedic surgery — A review on the state-of-the-art, *Clin. Mater.*, 1992, 10:75–80.

[2] K. P. Baidya, S. Ramakrishna, M. Rahman, A. Ritchie, and Z.-M. Huang, An investigation on the polymer composite medical device — External fixator, *J. Reinforced Plastics Compos.*, 2003, 22(6):563–590.

[3] P. Tormala, J. Vasenius, S. Vainionpaa, J. Laiho, T. Pohjonen, and P. Rokkanen, Ultra-high-strength absorbable self-reinforced polyglycolide (SR–PGA) composite rods for internal fixation of bone fractures: *In vitro* and *in vivo* study, *J. Biomed. Mater. Res.*, 1991, 25:1–22.

[4] K. B. Chandran and S. W. Shalaby, Soft tissue replacements, in *The Biomedical Engineering Handbook*, ed. J. D. Bronzino, (CRC Press, New York, USA, 1995), pp. 648–665.

[5] B. J-L. Moyen, P. J. Lahey, E. H. Weinberg, and W. H. Harris, Effects on intact femora of dogs of the application and removal of metal plates, *J. Bone Joint Surg.*, 1978, 60A(7):940–947.

[6] H. K. Uhthoff and M. Finnegan, The effects of metal plates on post-traumatic remodeling and bone mass, *J Bone Joint Surg.*, 1983, 65B(1):66–71.

[7] P. Christel, L. Claes, and S. A. Brown, Carbon reinforced composites in orthopedic surgery, in *High Performance Biomaterials: A Comprehensive Guide to Medical and Pharmaceutical Applications*, ed. M. Szycher, (Technomic Publishing Co., Inc., Lancaster, USA, 1991) pp. 499–518.

[8] J. S. Bradley, G. W. Hastings, and C. Johnson-Nurse, Carbon fiber reinforced epoxy as a high strength, low modulus material for internal fixation plates, *Biomaterials*, 1980, 1:38–40.

[9] G. B. McKenna, G. W. Bradley, H. K. Dunn, and W. O. Statton, Mechanical properties of some fiber reinforced polymer composites after implantation as fracture fixation plates, *Biomaterials*, 1980, 1:189–192.

[10] K. Tayton, C. Johnson-Nurse, B. Mckibbin, J. Bradleym, and G. W. Hastings, The use of semi-rigid carbon fiber reinforced plastic plates for fixation of human fractures, *J. Bone Joint Surg.*, 1982, 64B(1):105–111.

[11] G. Peluso, L. Ambrosio, M. Cinquegrani, L. Nicolis, S. Saiello, and G. Tajana, Rat peritoneal immune response to carbon fiber reinforced epoxy composite implants, *Biomaterials*, 1991, 12: 231–235.

[12] C. Morrison, R. Macnair, C. MacDonald, A. Wykman, I. Goldie, and M. H. Grant, *In vitro* biocompatibility testing of polymers for orthopedic implants using cultured fibroblasts and osteoblasts, *Biomaterials*, 1995, 16(13):987–992.

[13] S. Ramakrishna, J. Mayer, E. Wintermantel, and K. W. Leong, Biomedical applications of polymer-composite materials: A review, *Comp. Sci. Tech.*, 2001, 61(9):1189–1224.

[14] K. Fujihara, Z.-M. Huang, S. Ramakrishna, K. Satkunananthham, and H. Hamada, Development of braided carbon/PEEK composite bone plates, *Adv. Compos. Lett.*, 2001, 10(1):13–20.

[15] J. Choueka, J. L. Charvet, H. Alexander, Y. H. Oh, G. Joseph, N. C. Blumenthal, and W. C. LaCourse, Effect of annealing temperature on the degradation of reinforcing fibers for absorbable implants, *J. Biomed. Mater. Res.*, 1995, 29:1309–1315.

[16] M. Zimmerman, J. R. Parsons, and H. Alexander, The design and analysis of a laminated partially degradable composite bone plate

for fracture fixation, *J. Biomed. Mater. Res. Appl. Biomater.*, 1987, 21(A3):345–361.

[17] P. Tormala, S. Vainionpaa, J. Kilpikari, and P. Rokkanen, The effects of fiber reinforcement and gold plating on the flexural and tensile strength of PGA/PLA copolymer materials *in vitro*, *Biomaterials*, 1987, 8:42–45.

[18] A. Nazre and S. Lin, Theoretical strength comparison of bioabsorbable (PLLA) plates and conventional stainless steel and titanium plates used in internal fracture fixation, in *Clinical and Laboratory Performance of Bone Plates*, eds. J. P. Harvey Jr. and F. Games, ASTM, New York, USA, 1994, pp. 53–64.

[19] T. W. Lin, A. A. Corvelli, C. G. Frondoza, J. C. Roberts, and D. S. Hungerford, Glass peek composite promotes proliferation and osteocalcin production of human osteoblastic cells, *J. Biomed. Mater. Res.*, 1997, 36(2):137–144.

[20] J. Kettunen, A. Makela, H. Miettinen, T. Nevalainen, M. Heikkila, P. Tormala, and P. Rokkanen, Fixation of femoral shaft osteotomy with an intramedullary composite rod: An experimental study on dogs with a two-year follow-up, *J. Biomater. Sci. Polym. Ed.*, 1999, 10(1):33–45.

[21] M. van der Elst, C. P. A. T. Klein, P. Patka, and H. J. T. M. Haarman, Biodegradable fracture fixation devices, in *Biomaterials and Bioengineering Handbook*, ed. D. L. Wise, (Marcel Dekker, Inc., New York, 2000), pp. 509–524.

[22] N. Ashammakhi and P. Rokkanen, Absorbable polyglycolide devices in trauma and bone surgery, *Biomaterials*, 1997, 18:3–9.

[23] P. Tormala, P. Rokkanen, J. Laiho, *et al.*, Material for osteosynthesis devices, US Patent 4,743,257, 1988.

[24] S. Ramakrishna and Z. M. Huang, Biocomposite materials, in *Comprehensive Structural Integrity, Vol. 9: Bioengineering*, eds. S. H. Teoh and Y. W. Mai, (Elsevier Science Publisher, UK, 2003).

[25] S. Santavirta, Y. T. Konttinen, T. Saito, *et al.*, Immune response to polyglycolide acid implants, *J. Bone Joint Surg.*, 1990, 72(B):597–600.

[26] O. Bostman, E. K. Partio, E. Hirvensalo, *et al.*, Foreign-body reactions to polyglycolide screws, *Acta Ortop. Scand.*, 1992, 63:173–176.

[27] A. Ignatius, K. Unterricker, K. Wenger, M. Richter, and L. Claes, A new composite made of polyurethane and glass ceramic in a loaded implant model: A biomechanical and histological analysis, *J. Mater. Sci. Mater. Med.*, 1997, 8:753–756.

[28] L. Claes, M. Schultheiss, S. Wolf, H. J. Wilke, M. Arand, and L. Kinzl, A new radiolucent system for vertebral body replacement:

Its stability in comparison to other systems, *J. Biomed. Mater. Res. Appl. Biomater.*, 1999, 48(1):82–89.

[29] M. Marcolongo, P. Ducheyne, J. Garino, and E. Schepers, Bioactive glass fiber/polymeric composites bond to bone tissue, *J. Biomed. Mater. Res.*, 1998, 9(1):161–170.

[30] J. W. Brantigan, A. D. Steffee, and J. M. Geiger, A carbon fiber implant to aid interbody lumbar fusion mechanical testing, *Spine*, 1991, 16(6S):S277–S282.

[31] P. Ciappetta, S. Boriani, and G. P. Fava, A carbon fiber reinforced polymer cage for vertebral body replacement: A technical note, *Neurosurgery*, 1997, 41(5):1203–1206.

[32] Q. B. Bao, G. M. McCullen, P. A. Higham, J. H. Dumbleton, and H. A. Yuan, The artificial disc: Theory, design and materials, *Biomaterials*, 1996, 17:1157–1167.

[33] J. R. Urbaniak, D. S. Bright, and J. E. Hopkins, Replacement of intervertebral discs in chimpanzees by silicone–Dacron implants: A preliminary report, *J. Biomed. Mater. Res. Symp.*, 1973, 4:165–186.

[34] S. Ramakrishna, S. Ramaswamy, S. H. Teoh, and C. T. Tan, Development of a knitted fabric reinforced elastomeric composite intervertebral disc prosthesis, in *Proceedings of ICCM–11*, Vol. 1, (Conard Jupiters–Golad Coast, Australia, 1997), pp. 458–466.

[35] L. Ambrosio, P. A. Netti, S. Iannace, S. J. Huang, and L. Nicolais, Composite hydrogels for intervertebral disc prostheses, *J. Mater. Sci. Mater. Med.*, 1996, 7:251–254.

[36] K. H. Bridwell, R. L. DeWald, J. P. Lubicky, D. L. Spencer, K. W. Hammerberg, D. R. Benson, and M. G. Neuwirth, The textbook of spinal surgery, Book Reviews, (J. B. Lippincott Company, Philadelphia, USA, 1991).

[37] K. H. G. Schmitt-Thomas, Z. G. Yang, and T. Hiermer, Performace characterization of polymeric composite implant rod subjected to torsion, in *Proceedings of ICCM–11*, (Gold Coast, Australia, 1997), pp. V277–V286.

[38] N. Rushton and T. Rae, The intra-articular response to particulate carbon fiber reinforced high density polyethylene and its constituents: An experimental study in mice, *Biomaterials*, 1984, 5: 352–356.

[39] M. Deng and S. W. Shalaby, Properties of self-reinforced ultrahigh-molecular weight polyethylene composites, *Biomaterials*, 1997, 18:645–655.

[40] H. Gese, *et al.*, Relativbewegungen und stress-shielding bei zementfreien Hüftendoprothesen — eine Analyse mit der Methode der Finiten Elemente, in Die zementlose Hüftprothese, (Demeter Verlag, Gräfelfing, 1992), pp. 75–80.

[41] K. R. John St., in Applications of advanced composites in orthopedic implants. In *Biocompatible Polymers, Metals, and Composites*, ed. M. Szycher, (Technomic Publishing Co., Inc., Lancaster, USA, 1983), pp. 861–871.

[42] P. Christel, A. Meunier, and S. Leclercq, Development of a carbon-carbon hip prosthesis, *J. Biomed. Mater. Res.*, 1987, 21:191–218.

[43] F. K. Chang, J. L. Perez, and J. A. Davidson, Stiffness and strength tailoring of a hip prosthesis made of advanced composite materials, *J. Biomed. Mater. Res.*, 1990, 24:873–899.

[44] J. A. Simoes, A. T. Marques, and G. Jeronimidis, Design of a controlled-stiffness composite proximal femoral prosthesis, *Comp. Sci. Technol.*, 1999, 60:559–567.

[45] E. Wintermantel and J. Mayer, Anisotropic biomaterials strategies and developments for bone implants, in *Encyclopedic Handbook of Biomaterials and Bioengineering, Part B-1*, eds. D. L. Wise, D. J. Trantolo, D. E. Altobelli, J. D. Yaszemiski, J. D. Gresser, and E. R. Schwartz, (Marcel Dekker, New York, 1995), pp. 3–42.

[46] E. Wintermantel, A. Bruinink, K. Eckert, K. Ruffiex, M. Petitmermet, and J. Mayer, Tissue engineering supported with structured biocompatible materials: Goals and achievements, in *Materials in Medicine*, ed. M. O. Speidel, (ETH Zurich, Switzerland, 1998), pp. 1–136.

[47] M. Akay and N. Aslan, Numerical and experimental stress analysis of a polymeric composite hip joint prostheses, *J. Biomed. Mater. Res.*, 1996, 31:167–182.

[48] Q. Liu, J. R. de Wijn, and C. A. van Blitterwijk, Composite biomaterials with chemical bonding between hydroxyapatite filler particles and PEG/PBT copolymer matrix, *J. Biomed. Mater. Res.*, 1998, 40(3):490–497.

[49] S. Higashi, T. Yamamuro, T. Nakamura, Y. Ikada, S. H. Hyon, and K. Jamshidi, Polymer-hydroxyapatite composites for biodegradable bone fillers, *Biomaterials*, 1986, 7:183–187.

[50] W. Bonfield, M. D. Grynpas, A. E. Tully, J. Bowman, and J. Abram, Hydroxyapatite reinforced polyethylene — A mechanically compatible implant material for bone replacement, *Biomaterials*, 1981, 2:185–186.

[51] C. P. A. T. Klein, H. B. M. van der Lubbe, and K. de Groot, A plastic composite of alginate with calcium phosphate granules as implant material: An *in vivo* study, *Biomaterials*, 1987, 8:308–310.

[52] W. R. Krause, S. H. Park, and R. A. Straup, Mechanical properties of BIS–GMA resin short glass fiber composites, *J. Biomed. Mater. Res.*, 1989, 23:1195–1211.

[53] F. Issidor, P. Odman, and K. Brondum, Intermittent loading of teeth restored using prefabricated carbon fiber posts, *Int. J. Prosthodontics*, 1996, 9(2):131–136.

[54] S. Ramakrishna, V. K. Ganesh, S. H. Teoh, P. L. Loh, and C. L. Chew, Fiber reinforced composite product with graded stiffness, Singapore Patent No. 9800874-1, 1998.

[55] R. P. Kusy, A review of contemporary arch wires: Their properties and characteristics, *Angle Orthodontist*, 1997, 67(3):197–207.

[56] Z.-M. Huang, R. Gopal, K. Fujihara, S. Ramakrishna, P. L. Loh, W. C. Foong, V. K. Ganesh, and C. L. Chew, Fabrication of a new composite orthodontic arch wire and validation by a bridging micromechanics model, *Biomaterials*, 2003, 24(17):2941–2953.

[57] S. W. Zufall, K. C. Kennedy, and R. P. Kusy, Frictional characteristics of composite orthodontic arch wires against stainless steel and ceramic brackets in the passive and active configurations, *J. Mater. Sci. Mater. Med.*, 1998, 9:611–620.

[58] M. A. Tallent, C. W. Cordova, D. S. Cordova, and D. S. Donnelly, Thermoplastic fibers for composite reinforcement, in *International Encyclopedia of Composites*, Vol. 2, ed. S. M. Lee, (VCH Publishers, New York, 1990), pp. 466–480.

[59] Z.-M. Huang and S. Ramakrishna, Development of knitted fabric reinforced composite material for prosthetic application, *Adv. Compos. Lett.*, 1999, 8(6):289–293.

[60] M. N. Pradas and R. D. Calleja, Reproduction in a polymer composite of some mechanical features of tendons and ligaments, in *High Performance Biomaterials: A Comprehensive Guide to Medical and Pharmaceutical Applications*, ed. M. Szycher, (Technomic Publishing Co., Inc., Lancaster, USA, 1991), pp. 519–523.

[61] B. B. Seedham, Ligament reconstruction with reference to the anterior cruciate ligament of the knee, in *Mechanics of Human Joints: Physiology, Pathophysiology, and Treatment*, eds. V. Wright and E. L. Radin, (Marcel Dekker Inc., New York, USA, 1993), pp. 163–201.

[62] S. Iannace, G. Sabatini, L. Ambrosio, and L. Nicolais, Mechanical behavior of composite artificial tendons and ligaments, *Biomaterials*, 1995, 16(9):675–680.

[63] L. Ambrosio, R. De Santis, S. Iannace, P. A. Netti, and L. Nicolais, Viscoelastic behavior of composite ligament prostheses, *J. Biomed. Mater. Res.*, 1998, 42(1):6–12.

[64] B. Gershon, D. Cohn, and G. Marom, Utilization of composite laminate theory in the design of synthetic soft tissues for biomedical prostheses, *Biomaterials*, 1990, 11:548–552.

[65] B. Gershon, D. Cohn, and G. Marom, Compliance and ultimate strength of composite arterial prostheses, *Biomaterials*, 1992, 13: 38–43.

[66] N. Klein, M. L. Carciente, D. Cohn, G. Marom, G. Uretzky, and H. Peleg, Filament-wound composite soft tissue prostheses: Controlling compliance and strength by water absorption and degradation, *J. Mater. Sci. Mater. Med.*, 1993, 4:285–291.

[67] B. D. Agarwal and L. J. Broutman, *Analysis and Performance of Fiber Composites*, (John Wiley & Sons, Inc., New York, 1990).

[68] B. T. Astrom, *Manufacturing of Polymer Composites*, (Chapman & Hall, London, UK, 1997).

[69] K. K. Chawla, *Composite Materials Science and Engineering*, (Spinger–Verlag, New York, USA, 1998).

[70] Z. Maekawa, H. Hamada, A. Yokoyama, and S. Ueda, Tensile behavior of braided flat bar with a circular hole, *J. Jpn Soc. Compos. Mater.*, 1988, 14(3):116–123.

[71] Z.-M. Huang, On micromechanics approach for stiffness and strength of unidirectional composites, *J. Reinf. Plastics Comp.*, 2019, 38(4):167–196.

[72] S. Ryan, M. Wicklein, A. Mouritz, W. Riedel, F. Schäfer, and K. Thoma, Theoretical prediction of dynamic composite material properties for hypervelocity impact simulations, *Int. J. Impact Eng.*, 2009, 36: 899–912.

[73] R. Younes, A. Hallal, F. Fardoun, and F.H. Chehade, Comparative review study on elastic properties modeling for unidirectional composite materials, in *Composites and Their Properties*, ed. N. Hu, (IntechOpen, 2012), Chapter 17, pp. 391–408. http://dx.doi.org/10.5772/50362

[74] A. R. Ghasemi, M. M. Mohammadi, and M. Mohandes, The role of carbon nanofibers on thermo mechanical properties of polymer matrix composites and their effect on reduction of residual stresses, *Comp. Part B*, 2015, 77:519–527.

[75] L. L. Vignoli, M. A. Savi, P. M. C. L. Pacheco, and A. L. Kalamkarov, Comparative analysis of micromechanical models for the elastic composite laminae, *Comp. Part B*, 2019, 174: 106961.

[76] R. M. Guedes, Validation of trace-based approach to elastic properties of multidirectional glass fibre reinforced composites, *Comp. Struct.*, 2021, 257:113170.

[77] Z.-M. Huang, Mechanics theories for anisotropic or composite materials, *Adv. Appl. Mech.*, 2023, 56:1–137.

[78] Z.-M. Huang, C. C. Zhang, and Y. D. Xue, Stiffness prediction of short fiber reinforced composites, *Int. J. Mech. Sci.*, 2019, 161–162: 105068.

[79] H.B. Huang and Z.-M. Huang, Micromechanical prediction of elastic-plastic behavior of a short fiber or particle reinforced composite, *Compos. Part A*, 2020, 134:105889.

[80] J.D. Eshelby, The determination of the elastic field of an ellipsoidal inclusion and related Problems, *Proc. Royal Soc.*, 1957, A240: 367–396.

[81] Z.-M. Huang, Micromechanical strength formulae of unidirectional composites, *Mater. Lett.*, 1999, 40(4):164–169.

[82] D. B. Gundel and F. E. Wawner, Experimental and theoretical assessment of the longitudinal tensile strength of unidirectional SiC-fiber/titanium-matrix composites, *Comp. Sci. Technol.*, 1997, 57:471–481.

[83] Z.-M. Huang, Simulation of the mechanical properties of fibrous composites by the bridging micromechanics model, *Compos. Part A*, 2001a, 32(2):143–172.

[84] R. F. Gibson, *Principles of Composite Material Mechanics*, (McGraw–Hill, Inc., New York, 1994), pp. 201–207.

[85] Z.-M. Huang, Modeling strength of multidirectional laminates under thermo-mechanical loads, *J. Comp. Mater.*, 2001b, 35(4):281–315.

[86] Z.-M. Huang, The mechanical properties of composites reinforced with woven and braided fabrics, *Comp. Sci. Technol.*, 2000, 60(4):479–498.

[87] Z.-M. Huang and S. Ramakrishna, Towards automatic designing of 2D biaxial woven and braided fabric reinforced composites, *J. Compos. Mater.*, 2002, 36(13):1541–1579.

[88] Z.-M. Huang, Y. Z. Zhang, and S. Ramakrishna, Modeling progressive failure process of multilayer knitted fabric reinforced composite laminates, *Compos. Sci. Technol.*, 2001, 61(14):2033–2046.

[89] Z.-M. Huang, S. Ramakrishna, and A. A. O. Tay, A micromechanical approach to the tensile strength of a knitted fabric composite, *J. Compos. Mater.*, 1999, 33(19):1758–1791.

[90] Z.-M. Huang and S. Ramakrishna, Micromechanical modeling approaches for the stiffness and strength of knitted fabric composites: A review & comparative study, *Compos. Part A*, 2000, 31(5):479–501.

[91] T. E. Matikas and N. J. Pagano, Recent advances in composite science (editorial), *Compos. Part B*, 1998, 29B:91–92.

Chapter 10

Methods and Materials in Prosthetics for Rehabilitation of People with Lower Limb Amputations

Peter V. S. Lee[*,†] **and Hans A. Gray**[*]

*Department of Biomedical Engineering,
The University of Melbourne,
Australia
†pvlee@unimelb.edu.au*

Restoration of gait in people with lower limb amputations requires the aid of an artificial limb often referred to as a prosthesis. This chapter discusses the methods and materials related to lower limb prosthetics. Attention is paid particularly to the interface between the residual limb and the prosthesis, i.e., the prosthetic socket, where man interfaces with machine. The basic considerations, background, and constraints of various state-of-the-art techniques applied to prosthetics are discussed. These include the function and safety of prostheses, computer-aided design and fabrication methods, and prosthetic sockets. The field of prosthetics relies heavily on the innovative use of existing materials often found in other industries. The choice of materials is primarily derived from novel methods used in prostheses fabrication or component design, in order to achieve both function and safety for the person with an amputation. In the current edition of this book chapter, we have added a small section on bone-anchored percutaneous implants, an alternative method to sockets for attaching a prosthesis to a residual limb.

10.1   Introduction

Rehabilitation can be broadly defined as practices that lead to functional physical recovery. It encompasses a wide variety of professionals that can include counselors, therapists, doctors, and engineers, all working toward a similar goal. Rehabilitation engineering as Reswick [1] described is the application of science and technology to ameliorate the handicaps of individuals with disabilities. It applies methods and materials to design and manufacture devices suited to individuals in order to recover physical capabilities. A prosthesis or artificial limb is one such device that aims to substitute the loss of a limb with cosmetic and functional desirability to the person with an amputation. Lower extremity amputation continues to be a major problem due to motor vehicle and landmine accidents and vascular-related diseases.

A lower limb prosthesis can consist of an assembly of several component parts such as a socket, knee, shank, ankle, and foot as shown in Figure 10.1. It is no surprise that modern engineering methods and materials applicable to other industries, e.g., aerospace, have been used in the field of prosthetics. New technology has undoubtedly brought about many accomplishments. How the wooden artificial limb of the 1950s is being transformed into a leg with a flexible plastic socket, computer-controlled knee, carbon fiber shank, and energy-storing foot is certainly commendable. In the 1996 Paralympics in Atlanta, a person with a bilateral leg amputation, Tony Volpentest of the USA, set an athletic 100-meter record of 11.36 seconds — about two seconds behind the world record for able-bodied athletes.

This chapter focuses on the latest methods and materials that have impacted the field of prosthetics for the rehabilitation of people with a lower limb amputation. Prosthetics is only one of the many areas in rehabilitation. The other specialties would require chapters in their own rights.

10.2   Function and Safety

The motivation to introduce new methods and materials is to improve function and safety for people with amputations during walking. When a human walks, the position of the leg can be broken

(a)   (b)

(c)

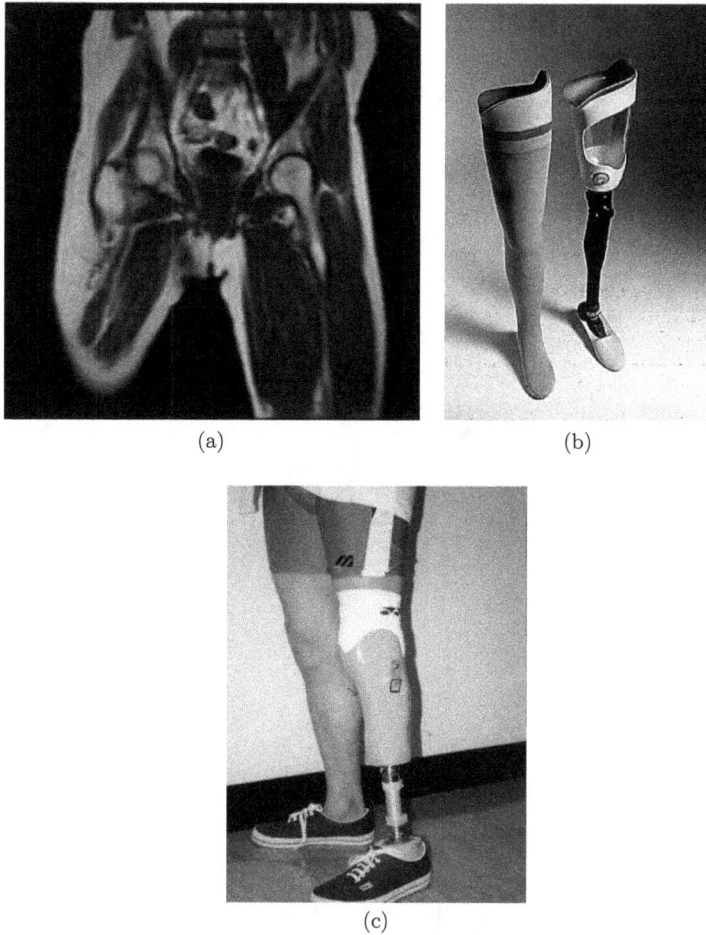

Figure 10.1. (a) MRI of a residual limb after trans-femoral (above-knee) amputation; (b) trans-femoral prostheses; (c) a person with trans-tibial (below-knee) amputation wearing a prosthesis.

down into repetitive cycles consisting of swing-and-stance phases. In the swing phase, the foot moves through the air; during the stance or support phase, the foot is in contact with the ground. The stance phase can then be further divided into heel contact, mid-stance, and toe-off or push-off phases (Figure 10.2).

Prosthetic components therefore have to be optimized for all phases of gait — for example, lightweight for the swing phase and high strength for the stance phase. To this end, the gait of

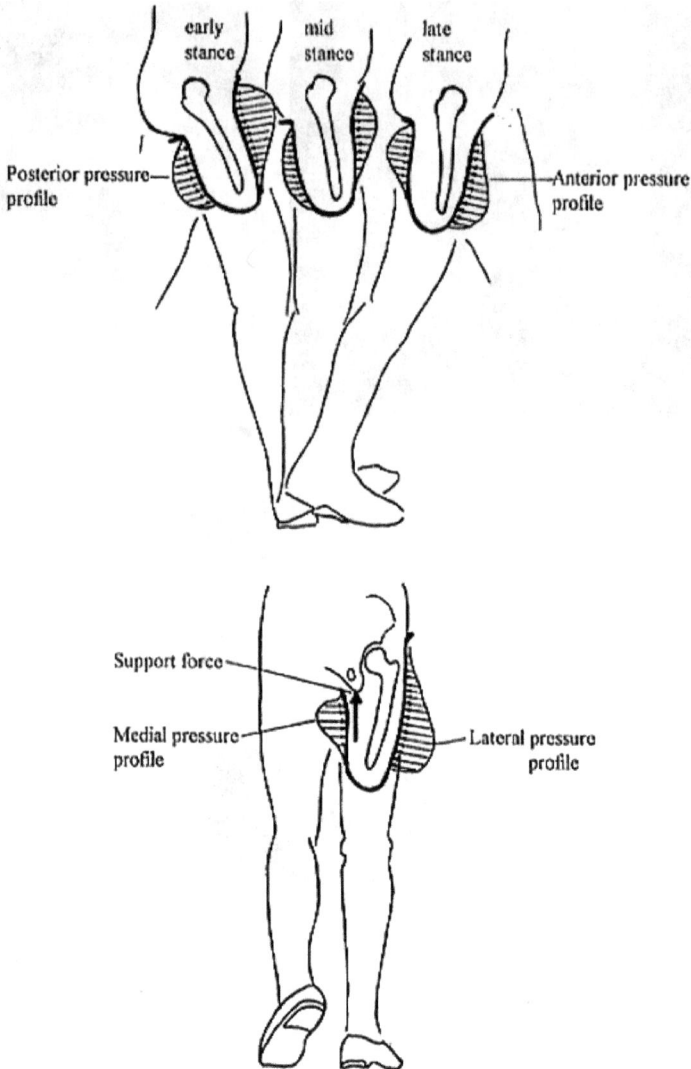

Figure 10.2. Interaction between the socket and residual limb during the stance phase of the gait cycle.

people with an amputation has been analyzed extensively to help design and evaluate prosthetic components. A complete gait analysis includes the study of temporal distance measurements, kinematics and kinetics analyses, energy factors, and muscular activities.

conditions, using a six-degree-of-freedom gait simulator that "walks" the foot to study both structure and function [7].

10.3   Methods and Materials

The process of implementing new methods and materials is slow due to the complexity of the man and machine interface, i.e., prosthesis–wearer interaction. In addition, the rehabilitation industry relies heavily on prosthetists' expertise and skills — which are derived from artisanal methods and which cannot be easily replaced with technology. New methods and materials — in terms of safety and function — are primarily guided by ISO safety standards and driven by patients' needs. Successful methods and component designs demonstrate excellence in balancing the two. The following sections thus discuss state-of-the-art techniques applicable to artificial limb components.

10.3.1   *Prosthetic Socket*

10.3.1.1   *Computer-aided design and manufacturing (CAD and CAM)*

The most important aspect of the artificial limb is the socket, which constitutes the critical interface between the residual limb and the prosthesis. The design and fitting of the socket are also the most difficult procedures due to the uniqueness of each person's residual limb. Every fitting requires much attention from the prosthetist. Although at present there exists a systemization of artisanal practices to design and fit sockets for different levels of amputation, a successful fitting is still highly dependent on the skill and experience of the prosthetist. Nevertheless, Computer-Aided Design and Computer-Aided Manufacturing (CAD and CAM) have emerged as methods that influence the design, manufacturing, and servicing of prosthetic sockets. CAD/CAM initiation arises from the need to automate procedures to increase productivity and the quality of products. The present CAD/CAM system is a much-simplified process compared to other mature engineering CAD/CAM operations. It basically comprises a computer (which controls a shape acquisition system) and a carving machine. The system processes closely copy the artisanal techniques

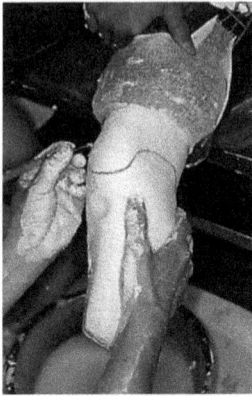

(a) **Shape acquisition using plaster cast.**

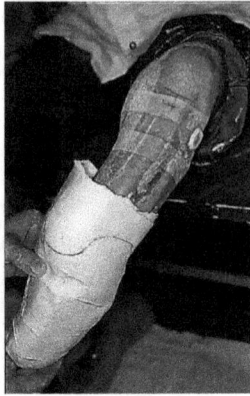

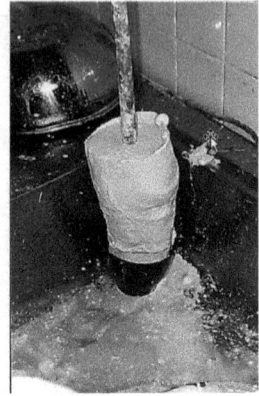

(b) **Plaster of Paris to create a positive model.**

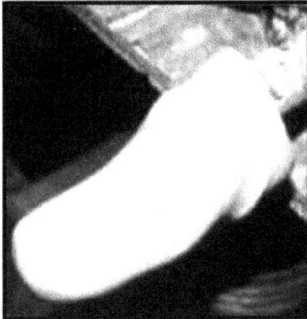

(c) **Shaping the positive model to form the socket; socket fabricated by draping plastic or laminating woven fabrics with resin over positive model.**

Figure 10.4. Artisanal techniques and stages of trans-tibial prosthetic socket fabrication.

(Figure 10.4) of making prosthetic sockets. A similar three-phase procedure is as follows (Figure 10.5):

1) Measurement of body contours where analogue measurements are converted to digital data recognized by computers;
2) Shape generation and manipulation — a shape rectification process controlled by the software user; and
3) Physical realization of socket design.

The initial shape of the residual limb is first recognized through shape measurement or acquisition techniques using a non-contact

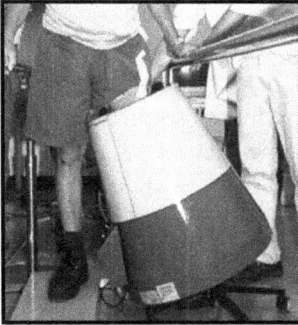

(a) **Shape acquisition using residual limb laser scanner.**

(b) **Rectify scanned model to socket shape.**

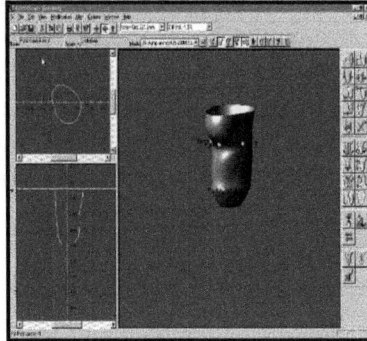

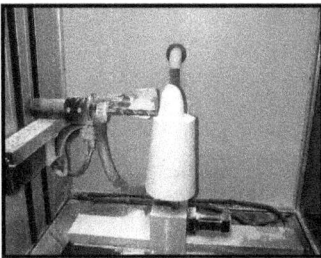

(c) **Milling machine fabricates rectified positive model.**

Figure 10.5. CAD/CAM process of socket design and fabrication.

laser scanner (Figure 10.5(a)). The acquired data are further interpreted by CAD software packages, which enable the residual limb shape to be displayed as computer graphics. The rectification phase of the software allows the acquired shape to be manipulated by decreasing or adding volume to it, moving and slicing it to any desired field of view (Figure 10.5(b)). Finally, a replica of the final socket shape is manufactured through computer codes sent to a numerically controlled milling machine which carves on plaster, foam, or wax

(Figure 10.5(c)). Depending on the final material of the socket, it can be vacuum-formed by draping heated thermoplastics or by applying layers of woven material with acrylic resin over the carved model. The latter is a time-consuming process and may require several days for the resin to cure, which severely hampers the CAD/CAM process's productivity. However, recent studies have shown that it is feasible to produce sockets directly without the need for any positive model. This is done by dispensing semi-molten polypropylene onto a machine table to form a prosthetic socket. Rovick *et al.* [8] and Ng *et al.* [9, 10] described the process using SQUIRT and RMM machines, which are capable of fabricating sockets within 30 minutes and three hours, respectively. The Rapid Manufacturing Machine (RMM) consists of two main components: the robotic system and the dispenser. Polypropylene filaments are fed into the heated dispenser and extruded in a semi-molten state. A filament is then dispensed onto the machine table according to the cross-sectional contour of the socket. The second layer is laid in a similar manner on top of the first. The process continues until the whole socket is built (Figure 10.6).

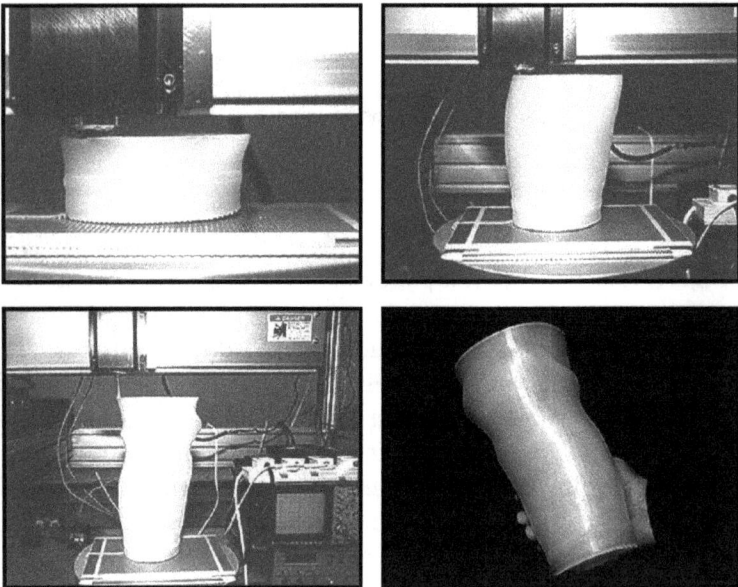

Figure 10.6. Rapid manufacturing machine (RMM), where a socket is fabricated by controlled layering of molten polypropylene.

Due to the layering process, concerns arose over the delamination of the socket materials. The socket materials were then tested using ASTM material test standards. Test results showed that they compared well with the polypropylene sheets used typically for socket fabrication. Moreover, the results indicated minimal strength loss [8, 9]. Ng *et al.* [9, 10] went on to successfully perform the ISO 10328 principal structure test on the socket.

10.3.1.2   *Intelligent CAD/CAM system*

The introduction of the CAD/CAM system for prosthetics has generated much debate. Pritham [11] suggested that until CAD/CAM reaches a product standard equivalent to that of the manual method, its application could not be justified. There are numerous studies comparing the outcome of CAD/CAM and manual sockets [12]. Nevertheless, it is clear a major technical disadvantage of the CAD/CAM system is that no new principles are introduced to optimize socket fit. The system offers only a controlled socket reproduction technique based on conventional principles. The system is still highly dependent on the skill of the prosthetist to produce a good-fitting socket. As described by Klasson [13], "a good fit is primarily not defined by a particular shape of socket, but by the accommodation of forces or pressure between the residual limb and the socket, to provide for comfortable and harmless weight bearing, stabilization and suspension." In line with this definition, residual limb/socket interface pressure is widely accepted as a quantitative way of evaluating socket fit.

As early as the 1960s, experimental studies on the residual limb/socket interface pressure measurement were attempted [14]. Only recently, the Finite Element (FE) method — a computation technique that enables the prediction of soft tissue displacement from input forces/pressures and vice versa — was recognized to have great potential in the field of lower limb prosthetics. By combining CAD/CAM with FE analysis, ideal pressure distribution over the residual limb/socket interface can be achieved and evaluation of different types of socket design can be made quantitatively. This could lead to a new generation of CAD/CAM systems — the intelligent CAD/CAM. A review of the use of the FE method for socket design can be found in a survey by Zhang *et al.* [15].

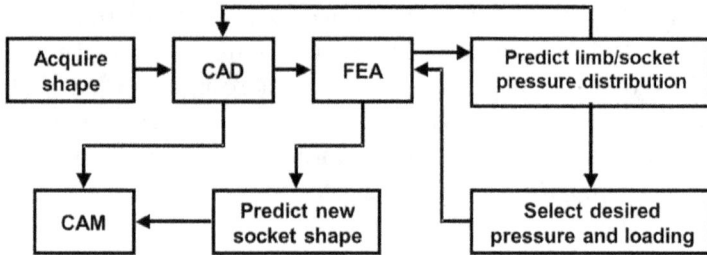

Figure 10.7. Concept of an intelligent CAD/CAM system for prosthetic socket fabrication.

Figure 10.7 describes the concept of an intelligent CAD/CAM process:

1) Acquire residual limb shape.
2) Input shape acquisition data to the CAD software so that an initial socket shape can be defined.
3) Transfer socket geometry data and other parameters required for an FE model to the FE analysis (FEA) program.
4) Calculate residual limb/socket interface pressure. (At this stage, an iterative loop can be formed — each time the CAD software recreates a new socket shape, the system recalculates the new pressure until a satisfactory pressure distribution over the residual limb is obtained.)
5) An alternative approach to step (4) is to define the desired pressure distribution as loading conditions for the FE model and thereby solve for a new socket shape.

The system described here can provide quantitative feedback information to the prosthetist recommending rectification in the CAD software, or even creating a new socket shape with a known and desired pressure distribution. In this manner, the CAD/CAM system can transition from being just a socket reproduction system to a genuine socket design and optimization technology.

Lee *et al.* [16] reported integrating a CAD system (CAPODCad, CAPOD Systems) with FE software (ANSYS, SAS IP Inc.). A volunteer with a trans-tibial amputation and an experienced prosthetist tested the integrated CAD–FE system. The residual limb geometry was captured using a non-contact optical scanner from CAPOD Systems. The residual limb shape was further rectified using the

CAD–FE process by the prosthetist to create a definitive socket shape. A customized program converted the CAD information to FE codes that automatically performed meshing of the residual limb geometry, followed by assigning suitable material properties, loading, and boundary conditions to create the FE model (Figure 10.8).

10.3.1.3 *Prosthetic socket design*

The previous sections described state-of-the-art technologies in prosthetic socket fabrications. With the advent of high-speed computers, SQUIRT, and RMM, productivity in socket fabrication should become less of a problem. However, what remains lacking are technologies that can provide the best or optimal socket fit for an individual patient, according to his/her unique biomechanical properties. The Optimal fit for a patient is an interesting research topic. Mak *et al.* [17] discussed various techniques that have been attempted to elucidate the biomechanics at the residual limb/socket interface. Factors affecting the acceptability of a socket fit can include the residual limb's external and internal geometry, tissue viability (pain, vascular response, lymphatic supply, skin temperature, and abrasion), the tissue's mechanical properties, the socket liner's geometrical and mechanical properties, and finally residual limb/socket interface mechanics generated via external loading (walking, running, and standing). These parameters are highly dependent on each other. For example, different socket materials would produce different residual limb/socket pressure patterns, resulting in different comfort levels and varying gait patterns.

A "good fit" is highly dependent on the skill of the prosthetist, his/her knowledge and experience. He/she must create a socket that will encourage muscle usage, relieve pressure at pressure-intolerant areas, distribute pressure around the residual limb to tolerant areas, and maintain suspension of the prosthesis throughout the gait cycle. All these are achieved through geometrical changes in the socket. Socket shapes or designs and their complementary materials have therefore evolved as one of the more controversial topics in prosthetics. The following sections illustrate some of their key developments.

Trans-femoral prosthetic socket: Currently, two main types of trans-femoral prosthetic sockets are in use: the quadrilateral (quad) socket developed in the 1950s [18] and the ischial containment (IC)

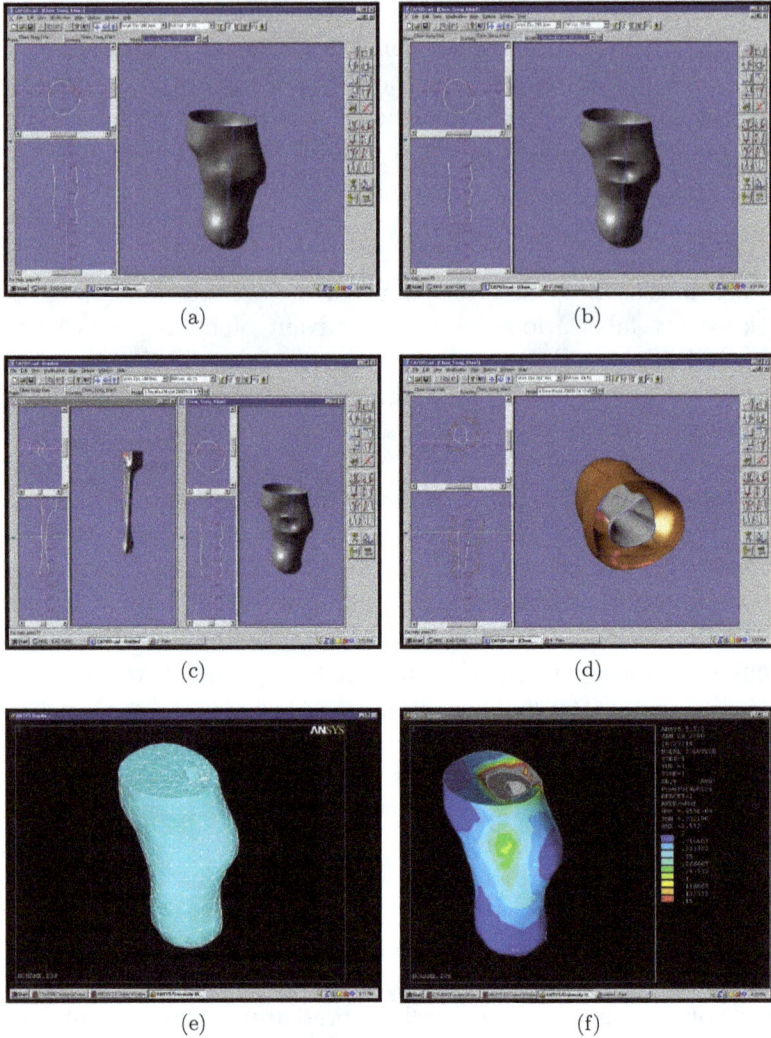

Figure 10.8. Example showing FE stress prediction on residual limb due to a localized compression introduced at the rectification stage: (a) original scanning obtained from AK/BK scanner; (b) prosthetist performed rectification to obtain rectified model; (c) imported generic bone scaled to the patient's anatomical landmarks; (d) bone positioned in the residual limb to form bone model; (e) transformed and combined data from residual limb and rectified bone model to create FE final model; (f) predicted residual limb/socket interface pressure, providing quantitative feedback to prosthetist.

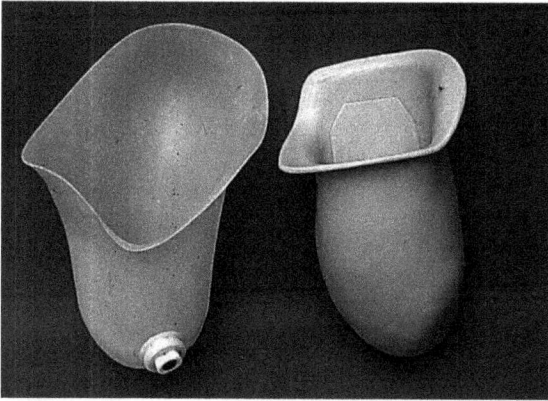

Figure 10.9.   Comparing Quad and IC socket designs.

socket developed in the 1980s [19]. The quad socket (Figure 10.9) takes its name from its shape when viewed in a transverse plane at the ischial tuberosity level. Four distinct walls make up the quad socket. At the proximal brim level of the posterior wall, there is a wide (25-mm) seat parallel to the ground, known as the ischial seat. A large percentage of body weight is directed to this ischial seat via the ischial tuberosity. The gluteal musculature also transmits vertical force onto this shelf. The newer socket design possesses an elliptical rather than a quadrilateral-shaped brim (Figure 10.9). The IC socket was initiated when Long [20] investigated the femoral angle of 100 patients with trans-femoral amputations with the quad socket. By using X-rays, he found 92 to have a difference in angle compared to the sound limb. However, the more significant revelation was that 91 of the patients experienced femoral abduction. Following this finding, new socket designs were attempted to maintain the femur in adduction. Instead of providing an ischial seat, the configuration encloses the ischial tuberosity and ramus within the socket. Hence, this design is generally termed the ischial containment socket or quite often the ischial ramal weight-bearing socket.

Clinical and laboratory evaluations of the IC socket have been carried out by various independent researchers. Gailey *et al.* [21] studied 10 subjects with unilateral amputation, each fitted alternately with quad and IC sockets. Oxygen consumption and heart rate were measured for two speeds of ambulation. The results showed a reduction in

the oxygen intake when the participants used the IC sockets, resulting in about 20 percent less energy. Lee *et al.* [22] measured the
pressure profile of two volunteers with trans-femoral amputations
fitted with both types of sockets. Comparison made between the two
sockets indicated that higher pressures were recorded at the proximal brim of the quad socket, whereas the IC socket produced a more
evenly distributed pressure profile. The pressure distributions on the
medial and lateral walls of both types of sockets were similar, but in
the anterior and posterior walls, significant differences were noted.

Trans-tibial prosthetic socket: The current trans-tibial socket of
choice is the Patellar Tendon-Bearing (PTB) socket that was developed in the late 1950s at the University of California [23]. The socket
design leverages the pressure-tolerant areas in the residual tibia, especially that of the patellar tendon and the posterior aspect of the
residual tibia. PTB socket advocates so determined that the patellar
tendon area could carry a substantial amount of the total load, therefore the patellar tendon bar was introduced to help relieve loading
at other regions of the socket. However, considerable skill is required
to generate a good PTB socket fit. Many prosthetists faced difficulties in consistently producing satisfactory socket fits. As early as
the 1960s, a technique known as pressure casting was introduced
to address these inconsistency problems. Gardner [24] introduced
a pneumatic pressure sleeve that wrapped the entire residual tibia
during cast-taking. Murdoch [25] described another pressure casting
concept where fluid was used as a medium to apply uniform pressure around the residual limb. The aim of these experiments was to
eliminate some factors related to manual dexterity during the casting
process, hence addressing the inconsistency problems.

The pressure casting concept was recently revived by Kristinsson [26], who used air as a medium. Using an air pressure chamber,
the socket shape was defined by casting plaster wrap over the residual limb while wearing a silicone liner. In addition to the silicone
liner, padding was placed over bony areas of the residual limb during the casting process. Casting was performed on the patient in
a non-weight-bearing fashion (i.e., not standing) in an air pressure
chamber. Figure 10.10 shows the commercial Icecast[®] air bladder
system from Ossur hf., derived from Kristinsson's work.

In a later study, Goh *et al.* [27] performed pressure casting
on five patients with trans-tibial amputations. Instead of using

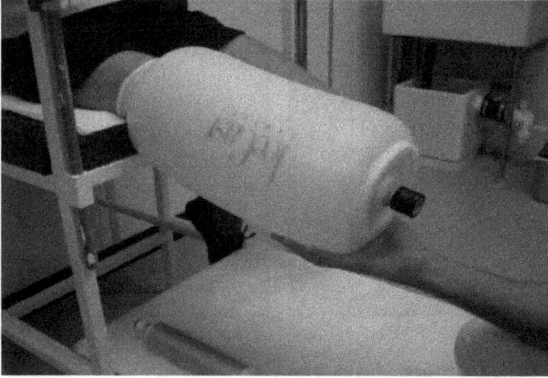

Figure 10.10. Icecast® pneumatic casting system for patient with trans-tibial amputation.

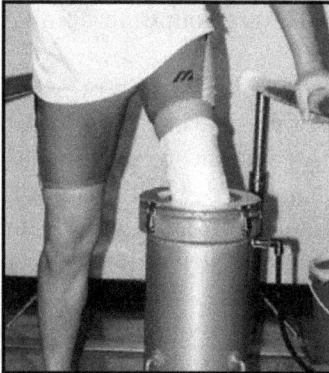

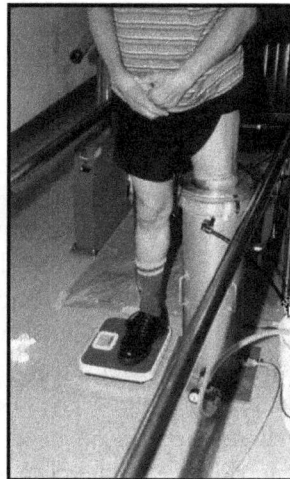

Figure 10.11. Pressure casting using a hydraulic medium.

air as a medium, pressure was applied to each residual limb in a tank separated from the hydraulic fluid medium by a diaphragm (Figure 10.11). Prior to placing the residual limb in the tank, a plaster wrap cast was applied over the residual limb. The patient was requested to stand without any aid, i.e., in a normal standing position under a weight-bearing situation, applying almost half of his/her body weight on the pressurized medium. Once the plaster wrap hardened, the system was depressurized and the plaster was

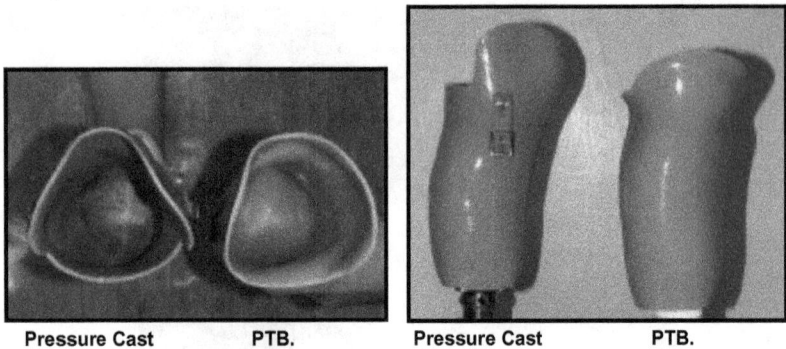

Pressure Cast   PTB.   Pressure Cast   PTB.

Figure 10.12.   Comparing PTB socket and pressure cast socket.

removed from the residual limb. A positive model was generated
from the wrap cast and, finally, a socket was fabricated using traditional lamination methods (Figure 10.12). A very important aspect
of this investigation was that none of the casts required any rectification. Pressure at the residual limb/socket interface was measured
for the five subjects, and socket fits were found acceptable by the
subjects.

The impact of generating an acceptable fit using pressure casting
methods is tremendous and worth investigating. The hypothesis in
pressure casting is "let nature dictate the most realistic and achievable pressure distribution." Such a method will remove all manual
dexterity and inter-prosthetist variances. In addition, an innovative
use of prosthetic socket materials can be derived. The commercial
Icex® system developed by Ossur hf. takes advantage of pressure
casting where there is no need for socket rectification and thus no
need for a positive model. Lee *et al.* [28] similarly reported the use
of a braided carbon fiber sock impregnated with quick-curing resin
prior to casting. The sock was donned directly on the residual limb,
instead of a plaster cast. The sock hardened within minutes to form
the final socket when pressure casting was completed (Figure 10.13).

10.3.2   *Bone-anchored Percutaneous Implants*

Bone-anchored   percutaneous   implants   often   referred   to   as
osseointegrated implants are an alternative to sockets for attaching

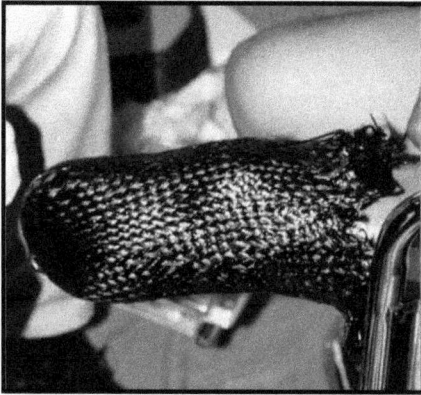

(a) **Resin-impregnated carbon fiber sock draped over residual limb.**

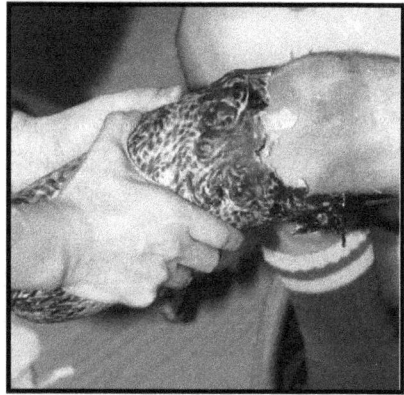

(b) **Sock hardened to form socket after pressure casting.**

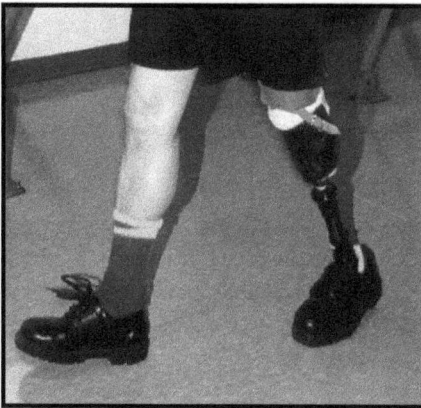

(c) **Socket fitted with the rest of the modular components.**

Figure 10.13. Direct socket casting used with pressure casting system.

a prosthetic limb to a residual limb. A metal implant is surgically attached to the residual limb bone in such a way that it protrudes out of the body through an opening made in the skin (Figure 10.14). The prosthesis is then attached to the part of the implant that protrudes via a connecting device. This technique has slowly gained popularity since its first implementation over three decades ago in Sweden [29]. The technique has several advantages over the use of sockets but is also associated with several challenges.

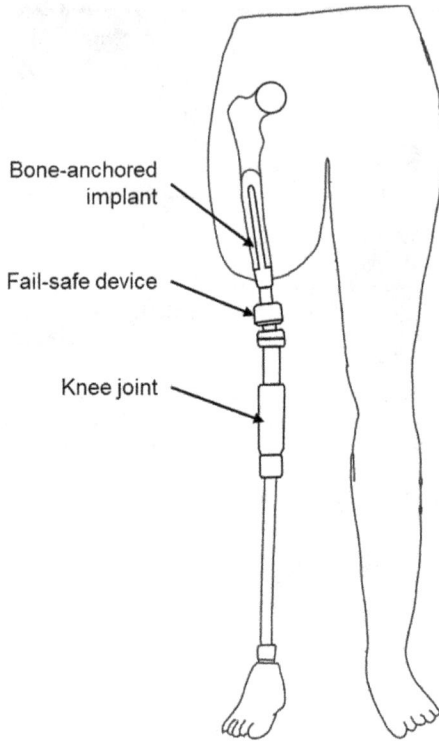

Figure 10.14. Bone-anchored percutaneous implant, fail-safe device, and prosthetic limb assembly for patient with transfemoral amputation.

10.3.2.1 *Advantages and challenges in bone-anchored implants*

The problems often associated with the use of a socket such as soreness, sweating, and poor or inconsistent fit [30] are eliminated through the use of a bone-anchored percutaneous implant. Other advantages of directly attaching the prosthetic limb to the bone are proprioception, osseoperception, and improved patient-reported functional outcomes [31]. Here, proprioception is the patient's ability to sense the movement and location of their prosthetic limb and osseoperception is the ability to feel tactile stimulations (for example, the ability to feel the ground contact through a prosthetic leg) [32]. Although these advantages have led to improved outcomes for patients, bone-anchored implants are associated with an increased risk of residual bone fracture. For example, a relatively large study found that 22 out of 347 (6%) residual femurs failed within 4 years of implantation of a bone-anchored implant [33]. The incidence of femoral fractures in people with transfemoral amputations using a socket is lower by comparison (2% to 3% fracture within the first year). This increase in fracture rate in patients with bone-anchored implants compared to socket users has led to the notion that the direct connection between the implant and bone may be responsible for overloading the bone. An adverse event such as a fall can generate large impact loads on the prosthetic limb. In the case of a socket user, the loads acting on the residual bone may be significantly reduced due to damping caused by the soft tissue between the socket and the underlying bone.

In the case of a bone-anchored implant, the total impact load may be transmitted to the implant–bone construct. Fail-safe devices that are meant to limit the load transmitted from the prosthetic limb to the implant have been in use to reduce residual bone fractures when a bone-anchored implant is used.

10.3.2.2 *Fail-safe devices and their limitations*

Fail-safe devices are fitted between the bone-anchored implant and the prosthetic limb (Figure 10.14). They function as a mechanical fuse that gives way when the loads applied on the implant exceed a predetermined threshold, thereby limiting the load transmitted to the implant. Loads acting on an implant during an adverse event such as a fall are three-dimensional in nature and comprise three force components and three moment components. Most fail-safe devices found in the market at present only protect against a single component of moments (e.g., BADAL X LUCI Connector, OTN Netherlands), while the other five force and moment components are ignored. This may be one reason for bone fracture despite the use of fail-safe devices. One of the reasons for this design limitation in fail-safe devices may be the poor understanding of implant–bone construct strength. A few studies have used cadaver specimens and finite element analysis to study the bone–implant construct [34,35]. However, more work is needed to completely characterize and understand the strength of the bone–implant construct. Such studies could lead to better-designed fail-safe devices as well as better-designed implants with improved outcomes for patients.

10.4 Conclusion

Highlighted in this chapter are the current research issues facing the prosthetic community on the utilization of novel methods and new materials. CAD/CAM has helped to increase productivity in socket fabrication, but currently faces new challenges to quantify socket fits and improve socket designs. However, the topic of designing an optimal socket fit is still being deliberated relentlessly. Simple pressure casting methods that aim to provide a consistent "perfect design" for every individual confront traditional concepts. Nevertheless, new quick-curing direct socket materials have emerged and are capable of achieving same-day prosthesis delivery. New socket fitting methods and components have indeed improved the lifestyle and capabilities of people with limb amputation. Nevertheless, their introduction will always be greeted with both excitement and skepticism. Bone-anchored percutaneous implants provide a viable alternative for overcoming some of the limitations associated with sockets but have other challenges such as increased risk of residual bone fracture that need to be overcome. Well-designed implants and fail-safe devices may provide improved outcomes for patients with amputations.

References

[1] J. B. Reswick, Rehabilitation engineering, *Annu. Rev. Rehabil.*, 1980, 1:55–79.

[2] M. L. van der Linden, S. E. Solomonidis, W. D. Spence, N. Li, and J. P. Paul, A methodology for studying the effects of various types of prosthetic feet on the biomechanics of trans-femoral amputee gait, *J. Biomech.*, 1999, 32:877–889.

[3] J. M. Czerniecki and A. J. Gitter, Gait analysis in amputee: Has it helped the amputee or contributed to the development of improved prosthetic components?, *Gait Posture*, 1996, 4:258–268.

[4] ISO Standards for lower limb prostheses, The Philadelphia Report, *International Society of Prosthetics and Orthotics*, Copenhagen, 1978.

[5]   ISO10328, Prosthetics — structural testing of lower limb prostheses, *International Standards Organization*, Geneva, 1996.

[6]   L. D. Neo, V. S. P. Lee, and J. C. H. Goh, Specimen preparation and principal structural testing of trans-tibial prosthetic assemblies, *Prosthet. Orthot. Int.*, 2000, 24:241–45.

[7]   P. M. Aubin, M. S. Cowley and W. R. Ledoux, Gait Simulation via a 6-DOF Parallel Robot With Iterative Learning Control, *IEEE Transactions on Biomedical Engineering*, 2008, 55:1237–1240.

[8]   S. Rovick, D. S. Childress, and R. Chan, An additive fabrication technique for the CAM of prosthetic sockets, *J. Rehab. Res. Dev., Progress Reports*, 1996, 33:1.

[9]   P. Ng, P. S. V. Lee, and J. C. H. Goh, Prosthetic socket fabrication using rapid prototyping technology, *Rapid Prototyping J.*, 2002, 8(1):53–59.

[10] J. C. Goh, P. V. Lee, and P. Ng, Structural integrity of polypropylene prosthetic sockets manufactured using the polymer deposition technique, *Proc. Inst. Mech. Eng. H.*, 2002, 216(6):359–368.

[11] C. H. Pritham, The application of advanced technology to the production of positive models: A sceptic's point of view, Report, ISPO workshop on CAD/CAM in prosthetics and orthotics, USA, 1988, 8–12th June.

[12] B. Klasson, Computer-aided design, computer-aided manufacture and other computer aids in prosthetics and orthotics, *Prosthet. Orthot. Int.*, 1985, 9(1):3–11.

[13] B. Klasson, Evaluation of CASD CAM, Report, ISPO workshop on CAD/CAM in prosthetics and orthotics, USA, 1988, 8–12th June.

[14] F. A. Appoldt and L. Bennett, Preliminary report on dynamic socket pressure, *Bull. Prosthet. Res.*, 1967, 10(8):20–55.

[15] M. Zhang, A. F. T. Mak, and V. C. Roberts, Finite element modeling of residual lower limb in prosthetic socket: a survey of the development in the first decade, Med. Eng. Phys., 1998, 20:360–373.

[16] V. S. P. Lee, S. K. Cheung, S. K. Pan, J. C. H. Goh, and S. DasDe, Computer Aided Design (CAD)-Finite Element Analysis (FEA) integration for prosthetic socket design, *10th Int. Conf. Biomed. Eng.*, Singapore, 2000, 415–416.

[17] A. F. T. Mak, M. Zhang, and D. A. Boone, State-of-the-art research in lower limb prosthetic biomechanics-socket interface, *J. Rehab. Res. Dev.*, 2001, 38(2):161–174.

[18] C. W. Radcliffe, Functional considerations in the fitting of above-knee prostheses, *Artificial Limbs*, 1955, 2(1):35–60.

[19] J. Sabolich, Contoured Adducted Trochanteric-Controlled Alignment Method (CAT-CAM): Introduction and basic principles, *Clin. Prosthet. Orthot.*, 1985, 9(4):15–26.

[20] I. A. Long, Allowing normal adduction of femur in above-knee amputations, *J. Orthot. Prosthet.*, 1975, 8(1):6–8.

[21] R. S. Gailey, D. Lawrence, H. C. Burdi, P. Spyropoulos, C. Newell, and M. S. Nash, The CAT-CAM socket and quadrilateral socket: A comparison of energy cost during ambulation, Prosthet. *Orthot. Int.*, 1993, 17:95–100.

[22] V. S. P. Lee, W. D. Spence, and S. E. Solomonidis, Stump/socket interface pressure as an aid to socket design in prostheses for transfemoral amputees — A preliminary study, *Proc. Inst. Mech. Eng. H.*, 1997, 211:167–180.

[23] C. W. Radcliffe, The biomechanics of below-knee prostheses in normal level, bipedal walking, *Artificial Limbs*, 1961, 6:16–24.

[24] H. Gardner, A pneumatic system for below-knee casting, *Prosthetic International*, 1968, 3(4/5):12–14.

[25] G. Murdoch, The Dundee socket for below-knee amputation, *Prosthetic International*, 1965, 3(4/5):15–21.

[26] O. Kristinsson, Pressurized casting instruments, 7th *World Congress ISPO*, Chicago, 1992, 43.

[27] J. C. H. Goh, P. V. S. Lee, and S. Y. Chong, Stump/socket pressure profile of the pressure cast (PCast) prosthetic socket, *Clin. Biomech.*, 2003, 18(3):237–243.

[28] P. Lee, J. Goh, and V. Tong (2000), Biomechanical evaluation of the pressure cast (PCast) prosthetic socket for trans-tibial amputee, *World Congress on Medical Physics and Biomedical Eng.*, Chicago, 2000, 23rd July.

[29] Y Li, and R. Brånemark, Osseointegrated prostheses for rehabilitation following amputation : The pioneering Swedish model, *Unfallchirurg.* 2017:120:285–92.

[30] K Hagberg, Jahani SA Ghassemi, K Kulbacka-Ortiz, P Thomsen, H Malchau, and C. A. Reinholdt, 15-year follow-up of transfemoral amputees with bone-anchored transcutaneous prostheses: Mechanical complications and patient-reported outcomes. *Bone Jt J.*, 2020, 102 B:55–63.

[31] J. Sullivan, M. Uden, K. P. Robinson, and S. Sooriakumaran, Rehabilitation of the trans-femoral amputee with an osseointegrated prosthesis: The United Kingdom Experience, *Prosthet Orthot Int.*, 2003, 27:114–20.

[32] V.M. Bhatnagar, J. T. Karani, A. Khanna, P. Badwaik, and A. Pai, Osseoperception: An Implant Mediated Sensory Motor Control- A Review, *J Clin Diagn Res.*, 2015, 9:ZE18–20.

[33] J. S. Hoellwarth, K. Tetsworth, J. Kendrew, N. V. Kang, O. Van Waes, Q. Al-Maawi, *et al.*, Periprosthetic osseointegration fractures are infrequent and management is familiar, *Bone Jt J.*, 2020, 102 B:162–9.

[34] K. Ahmed, R. J. Greene, W. Aston, T. Briggs, C. Pendegrass, M. Moazen, *et al.*, Experimental validation of an ITAP numerical model and the effect of implant stem stiffness on bone strain energy, *Ann Biomed Eng.*, 2020, 48:1382–95.

[35] D. L. Robinson, L. Safai, V. J. Harandi, M. Graf, L. E. C. Lizama, P. Lee, *et al.*, Load response of an osseointegrated implant used in the treatment of unilateral transfemoral amputation: An early implant loosening case study, *Clin Biomech.*, 2020, 73:201–12.

Chapter 11

Chitin-Based Biomaterials

Eugene Khor

Department of Chemistry, National University of Singapore, Singapore
chmkhore@nus.edu.sg

Chitin is a unique biopolymer based on the N–acetyl–glucosamine monomer. Over the years, there has been much interest in exploiting this biopolymer and its variants for a myriad of biomedical applications. Chitin and its derivatives have been shown to be useful as wound dressing materials, drug delivery vehicles, and increasingly as candidates for tissue engineering. The potential for this biomaterial is immense and will continue to increase. Studies are underway to explore its utilization in new biomedical applications and investigate the chemistry of extending its capability.

11.1   Introduction

Traditionally, implants or "body part" replacements were fabricated from inert biomaterials such as metals, ceramics, and synthetic polymers. In recent years, science and technology trends in medical devices have been directed at more "temporal" tissue-engineered implants, which are fabricated using a combination of cells and biodegradable biomaterials. These implants are expected to perform transient roles without upsetting the body's functions and will eventually be replaced by the body's own cells with the biodegradable property (which permits the biomaterial to be removed in a non-toxic manner). The use of biopolymers as biomaterials for such purposes is becoming increasingly popular as materials derived from nature are

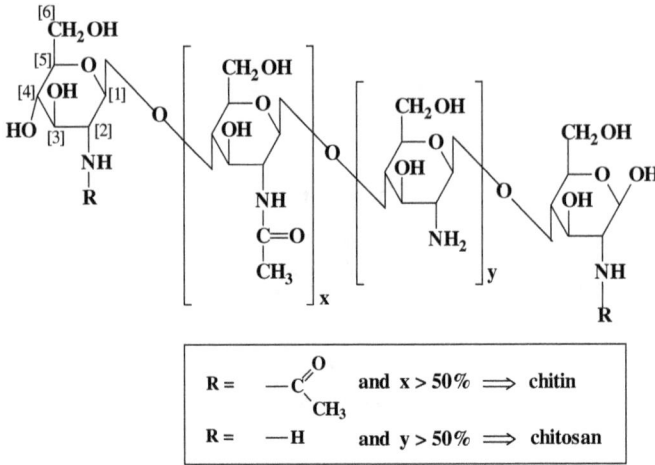

Figure 11.1. Chemical structure of the biopolymer chitin and its derivative, chitosan. Reprinted with permission from Khor [6].

expected to exhibit greater compatibility with humans and may be bioactive and biodegradable. Among the candidate biopolymers for this purpose is chitin.

11.2 Chitin Occurrence and Isolation

Chitin is a co-polymer of N–acetyl–glucosamine and N–glucosamine units (Figure 11.1) randomly or block distributed throughout the biopolymer chain — depending on the processing method used to derive the biopolymer. When the number of N–acetyl–glucosamine units is higher than 50 percent, the biopolymer is termed chitin. Conversely, when the number of N–glucosamine units is higher, the term chitosan is used. Chitin chains are strongly hydrogen bonded, making the biopolymer insoluble in common solvents. Chitosan is the deacetylated chemical derivative of chitin and has been the more prevalent version of the biopolymer because of its ready solubility in dilute acids — rendering chitosan more accessible for chemical reactions and a preferred choice for utilization.

Chitin is a biopolymer found in nature — primarily in the shells of crustaceans and mollusks, in the backbone of squids, and in the cuticle of insects [1]. Chitin is also present in the algae commonly known as marine diatoms, in protozoa, and in the cell walls of several fungal species [2]. Chitin from the diatom spines — such as *Cyclotella cryptica* and *Thalassiosira fluviatilis* — is the only form reported to be 100% poly–N–acetyl–glucosamine; that is, it is not associated with proteins and is termed chitan [3]. A small number of fungal strains are known to produce chitosan in preference to chitin [4]. Chitosan is not native to animal sources and is normally obtained by the deacetylation of shellfish-derived chitin using sodium hydroxide [5].

The primary biological function of crustacean chitin and fungal chitin is to provide a structural scaffold to support the animal exoskeleton or fungal cell wall. While this is achieved differently in animals and plants, the common feature is an intimate link between the biopolymer and the biological system in which it is found. Isolation of the biopolymer involves a systematic destruction of its links with the biological system as well as the removal of components such as proteins, calcium carbonate, and β-glucans. The efficiency of the methods used to remove these components has a significant bearing on the final quality of chitin and chitosan materials [6]. Presently, the chemical method using hydrochloric acid for decalcification and sodium hydroxide for deproteination is practiced on shellfish, although milder enzymatic methods are beginning to make inroads.

11.3   Chitin as a Biomaterial

The potential for chitin as a biomaterial has been reported in scientific literature for more than 40 years. Chitin and chitosan have been shown to be useful materials in biomedical applications such as wound dressings, hemocompatible coatings, drug delivery, tissue engineering, and cell encapsulation. Wound dressings and hemocompatibility coatings are normally external device applications, while tissue engineering and drug delivery are intended for internal use that requires biodegradability — except possibly when drug delivery is *per os*. In this chapter, chitin as a biomaterial in wound dressings, tissue engineering, and drug delivery will be discussed to illustrate its huge potential in biomedical applications.

11.3.1 *Wound Healing*

Prudden *et al.* were the first to use chitin as a wound dressing material. Chitin obtained from shrimp and fungal sources was ground into topical powders and applied to wounds. It was found to accelerate wound healing. The rationale was such that the lysozyme enzyme — which is abundantly present in fresh and healing wounds — acted to break down the chitin powder to release the N–acetyl–glucosamine required for wound healing [7]. Soon after, reports followed in which chitin was cited to be used as a wound dressing material in more conventional ways like as a film or in a woven form. For example, in a report published in the 1980s, chitosan films of differing molecular weights were assessed in wound model studies in which animal models were used. In some instances, the films were even coated with a silver antibiotic. It was demonstrated that animals covered with the chitosan films had a better chance of survival [8].

As for non-woven, fabric-type chitin dressing, the first step in its preparation was to make the chitin fiber. The fiber was then cut into segments of the desired length, followed by dispersing the cut segments in water and binders, thereby giving rise to non-woven sheets. These non-woven chitin sheets have been shown to be effective in treating burns, skin ulcers, and skin graft areas as that wounds are kept dry and the dressing adheres to the wounds well [9]. Another chitin source for this dressing method is from fungal mycelia, which when applied directly as a wound dressing led to favorable results in rat model studies [10].

Fluid-absorbing chitin beads and a bi-layered chitosan membrane obtained by "immersion-precipitation phase inversion" have also been proposed as a wound dressing material [11–13]. In the fluid-absorbing chitin bead, the primary feature was an external layer of carboxymethyl–chitin (CM–chitin) with a chitin core (Figure 11.2). The bi-layered membrane was a thin layer of chitosan that acted as an antibacterial and moisture control barrier and was affixed to a sponge layer to absorb wound exudates. N–carboxybutyl–chitosan has also been developed as wound dressing. The water-soluble, gel-forming ability and ease of sterilization are advantages of this chitosan derivative. Favorable wound healing observations, such as the formation of repair tissue and the absence of scar formation and

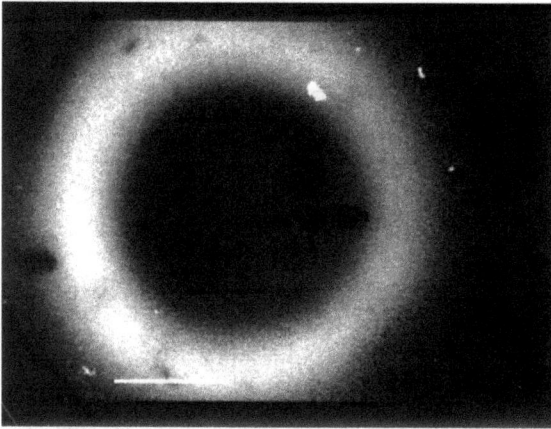

Figure 11.2. Confocal microscope image of chitin bead showing outer core of CM–chitin (light ring) and inner core of chitin (dark circle). Reprinted with permission from Yusof [12], Copyright 2001 from John Wiley & Sons, Inc.

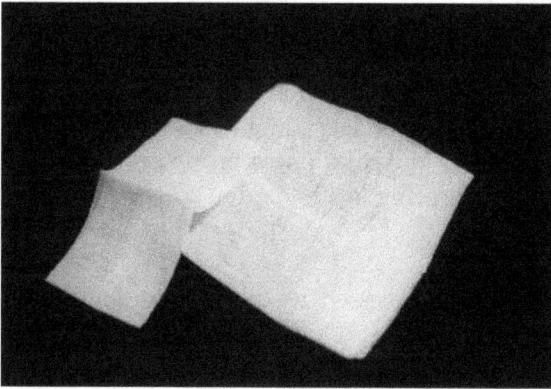

Figure 11.3. Chitosan gauze.

contraction, were noted in animal model studies and human patients [14–16].

Instead of being the only material in wound dressing applications, chitosan materials have been combined with other materials such as collagen and glycosaminoglycans (GAGs). Under such compositions, wound healing was found to be comparable, if not better, than with only single materials [17, 18]. The inclusion of anti-microbial agents (such as silver sulfadiazine and chlorhexidine) into wound dressings has also been shown to be promising [19, 20]. Both instances exhibited favorable infection control or antibacterial activity.

Today, chitosan gauze (Figure 11.3) is widely used in wound dressing applications. However, given the extensive scientific studies devoted to investigating the candidacy of chitin and chitosan as wound dressings, the full potential of these biopolymers is just waiting to be tapped.

11.3.2 *Tissue Engineering*

Tissue Engineering (TE) is defined as "an interdisciplinary field that applies the principles of engineering and life sciences toward the development of biological substitutes that restore, maintain, and improve the function of damaged tissues and organs" [21]. Biomaterials are required in tissue engineering to provide a structure termed "scaffold" onto which cells are seeded and allowed to proliferate to form a "tissue system." Normally, included under the tissue engineering concept is the encapsulation of bioactive substances such as pancreatic β cells that can secrete insulin at a controlled rate. In many instances, biodegradable polymers are used for the scaffolds as they have the advantage of degrading *in vivo* into non-toxic products.

Chitosan is one of the candidates proposed as a suitable polymer to form tissue engineering scaffolds due to the following advantages [22]:

- Chitosan is easily processed as dilute acid solutions into various shapes, films, and fibers. This thus allows scaffolds to be prefabricated in all forms and sizes, including three-dimensional assemblies.
- Since chitosan is insoluble at the physiological pH of 7, the structure once formed is maintained. Moreover, its monomeric unit N–glucosamine that is found in human extracellular matrices gives non-toxic residues upon biodegradation.
- Chitosan can be chemically modified at its C–6 and N–2 positions to give new derivatives, hence extending its versatility.

Porous chitosan scaffolds are commonly prepared in two steps. First, controlled freezing of chitosan solutions and gels to yield pore sizes ranging from 1 μm to 250 μm. Subsequently, it is lyophilization that produces the freeze-dried construct. From this simple two-step process, variously shaped scaffolds that fit the desired applications can be fabricated. The porous nature of the scaffolds makes them behave like composite materials where low-modulus and high-modulus regions — which are dependent on pore size and orientation — are present.

Using similar strategies of freezing and lyophilization, chitin scaffolds with pore sizes ranging from < 10 μm to 500 μm have been reported (Figures 11.4(a) to 11.4(d)) [23]. Any open-pore architecture with pore sizes above 500 μm has been prepared using a novel chemical method (Figure 11.4(e)) [24]. This novel chemical method included calcium carbonate in the chitin gel. Depending on the amount of calcium carbonate particles used, a reaction with dilute HCl then resulted in a homogeneous open-pore system of 100–500 μm pore size with ~76% porosity and another one of 500–1000 μm pore size with 81% porosity.

Several studies have demonstrated the usefulness of chitosan matrices as tissue engineering scaffolds. For example, Mathew *et al.* reported the use of chitosan in cartilage regeneration [25]. In this study, the cationic character of chitosan enabled an interaction with anionic polymers (such as chondroitin–4–sulfate–A (CSA) basis) to form insoluble complexes for membrane fabrication. The membranes are then used to grow bovine articular chondrocytes with retention of phenotype expression both in morphology and mitosis [26]. Hence, this biomaterial could be useful as a carrier for autologous chondrocytes or as a scaffold for the generation of cartilage-like "tissue systems." Frondoza *et al.* reported similar observations, however, with chitosan only. When in contact with human osteoblasts and chondrocytes, chitosan assisted the continued expression of type I collagen in osteoblasts and type II collagen in chondrocytes, suggesting that chitosan has potential applications in bioengineering repair of cartilage and bone defects [27].

Ma *et al.* [28] poured a porogen-containing chitosan solution onto a prefabricated chitosan film. The chitosan film was then freeze-dried and eventually soaked (to dissolve the porogen) in order to produce a bi-layered chitosan film-sponge. Human neofetal dermal fibroblast cells were seeded on this chitosan film-sponge. The growth and proliferation of the cells on the chitosan substrate implied the latter's potential as a tissue-engineered skin substitute.

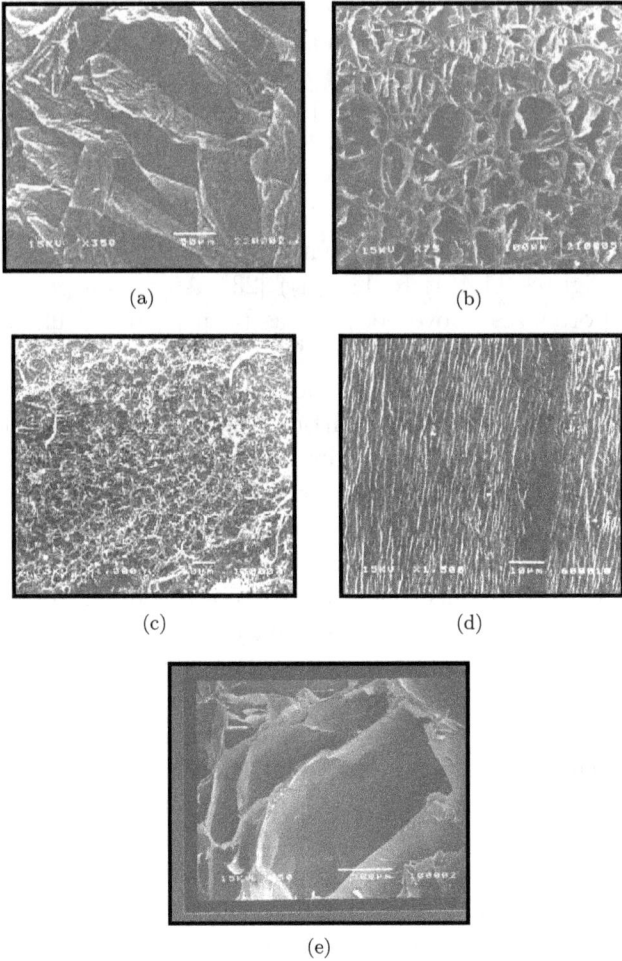

Figure 11.4. Scanning electron photomicrographs showing pore size morphology of variously frozen/lyophilized gels: (a) dry ice/acetone; (b) liquid nitrogen; (c) freezer; (d) air-dried chitin gel; (e) calcium carbonate-produced matrix. Reprinted with permission from Chow *et al.* [23] Copyright 2001, from Kluwer Academic Publishers.

Using simple methods as described, chitin and chitosan biomaterials can be manipulated into various shapes to produce scaffolds suitable for tissue engineering. On this note, the potential of chitin and chitosan as biomaterials in tissue engineering is just beginning to be realized.

11.3.3 *Drug Delivery*

In drug delivery, the drug is normally combined with a polymeric material that serves two purposes: to protect the drug from the biological environment prior to its therapeutic action and to make the drug available to the body.

In today's context, the indispensable requirements of controlled release, sustained release, and site-specific delivery demand more sophisticated delivery systems. This is because a regular dosage of a drug is delivered for an extended period of time at the target site to attain a specific beneficial, therapeutic effect.

For an intravenous application, the polymer normally deteriorates *in vivo*, preferably at a constant rate, releasing the drug or functioning as a semi-permeable membrane in the release of the drug. The polymeric material has to be compatible with the drug. In other words, the material must be non-toxic, stable, sterilizable, and biodegradable — the very qualities discovered of chitin and chitosan, hence justifying studies of these materials as drug carriers.

Chitosan is an important drug delivery vehicle. It has been shown to enhance drug absorption, controlled release, and bioadhesion [29]. In terms of delivery methods, oral, parenteral, nasal, and ocular routes are available, as well as others such as encapsulation for gene therapy and gel systems. If it is by oral delivery, chitosan can be devised in various forms: microparticulate, liposomal, buccal disk, solution, vesicle, coated film, tablet, or capsule. If it is by a parenteral route, chitosan will be delivered in the form of microspheres or solutions.

Early studies utilized gel-based chitin and chitosan for drug delivery applications. For example, the drugs indomethacin and papaverine hydrochloride were included in various chitin or chitosan solutions. Once the solvent evaporated and dried up, the final product was a drug containing chitin or chitosan gel [30]. Steroids, specifically β–oestradiol, progesterone, and testosterone have also been incorporated into chitosan films and beads [31]. Release studies indicated the potential of these chitin and chitosan gels, films, and beads as sustained release agents. Furthermore, dissolution studies on the chitosan films and beads showed no degradation over 30 days, suggesting their usefulness as controlled release systems if degradation of the carrier is not required. Chitosan films containing diazepam have also been prepared for oral administration in rabbit model studies, through which it was shown that film formulations were a suitable alternative to tablet forms [32].

Chitosan and hydroxypropyl–chitosan have been developed for implantable, sustained anticancer drug delivery systems suitable for zero-order drug release [33]. In one preparation, the anticancer agent, uracil, was mixed with chitosan and hydroxypropyl–chitosan powders. The mixture was then dissolved using water and acetic acid. The resulting solution was either cast and dried to give a membrane or extruded through a nozzle into dry air and neutralized with ammonia gas to give stick forms. *In vitro* and *in vivo* studies showed sustained release of uracil.

The pro-drug behavior is further demonstrated when the amino functionality of hydroxypropyl–chitosan interacts with the anti-tumor agent cis–diamino–dichloroplatinum (CDDP) [34]. CDDP containing hydroxypropyl–chitosan was prepared as a cotton mesh and implanted onto the tumor surface of mice. The results indicated that this method of drug delivery provided anti-tumor efficacy with no nephrotoxic side effects normally encountered with systemic delivery. In another study, the pro-drug behavior was demonstrated using the carminomycin–chitosan system where a dialdehyde was employed as the linking agent [35]. An aqueous solution of hydroxypropyl–chitosan containing basic fibroblast growth factors (bFGF) was impregnated into Gore Tex® vascular grafts, entrapping the growth factors as they were deposited by the biopolymer in the pores of the graft [36]. The hydroxypropyl–chitosan slowly dissolved, resulting in the sustained release of bFGF.

The anionic carboxymethyl–chitin (CM–chitin) is another chitin-based candidate for drug delivery in pro-drug platforms, in adsorption and entrapment materials or in methods that combine both adsorption and entrapment [36]. Watanabe *et al.* incorporated 30% doxorubicin in a CM–chitin gel and demonstrated the time-dependent release of the drug from the gel as the lysozyme enzyme hydrolyzed the CM–chitin [37].

Combination systems are another popular channel to achieve drug delivery. For example, the simple mixing of chitosan, sodium alginate, and drug powders, followed by compaction into a tablet form gives good bioadhesion to the buccal and sublingual mucosa — justifying the fact that this method is suitable for intraoral drug delivery [39]. Another demonstration of chitosan as a drug delivery vehicle is through semi-interpenetrating polymer network (semi-IPN) membranes for pH-sensitive drug delivery applications [40]. *In vitro* results indicated that chitosan gels were sensitive to simulated gastric fluid of low pH, hence swelling significantly, whereas in simulated intestinal fluid at neutral pH, the swelling was nominal.

Other examples include a poly(ethylene–vinylacetate) (PE–VAc) copolymer-chitosan co-matrix developed by Chandy *et al.* [41]. Aspirin was first loaded onto chitosan beads, which were in turn exposed to a PE–VAc solution. The solvent was left to evaporate to generate the co-matrix. Release studies showed a burst effect that could be attenuated by an additional polystyrene butadiene barrier membrane. Chitosan–gelatin sponges are another system that has been shown to provide a controlled release of prednisolone [42]. Finally, a new pH-sensitive system utilizing an inorganic material tetra-ethyl–orthosilicate (TEOS) with chitosan in a transparent IPN membrane (that swells at low pH and shrinks at physiological pH) can be useful as a delivery system [43].

Microspheres and their more recent descendant nanospheres, well liked for their better drug release profiles or the ability to protect body tissue from harmful side effects of the drug, are another popular method of effecting drug delivery.

In a series of papers, Nishioka *et al.* described a simple method of preparing CDDP that contains chitosan microspheres. First, the drug cis–diamino–dichloroplatinum (CDDP) was dispersed in a chitosan solution to be followed by vortexing until the desired sizes of particles were attained. The particles were crosslinked with glutaraldehyde to derive consolidated microspheres. Finally, lyophilization gave rise to the drug-containing chitosan microspheres [44–46]. The authors found that increasing the amount of chitosan or adding chitin to the mixture prior to forming the microspheres led to an increase in CDDP incorporation, while at the same time the release rate of CDDP became more regulated with no initial burst effect. The improvement was attributed to better consolidation of the microspheres arising from the higher amount of biopolymers.

In another technique, diclofenac sodium (DS) was dispersed in a chitosan solution followed by dropping via a syringe/needle assembly into a non-solvent tripolyphosphate. This gave rise to microspheres that were roughly $750\,\mu$m in diameter with a very narrow

size distribution [47]. A slow release of the drug was obtained over
six hours *in vitro*, while *in vivo* studies demonstrated effective protection of the gastric mucosa. Other drugs that have been incorporated using similar techniques include 5–fluorouracil, where the drug
release characteristics were in turn modified with other substances
such as alginic acid, chitin, and agar. Bisphosphonates were used
for treating pathological bone conditions and gadolinium–DTPA for
neutron capture cancer therapy [48–50]. As for oral vaccination applications, microparticles of chitosan were prepared from a surfactant
containing chitosan solution, which was subjected to stirring and son-
ication. The chitosan microspheres were then loaded with a model
antigen, ovalbumin [51]. The experimental results indicated good
uptake of ovalbumin, and release studies using Balb/c mice showed
good uptake based on Peyer's patches, hence indicating the potential
of chitosan microspheres as a vaccine delivery system. The versatility
of chitosan microspheres is also extended to nasal administration systems. This application method was exemplified when chitosan containing the luteinizing hormone-releasing hormone (LHRH) agonist
was used in prostate and advanced breast cancer treatment prepara-
tions [52].

In gene delivery, polycationic systems bound to DNA via ionic
interactions have been proposed as one delivery route with chitosan as a convenient candidate biomaterial. Leong *et al.* reported
the possible benefits of using chitosan as a delivery system for
DNA-polycation nanospheres [53]. Chitosan was found to readily
form nanospheres with the possibility of conjugating ligands to the
nanospheres for targeting and protecting the DNA during transit and
lyophilization for storage.

To enhance recognition of the cellular target, Murata *et al.*
have synthesized pendant galactose-containing chitosan [54]. Using
N–trimethyl–chitosan (TM–chitosan), galactose units were attached
to the C–6 position of the chitosan monomer. The TM–chitosan
demonstrated low cytotoxicity while the DNA–galactose conjugate
demonstrated receptor recognition. Subsequently, a tetragalactose
group was shown to further improve target recognition [55].

Chemical derivatives of chitin have also been used. For example, the complex coacervation of the anionic carboxymethyl–chitin
with 6–mercaptopurine (an anticancer agent) in the presence of iron
(III) chloride solution produced an ionically crosslinked microsphere

system [56]. On the other hand, Genta *et al.* utilized a spray-drying technique to prepare ampicillin containing methylpyrrolidinone–chitosan microspheres [57]. Although release studies have indicated unsatisfactory profiles as a drug release agent, the chitosan microspheres retain their utility in wound treatment [58].

In summary, there are many ways to utilize chitin, chitosan, and their derivatives for drug delivery. Forms such as tablets, films, and gels do not require sophistication in formulation, while microspheres and nanospheres intended for internal use require proper fabrication that takes biodegradability into consideration. The present emphasis is on efforts to better understand the modulating effects of chitosan on drug transport, as well as mechanisms such as muco-adhesion and action at the tight epithelial cells' junction. As these issues get resolved and become better understood, the vast potential for chitin and chitosan in the drug delivery field will increase.

11.4 Processing

When it comes to biomedical applications, it is mandatory that chitin and chitosan be produced under some form of GMP (Good Manufacturing Practice) guidelines. This is because GMP ensures consistency and verifiable characteristics of the chitin-based materials. Some characteristics that must be consistent and verifiable are molecular weight and degree of acetylation — a regulatory requirement of the material if it is to be incorporated as a component of a medical device, drug, or other medical products. Several companies have started to actively produce GMP "medical-grade" chitosan. Riding on this trend, it is likely that medical-grade chitin and other chitin/chitosan derivatives will soon follow in the not-too-distant future [59].

One of the forerunner examples is the process reported by Dornish *et al.* on producing ultra-pure chitosan salts for biomedical and pharmaceutical use [60]. In the Protosan^{TM} process to produce the ultra-pure chitosan salts, the chitin was first isolated from shellfish sources and deacetylated to give crude chitosan. Subsequently, the chitosan was depyrogenized to remove endotoxins, followed by microfiltration and ultrafiltration to remove insoluble materials and low-molecular-weight compounds, respectively.

Several grades of the Protosan^{TM} material were evaluated for oral, intravenous, and intraperitoneal toxicities using a rat model. No observable toxicological effects were found in all three studies. Several other safety evaluations including hypersensitization studies and the Ames test gave acceptable results.

In summary, the processing of chitin and chitosan has come a long way from crude treatment with acids and bases to produce chitin and chitosan flakes to refined methods that are more regulatory compliant for biomedical applications. The proliferation of "medical-grade" chitin-based biomaterials in the first decade of the 21st century will certainly springboard these biomaterials as a significant resource for a wide variety of biomedical applications.

11.5   Chitin or Chitosan

Chitosan is the more often cited form of chitin whenever it comes to demonstrating the utility of this biopolymer in biomedical applications. In contrast, the intractability tag has been the cause for the lag in exploiting chitin, although the advent of the solvent system N, N', dimethylacetamide/5% lithium chloride is changing this trend. The importance of chitin should be underscored — chitin is the first isolate, while chitosan is chemically derived from chitin. This suggests that chitin is more natural, a fact that may be significant where biomedical applications are concerned.

The utilization of chitin or chitosan — as noted in the survey of biomedical applications — is likely to proliferate, in particular with applications that require the biodegradability property. Increasingly, there will be a need to look at this property more thoroughly. The true biodegradability or bioassimilation of chitin, chitosan, and their derivatives over a defined time period, as well as the consequences of bioaccumulation, must be fully addressed before chitin-based biomaterials receive general acceptability for biomedical applications.

11.6   Future Outlook

Chitin-based biomaterials are poised to be important biopolymers for the present and future needs of biomaterials [61, 62]. The survey in this chapter gives a flavor of the wide-ranging application potential of this biopolymer and its variants. The eventual realization of biomedical products from this biomaterial will vindicate the foresight and hopes currently pinned on this biomaterial, based on its potential and versatility in utilization.

References

[1] G. A. F. Roberts, *Chitin Chemistry*, (Macmillan Press Ltd., UK, 1992) Ch. 1.

[2] E. P. Feofilova, D. V. Nemtsev, V. M. Tereshina, and V. P. Kozlov, Polyaminosaccharides of mycelial fungi: New biotechnological use and practical implications (review), *Appl. Biochem. Microbio.*, 1996, 32:437–445.

[3] J. McLachlan, A. G. McInnes, and M. Falk, Studies on the chitan (Chitin: Poly-N–acetylglucosamine) fibers of the diatom *thalassiosira fluviatilis hustedt*, 1. Production and isolation of chitin fibers, *Can. J. Botany*, 1965, 43:707–713.

[4] S. Arcidiacono, S. J. Lombardi, and D. L. Kaplan, Fermentation, processing and enzyme characterization for chitosan biosynthesis by *Mucor Rouxii*, in *Chitin and Chitosan: Sources, Chemistry, Biochemistry, Physical Properties and Applications*, eds. G. Skjåk-Bræk, T. Anthonsen, and P. Sanford, (Elsevier Appl. Sci., UK, 1989) pp. 319–332.

[5] H. K. No and S. P. Meyers, Preparation of chitin and chitosan, *Chitin Handbook*, eds., R. A. A. Muzzarelli and M. G. Peters, (Atec Edizioni, Italy, 1997) pp. 475–489.

[6] E. Khor, *Chitin: Fulfilling a Biomaterial's Promise*, (Elsevier Sci. Pub., UK, 2001) Ch. 5.

[7] J. F. Prudden, P. Migel, P. Hanson, L. Freidrich, and L. Balassa, The discovery of a potent pure chemical wound-healing accelerator, *Amer. J. Surg.*, 1970, 119:560–564.

[8] G. G. Allan, L. C. Altman, R. E. Bensinger, D. K. Ghosh, Y. Hirabayashi, A. N. Neogi, and S. Neogi, Biomedical applications of chitin and chitosan, in *Chitin, Chitosan and Related Enzymes*, ed., J. P. Zikakis, (Academic Press Inc., Orlando, FL, USA, 1984) pp. 119–133.

[9] Y. Oshshima, K. Nishino, Y. Yonekura, S. Kishimoto, and S. Wakabayashi, Clinical applications of chitin non-woven fabric as wound dressing, *Europ. J. Plast. Surg.*, 1987, 10:66–69.

[10] C. H. Su, C. S. Sun, S. W. Juan, C. H. Hu, W. T. Ke, and M.
      T. Sheu, Fungal mycelia as the source of chitin and polysaccharides
      and their applications as skin substitutes, *Biomaterials*, 1997, 18:
      1169–1174.

[11] Y. W. Cho, Y. N. Cho, S. H. Chung, G. Yoo, and S. W. Ko, Water-
      soluble chitin as a wound healing accelerator, *Biomaterials*, 1999,
      20:2139–2145.

[12] N. L. B. M. Yusof, L. Y. Lim, and E. Khor, Preparation and charac-
      terization of chitin beads as a wound dressing precursor, *J. Biomed.
      Matls. Res.*, 2001, 54:59–68.

[13] F. L. Mi, S. S. Shyu, Y. B. Wu, S. T. Lee, J. Y. Shyong, and
      R. N. Huang, Fabrication and characterization of a sponge-like asym-
      metric chitosan membrane as a wound dressing, *Biomaterials*, 2001,
      22:165–173.

[14] G. Biagini, A. Pugnaloni, A. Damadei, A. Bertani, A. Belligolli,
      V. Bicchiega, and R. Muzzarelli, Morphological study of the capsular
      organization around tissue expanders coated with N−carboxybutyl
      chitosan, *Biomaterials*, 1991, 12:287–291.

[15] G. Biagini, A. Bertani, R. Muzzarelli, A. Damadei, G. Diben-
      edetto, A. Belligolli, and G. Riccotti, Wound management with
      N−carboxybutyl chitosan, *Biomaterials*, 1991, 12:281–286.

[16] G. Biagini, R. A. A. Muzzarelli, R. Giardino, and C. Castaldini, Bio-
      logical materials for wound healing, *Advances in Chitin and Chitosan*,
      eds., C. J. Brine, P. A. Sandford, and J. P. Zikakis, (Elsevier Appl.
      Sci, New York, 1992) pp. 16–24.

[17] O. Damour, P. Y. Gueugniaud, M. Berthin-Maghit, P. Rousselle, F.
      Berthod, F. Sahuc, and C. Colombel, A dermal substrate made of
      collagen–GAG–chitosan for deep burn coverage: First clinical uses,
      Clin. Matls., 1994, 15:273–276.

[18] G. Kratz, C. Arnander, J. Swedenborg, M. Back, C. Falk, I. Gouda,
      and O. Larm, Heparin–chitosan complexes stimulate wound heal-
      ing in human skin, *Scand. J. Plast. Recon. Hand Surg.*, 1997, 31:
      119–123.

[19] Y. M. Lee, S. S. Kim, M. H. Park, K. W. Song, Y. K. Sung, and
      I. K. Kang, β-Chitin-based wound dressing containing sulfurdiazine,
      J. Matls. Sci.: Mats. Med., 2000, 11:817–823.

[20] W. K. Loke, S. K. Lau, L. Y. Lim, E. Khor, and K. S. Chow, Wound
      dressing with sustained anti-microbial capability, *J. Biomed. Matls.
      Res.*, 2000, 53:8–17.

[21] B. E. Chaignaud, R. Langer, and J. P. Vacanti, The history of tis-
      sue engineering using synthetic biodegradable polymer scaffolds and

cells, in *Synthetic Biodegradable Polymer Scaffolds*, eds., A. Atala, D. Mooney, R. Langer, and J. P. Vacanti, (Birkhauser, Boston, USA, 1997) p. 1.

[22] S. V. Madihally and H. W. T. Matthew, Porous chitosan scaffolds for tissue engineering, *Biomaterials*, 1999, 20:1133–1142.

[23] K. S. Chow, E. Khor, and A. C. A. Wan, Porous chitin matrices for tissue engineering: Fabrication and *in vitro* cytotoxic assessment, *J. Polym. Res.*, 2001, 8:27–35.

[24] K. S. Chow and E. Khor, Novel fabrication of open-pore chitin matrixes, *Biomacromol.*, 2000, 1:61–67.

[25] J. K F. Suh and H. W. T. Matthew, Application of chitosan-based polysaccharide biomaterials in cartilage tissue engineering: a review, *Biomaterials*, 2000, 21:2589–2598.

[26] V. F. Sechriest, Y. J. Miao, C. Niyibizi, A. Westerhausen-Larson, H. W. Matthew, C. H. Evans, F. H. Fu, and J. K. Suh, GAG-augmented polysaccharide hydrogel: A novel biocompatible and biodegradable material to support chondrogenesis, *J. Biomed. Matls. Res.*, 2000, 49:534–541.

[27] A. Lahiji, A. Sohrabi, D. S. Hungerford, and C. G. Frondoza, Chitosan supports the expression of extracellular matrix proteins in human osteoblasts and chondrocytes, *J. Biomed. Matls. Res.*, 2000, 51:586–595.

[28] J. Ma, H. Wang, B. He, and J. Chen, A preliminary *in vitro* study on the fabrication and tissue engineering applications of a novel chitosan bi-layer material as a scaffold of human neofetal dermal fibroblasts, *Biomaterials*, 2001, 22:331–336.

[29] V. Dodane and V. D. Vilivalam, Pharmaceutical applications of chitosan, *Pharm. Sci. Tech. Today*, 1998, 1:246–253.

[30] S. Miyazaki, K. Ishii, and T. Nadai, The use of chitin and chitosan as drug carriers, *Chem. Pharm. Bull.*, 1983, 31:2507–2509.

[31] T. Chandy and C. P. Sharma, Biodegradable chitosan matrix for the controlled release of steroids, *Biomat. Artif. Cells Imm. Biotech.*, 1991, 19:745–760.

[32] S. Miyazaki, H. Yamaguchi, M. Takada, W. M. Hou, Y. Takeichi, and H. Yasubuchi, Pharmaceutical application of biomedical polymers XXIX, Preliminary study of film dosage form prepared from chitosan for oral drug delivery, *Acta Pharm. Nordica*, 1990, 2:401–406.

[33] Y. Machida, T. Nagai, M. Abe, and T. Sannan, Use of chitosan and hydroxypropylchitosan in drug formulations to effect sustained release, *Drug Design Del.*, 1986, 1:119–130.

[34] K. Suzuki, T. Nakamura, H. Matsuura, K. Kifune, and R. Tsurutani, A new drug delivery system for local cancer chemotherapy using cis-platin and chitin, *Anticancer Res.*, 1995, 15:423–426.

[35] N. Todorova, M. Krysteva, K. Maneva, and D. Todorov, Carminomycin–chitosan: A conjugated antitumor antibiotic, *J. Bioact. Compat. Polym.*, 1999, 14:178–184.

[36] K. Yamamura, T. Sakurai, K. Yano, T. Nabeshima, and T. Yot-suyanagi, Sustained release of basic fibroblast growth factor from the synthetic vascular prosthesis using hydroxypropylchitosan acetate, *J. Biomed. Matls. Res.*, 1995, 29:203–206.

[37] S. Tokura, Y. Miura, Y. Kaneda, and Y. Uraki, Drug delivery system using biodegradable carrier, in *Polymeric Delivery Systems: Proper-ties and Applications*, eds., M. A. El-Nokaly, D. M. Platt, and B. A. Charpentier, (ACS Symposium Series 520, 1993) pp. 351–361.

[38] K. Watanabe, I. Saiki, Y. Uraki, S. Tokura, and I Azuma, 6–O–Carboxymethyl–chitin (CM–chitin) as a drug carrier, *Chem. Pharm. Bull.*, 1990, 38:506–509.

[39] S. Miyazaki, A. Nakayama, M. Oda, M. Takada, and D. Attwood, Chitosan and sodium alginate based bioadhesive tablets for intraoral drug delivery, *Bio. Pharm. Bull.*, 1994, 17:745–747.

[40] V. R. Patel and M. M. Amiji, pH-sensitive swelling and drug-release properties of chitosan-poly(ethylene oxide) semi-interpenetrating polymer network, eds., R. M. Ottenbrite, S. J. Huang, and K. Park, *Hydrogels and Biodegradable Polymers for Bioapplications* (ACS Symposium Series 627, 1996) pp. 209–220.

[41] S. C. Vasudev, T. Chandy, and C. P. Sharma, Development of chitosan/polyethylene vinyl acetate co-matrix: controlled release of aspirin–heparin for preventing cardiovascular thrombosis, *Biomate-rials*, 1997, 18:375–381.

[42] C. C. Leffler and B. U. W. Müller, Chitosan–gelatin sponges for controlled drug delivery: the use of ionic and non-ionic plasticizers, *S. T. P. Pharma Sci.*, 2000, 10:105–111.

[43] S. B. Park, J. O. You, H. Y. Park, S. J. Haam, and W. S. Kim, A novel pH-sensitive membrane from chitosan–TEOS IPN: preparation and its drug permeation characteristics, *Biomaterials*, 2001, 22:323–330.

[44] Y. Nishioka, S. Kyotani, M. Okamura, Y. Mori, M. Miyazaki, K. Okazaki, S. Ohnishi, Y. Yamamoto, and K. Ito, Preparation and evaluation of albumin microspheres and microcapsules containing cis-platin, *Chem. Pharm. Bull.*, 1989, 37:1399–1400.

[45] Y. Nishioka, S. Kyotani, H. Masui, M. Okamura, M. Miyazaki, K. Okazaki, S. Ohnishi, Y. Yamamoto, and K. Ito, Preparation and release characteristics of cisplatin albumin microspheres containing

chitin and treated with chitosan, *Chem. Pharm. Bull.*, 1989, 37:3074–3077.

[46] Y. Nishioka, S. Kyotani, M. Okamura, M. Miyazaki, K. Okazaki, S. Ohnishi, Y. Yamamoto, and K. Ito, Release characteristics of cisplatin chitosan microspheres and effect of containing chitin, *Chem. Pharm. Bull.*, 1990, 38:2871–2873.

[47] M. Açikgöz, H. S. Kaş, Z. Hasçelik, Ü. Milli, and A. A. Hincal, Chitosan microspheres of diclofenac sodium, II: *In vitro* and *in vivo* evaluation, *Pharmazie*, 1995, 50:275–277.

[48] J. Akbuğa and N. Bergişadi, 5–Fluorouracil-loaded chitosan microspheres: preparation and release characteristics, *J. Microencap.*, 1996, 13:161–168.

[49] S. Patashnik, L. Rabinovich, and G. Golomb, Preparation and evaluation of chitosan microspheres containing bisphosphonates, *J. Drug Targeting*, 1997, 4:371–380.

[50] H. Tokimitsu, H. Ichikawa, T. K. Saha, Y. Fukumori, and L. H. Block, Design and preparation of gadolinium-loaded chitosan particles for cancer neutron capture therapy, *S. T. P. Pharma Sci.*, 2000, 10:39–49.

[51] I. M. van der Lubben, J. C. Verhoef, A. C. can Aelst, G. Borchard, and H. E. Junginger, Chitosan microparticles for oral vaccination: preparation, characterization and preliminary *in vivo* uptake studies in murine Peyer's patches, *Biomaterials*, 2001, 22:687–694.

[52] L. Illum, P. Watts, A. N. Fischer, I. Jabba Gill, and S. S. Davis, Novel chitosan-based delivery systems for the nasal administration of a LHRH-analog, *S. T. P. Pharma Sci.*, 2000, 10:89–94.

[53] K. W. Leong, H. Q. Mao, V. L. Troung-Le, K. Roy, S. M. Walsh, and J. T. August, DNA-polycation nanospheres as non-viral gene delivery vehicles, *J. Cont. Rel.*, 1998, 53:183–193.

[54] J. Murata, Y. Ohya, and T. Ouchi, Possibility of application of quaternary chitosan having pendant galactose residues as a gene delivery system, *Carbohydrate Polym.*, 1996, 29:69–74.

[55] J. Murata, Y. Ohya, and T. Ouchi, Design of quaternary chitosan conjugate having antennary galactose residues as a gene delivery tool, *Carbohydrate Polym.*, 1997, 32:105–109.

[56] F. L. Mi, C. T. Chen, Y. C. Tseng, C. Y. Kuan, and S. S. Shyu, Iron(III)–carboxymethylchitin microsphere for the pH-sensitive release of 6–mercaptopurine, *J. Control. Rel.*, 1997, 44:19–32.

[57] P. Giunchedi, I. Genta, B. Conti, R. A. A. Muzzarelli, and U. Conte, Preparation and characterization of ampicillin loaded

methyl—pyrrolidinone chitosan and chitosan microspheres, *Biomaterials*, 1998, 19:157–161.

[58] B. Conti, P. Giunchedi, I. Genta, and U. Conte, The preparation and *in vivo* evaluation of the wound-healing properties of chitosan microspheres, *S. T. P. Pharma Sci.*, 2000, 10:101–104.

[59] E. Khor, Chitin: a biomaterial in waiting, *Current Opinion in Solid State & Materials Science*, 2002, 6:313–317.

[60] M. Dornish, A. Hagen, E. Hansson, C. Pecheur, F. Verdier, and Ø. Skaugrud, Safety of Protosan^{TM}: Ultrapure chitosan salts for biomedical and pharmaceutical use, *Advances in Chitin Science*, Volume II, eds., A. Domard, G. A. F. Roberts, and K. M. Vårum, (Jacques Andre Publisher, Lyon, 1997) pp:664–670.

[61] A. C. A. Wan and B. C. U. Tai, Chitin — A promising biomaterial for tissue engineering and stem cell technologies, *Biotechnology Advances*, 2013, 31:1776–1785.

[62] J. Lv, X. H. Lv, M. H. Ma. D-H. Oh, Z. Q. Jiang, and X. Fu, Chitin and chitin-based biomaterials: A review of advances in processing and food applications, *Carbohydrate Polymers*, 2023, 299: 120142–120155.

Chapter 12

Regulatory Requirements for Medical Devices

Jack Wong[*,‡] **and S. H. Teoh**[†,§]

*Founder of Asia Regulatory Professionals Association (ARPA)
National University of Singapore, Singapore
†Center for Advanced Medical Engineering (CAME)
College of Materials Science and Engineering, Hunan University,
#2 South Lushan Road, Changsha 410082, China
‡jackwong@nus.edu.sg
§teohsh@hnu.edu.cn*

The aim of regulation for medical devices is to ensure that the device is safe and efficacious for human beings. The regulations also improve access of countries to good-quality and safe medical devices by offering step-by-step guidance on strengthening their regulatory controls. All countries seeking to develop their regulatory capacity can apply these steps, protect the consumer, and provide a means for international trade. Most developed regions like the United States, China, and countries in the European Union have strict regulatory standards to protect the well-being of their citizen. The introduction to regulatory requirements for medical devices will give the reader and overview with case studies to understand how to apply regulatory knowledge.

12.1 Introduction

Medical devices are an essential component of healthcare, providing important diagnostic and therapeutic benefits to patients. However, the development and use of medical devices are subject to regulatory requirements [1–3], which aim to ensure patient safety, efficacy, and compliance with legal and ethical standards.

First and foremost, the primary reason for medical device regulation is to ensure patient safety. Medical devices can have a significant impact on a patient's health, and it is important that they are safe and effective. Regulatory requirements establish standards for the design, manufacture, and use of medical devices, including safety and performance requirements. By studying these requirements, manufacturers can ensure that their devices meet the necessary safety and efficacy standards before they are released onto the market. This can help minimize the risk of adverse events and ensure that patients receive the best possible care.

In addition to patient safety, compliance with laws and regulations is also a critical aspect of medical device development. Medical device regulation is a legal requirement in many regions, including the United States, the European Union, and Japan. Regulatory agencies such as the US Food and Drug Administration (FDA) and the European Medicines Agency (EMA) are responsible for enforcing these regulations and ensuring that medical devices meet the necessary safety and efficacy standards. By studying regulatory requirements, manufacturers can ensure that they are following the laws and regulations that apply to their devices. The failure to comply with these requirements can result in legal penalties, including fines and product recalls.

Another important reason to study medical device regulatory requirements is to enhance market access. In many cases, compliance with regulatory requirements is a prerequisite for market access. By studying regulatory requirements, manufacturers can ensure that their devices meet the necessary standards for market approval. This can help streamline the approval process and enhance market access, which can be critical to the success of a medical device. Failure to comply with regulatory requirements can delay or prevent market access, which can have significant financial and reputational consequences for manufacturers.

Finally, studying medical device regulatory requirements can also facilitate international trade. Medical device regulation is often harmonized across different countries, particularly in regions such as the European Union. By studying regulatory requirements, manufacturers can ensure that their devices meet the necessary standards for international trade. This can help facilitate the export of medical devices and open up new markets for manufacturers. Compliance with regulatory requirements can also help build trust and confidence in medical devices, which can be critical to success in the global marketplace.

12.1.1 *Key Terms and Definitions in Medical Device Regulation*

Medical device regulation is a complex and highly specialized field that involves a wide range of terms and definitions. The following are some key terms and definitions that are commonly used in medical device regulation:

510(k): The 510(k) process is a regulatory pathway in the United States for certain medical devices that are considered to be moderate to low risk. It requires a manufacturer to demonstrate that their device is substantially equivalent to a legally marketed device that is already on the market.

CE mark: The CE mark is a symbol indicating that a medical device complies with the European Union's regulatory requirements for medical devices.

Classification: Medical devices are classified into different classes based on their risk level. Class I devices have the lowest risk, while Class III devices (Class IV devices in some countries) have the highest risk.

Conformity assessment: Conformity assessment is the process of evaluating a medical device to ensure that it complies with the applicable regulatory requirements.

De Novo classification: The De Novo classification is a regulatory pathway in the United States for certain medical devices that are considered to be low to moderate risk and for which no legally marketed predicate device exists.

Human factors: Human factors refers to the study of how people interact with technology, including medical devices. It is an important consideration in medical device design and development, as it can impact the safety and effectiveness of a device.

***In vitro* diagnostic device (IVD):** An IVD is a medical device that is used for testing human samples (such as blood, urine, or tissue) outside of the body to diagnose or monitor medical conditions.

Medical device: A medical device is any instrument, apparatus, machine, software, or other similar article that is intended to be used in the diagnosis, treatment, or prevention of disease or other medical conditions.

Pre-market approval: Pre-market approval (PMA) is a regulatory process in which a medical device manufacturer must demonstrate the safety and efficacy of a new medical device before it can be marketed in the United States.

Post-market surveillance: Post-market surveillance is the ongoing monitoring of medical devices after they have been approved and released onto the market. The goal of post-market surveillance is to identify and address any safety or performance issues that may arise.

Quality management system: A quality management system (QMS) is a set of policies, processes, and procedures designed to ensure that a medical device manufacturer produces products that meet the necessary regulatory requirements.

Regulatory agency: A regulatory agency is a government agency responsible for overseeing and enforcing laws and regulations related to medical devices. Examples include the China National Medical Products Administration (NMPA), the US Food and Drug Administration (FDA), and the European Medicines Agency (EMA).

Risk management: Risk management is the process of identifying, assessing, and mitigating risks associated with the use of a medical device. It is an important aspect of medical device design, development, and regulatory compliance.

Unique device identifier (UDI): A UDI is a unique identifier assigned to a medical device to help track and trace the device throughout its life cycle, including manufacturing, distribution, and use.

12.1.2 *Criteria to get Product Registration Approvals*

The product registration approval criteria involve three components: 1) safety, 2) performance of the devices, and 3) quality. These can sometimes be expressed by the following formula:

$$\text{Product Registration approval criteria}$$
$$= \text{Safety} \times \text{Performance} \times \text{Quality}$$

The regulatory approval process for medical devices is complex and involves several criteria that manufacturers must meet to obtain market authorization. These criteria vary depending on the regulatory agency and the country where the device will be marketed, but they generally include safety, performance, and quality.

Safety is a top priority when it comes to medical devices. The device must be designed, manufactured, and controlled in a way that ensures it is safe for patients, users, and anyone who may come into contact with it. This means that the device should not cause harm or injury when used according to its intended purpose. The typical way to demonstrate product safety is data from product testing and clinical studies.

Performance is another key criterion for obtaining regulatory approval. The device must perform its intended function as described by the manufacturer. It should be effective in diagnosing, treating, or preventing the medical condition it is designed for. In addition, the device must be reliable and consistent in its performance. The typical way to demonstrate product performance is data from clinical studies.

Quality is also an important consideration for regulatory approval. The device must be manufactured and controlled in a way that ensures consistent quality and reliability. This includes adherence to the ISO standard on good manufacturing practices, e.g., the ISO 13485 certificate. Quality is critical for ensuring that the device performs as intended and that it is safe for use. The typical way to demonstrate product quality is data from product testing and an ISO 13485 certificate.

12.2   Regulatory system of Key Reference Countries and Key Asia countries

Each country has its own special requirements and Table 12.1 summarizes some of the medical device requirements in the United States, European Union, Japan, Canada, and Australia.

12.2.1   *Regulatory System of the United States of America (USA)*

The regulatory approval system for medical devices in the United States is overseen by the Food and Drug Administration (FDA). The FDA is responsible for ensuring that medical devices are safe and effective for their intended use.

The FDA uses a risk-based classification system to determine the level of regulatory oversight required for each device. This system categorizes medical devices into three classes based on the level of risk they pose to patients: Class I (low risk), Class II (moderate risk), and Class III (high risk).

For Class I devices, which include items such as bandages and tongue depressors, the manufacturer must register their establishment with the FDA, and the device must be labeled with the manufacturer's name and contact information. These devices are generally exempt from pre-market review and clearance by the FDA.

Class II devices, which include items such as hearing aids and X-ray machines, require a pre-market clearance process known as a 510(k) submission. This process requires the manufacturer to demonstrate that the device is substantially equivalent to a device already on the market, known as a predicate device. The manufacturer must provide data and evidence to support the safety and effectiveness of the device.

Class III devices, which include items such as heart valves and implantable pacemakers, require pre-market approval (PMA) from the FDA. This process is more rigorous than the 510(k) clearance process and requires the manufacturer to provide clinical data demonstrating the safety and effectiveness of the device.

In addition to pre-market review, the FDA also conducts post-market surveillance of medical devices. This includes monitoring adverse events and conducting inspections of manufacturing facilities to ensure ongoing compliance with regulatory requirements.

Table 12.1. Summary of the medical device requirements in the United States, European Union, Japan, Canada, and Australia.

Regulation	United States (US)	European Union (EU)	Japan	Canada	Australia
Regulatory Body	FDA (Food and Drug Administration)	European Commission and Notified Bodies	PMDA (Pharmaceuticals and Medical Devices Agency)	Health Canada	Therapeutic Goods Administration (TGA)
Regulatory Framework	FDA 510(k), PMA, De Novo, and Humanitarian Device Exemption (HDE)	Medical Devices Directive (MDD) and Medical Devices Regulation (MDR)	Pharmaceutical Affairs Law (PAL) and the Medical Device Act (MDA)	Medical Devices Regulations	Therapeutic Goods Act and Therapeutic Goods Regulations
Risk Classification	Class I, II, and III	Class I, IIa, IIb, and III	Class I, II, III, and IV	Class I, II, III, and IV	Class I, IIa, IIb, III, and IV
Premarket Approval	510(k) notification or Premarket Approval (PMA)	Conformité Européene (CE) Marking and Notified Body Certification	Pre-market Certification	Medical Device License (MDL) or Medical Device Establishment License (MDEL)	Australian Register of Therapeutic Goods (ARTG)
Quality System	FDA Quality System Regulation (QSR)	ISO 13485 and Notified Body Audits	ISO 13485 and QMS inspections	ISO 13485 and Canadian Medical Devices Conformity Assessment System (CMDCAS)	ISO 13485 and QMS inspections
Post-Market Surveillance	Medical Device Reporting (MDR) and Post-Market Surveillance (PMS)	Post-Market Clinical Follow-up (PMCF), Post-Market Surveillance (PMS), and Vigilance Reporting	Post-Marketing Safety Reporting (PMSR) and Adverse Event Reporting (AER)	Mandatory Problem Reporting and Post-Market Surveillance	Post-Market Review and Monitoring

12.2.2   *Regulatory System of the European Union (EU)*

The regulatory approval system for medical devices in Europe is overseen by the European Medicines Agency (EMA). The EMA is responsible for ensuring that medical devices are safe and effective for their intended use.

The European regulatory system for medical devices is based on the Medical Device Regulation (MDR) and the *In Vitro* Diagnostic Regulation (IVDR), which replaced the previous Medical Device Directives in May 2021. The MDR and IVDR introduce more rigorous requirements for medical devices, including stricter pre-market evaluation and post-market surveillance.

Under the new regulations, medical devices are classified based on their risk to patients. There are four classes of medical devices, ranging from Class I (low risk), Class IIa, and Class IIb to Class III (high risk). Class I devices are generally subject to self-certification by the manufacturer, while higher-risk devices require a conformity assessment by a Notified Body.

The conformity assessment process involves an evaluation of the manufacturer's quality management system, as well as testing and evaluation of the device itself. For Class III devices, which include items such as implantable pacemakers and heart valves, the Notified Body must also review clinical data demonstrating the safety and effectiveness of the device.

In addition to pre-market review, the European regulatory system also includes post-market surveillance of medical devices. This includes monitoring adverse events and conducting inspections of manufacturing facilities to ensure ongoing compliance with regulatory requirements.

The MDR and IVDR also introduce new requirements for labeling and traceability of medical devices, as well as enhanced transparency and information sharing between regulatory authorities and manufacturers.

12.2.3   *Regulatory System of Japan*

The regulatory approval system for medical devices in Japan is overseen by the Pharmaceuticals and Medical Devices Agency (PMDA).

The PMDA is responsible for ensuring that medical devices are safe and effective for their intended use.

The Japanese regulatory system for medical devices is based on the Pharmaceutical and Medical Device Act (PMD Act) and related regulations. The PMD Act applies to both medical devices and pharmaceuticals.

Under the PMD Act, medical devices are classified into three classes based on their level of risk to patients. Class I devices are low risk, Class II devices are moderate risk, and Class III devices are high risk.

For Class I devices, the manufacturer must submit a notification to the PMDA before marketing the device. The notification should include information about the device's safety and effectiveness, as well as its manufacturing and quality control processes.

Class II devices require a pre-market review process, known as a "Shonin" application, similar to the 510(k) process in the United States. The manufacturer must demonstrate that the device is safe and effective for its intended use, and provide data and evidence to support the safety and effectiveness of the device.

Class III devices require a more rigorous pre-market review process, known as a "Shonin" application with clinical data, similar to the pre-market approval (PMA) process in the United States. The manufacturer must provide clinical data demonstrating the safety and effectiveness of the device.

In addition to pre-market review, the Japanese regulatory system also includes post-market surveillance of medical devices.

12.2.4 *Regulatory System of Canada*

Canada's medical device regulatory system is structured to ensure that medical devices available on the market are safe, effective, and of high quality. The system is managed by Health Canada under the Medical Device Regulations (MDR) of the Food and Drugs Act and is comprehensive, covering various stages from pre-market evaluation to post-market surveillance.

The basis of the regulatory framework is a classification system that categorizes medical devices into four classes based on the degree of risk they pose. Class I devices such as bandages and thermometers pose the lowest risk, while Class IV devices such as heart valves and nerve stimulators pose the highest risk. This classification determines the regulatory requirements for each device, with higher-risk devices subject to more rigorous testing.

The licensing process varies by device class. Class I devices do not require a medical device license but must meet safety and effectiveness standards. In contrast, Class II, III, and IV devices must obtain a medical device license before entering the Canadian market. Applying for these licenses requires detailed submissions that demonstrate the safety, effectiveness, and quality of the device and are tailored to the complexity and risk level of the device.

An important aspect of compliance for Class II, III, and IV devices is the implementation of a quality management system "QMS." This corresponds to ISO 13485: 2016. This international standard describes the requirements for a QMS specifically for the medical device industry and helps manufacturers maintain the consistent quality of their products. Canada's Medical Device Conformity Assessment System "CMDCAS" was replaced by MDSAP in January 2019. The Medical Device Single Audit Program (MDSAP) is an initiative that allows a medical device manufacturer to meet the requirements of multiple regulatory agencies with a single regulatory audit of his QMS. Health Canada is participating in the program, as well as regulatory authorities in the United States, Australia, Brazil, and Japan. Under MDSAP, manufacturers are audited by accredited audit organizations (AOs) and the results of these audits are recognized by participating regulatory authorities.

Post-market surveillance is an important part of the regulatory framework. Once a device is on the market, manufacturers must continually monitor its performance and report any adverse events to Health Canada. This continued vigilance helps identify potential problems early and quickly take corrective action to protect public health.

Canada's Medical Device Regulatory System, administered by Health Canada, is a robust framework designed to ensure that medical devices are safe, effective, and of high quality. Complying with these regulations allows manufacturers to navigate the complex Canadian market and ensure that their products meet the rigorous standards necessary to protect public health.

12.2.5   *Regulatory System of Australia*

The regulatory approval system for medical devices in Australia is overseen by the Therapeutic Goods Administration (TGA). The TGA is responsible for ensuring that medical devices are safe and effective for their intended use.

The Australian regulatory system for medical devices is based on the Therapeutic Goods Act 1989 (the Act) and the related regulations. Under the Act, medical devices are classified based on their risk to patients. There are four classes of medical devices, ranging from Class I (low risk) to Class III (high risk).

Class I devices are generally subject to self-certification by the manufacturer, while higher-risk devices require an evaluation by the TGA. For Class IIa, IIb, III, and Active Implantable devices, the TGA must assess and certify the device before it can be sold in Australia.

The certification process involves an evaluation of the manufacturer's quality management system, as well as testing and evaluation of the device itself. For higher-risk devices, the TGA may also review clinical data demonstrating the safety and effectiveness of the device.

In addition to pre-market review, the Australian regulatory system also includes post-market surveillance of medical devices. This includes monitoring adverse events and conducting inspections of manufacturing facilities to ensure ongoing compliance with regulatory requirements.

The TGA also maintains a database of medical devices that have been certified for use in Australia, known as the Australian Register of Therapeutic Goods (ARTG). All medical devices marketed in Australia must be included in the ARTG.

12.2.6   *Regulatory System of Asia*

The regulatory approval system for medical devices in Asia varies depending on the country, but many countries have similar regulatory frameworks. The following are some examples of regulatory approval systems in Asian countries and a Table 12.2 to summarize their system:

China: In China, the regulatory authority for medical devices is the National Medical Products Administration (NMPA). Medical devices are classified into three classes based on their risk level. For Class I devices, manufacturers are required to obtain a "product registration certificate" from the NMPA. For Class II and III devices, manufacturers must submit a registration application and undergo a review process that includes an evaluation of the device's safety and effectiveness.

South Korea: In South Korea, the regulatory authority for medical devices is the Ministry of Food and Drug Safety (MFDS). Medical devices are classified into four classes based on their risk level. For Class I devices, manufacturers are required to obtain a "notification of manufacturing and sales" from the MFDS. For higher-risk devices, manufacturers must submit a pre-market

Table 12.2. Summary of regulatory requirements in Asia.

Regulation	China	India	South Korea
Regulatory Body	NMPA (National Medical Products Administration)	CDSCO (Central Drugs Standard Control Organization)	MFDS (Ministry of Food and Drug Safety)
Regulatory Framework	Medical Device Classification Rules and Registration Regulations	Medical Device Rules (MDR) and Registration Process	Medical Device Act and Registration Process
Risk Classification	Class I, II, III, and IV	Class A, B, C, and D	Class I, II, III, and IV
Pre-Market Approval	Medical Device Registration Certificate	Medical Device Registration Certificate	Medical Device Approval (MFDS Approval)
Quality System	Good Manufacturing Practice (GMP) Regulations	ISO 13485 and QMS inspections	ISO 13485 and QMS inspections
Post-Market Surveillance	Adverse Event Reporting (AER) and Post-Market Inspections	Adverse Event Reporting (AER) and Post-Market Surveillance	Adverse Event Reporting (AER) and Post-Market Surveillance

approval application and undergo a review process that includes evaluation of the device's safety and effectiveness.

India: In India, the regulatory authority for medical devices is the Central Drugs Standard Control Organization (CDSCO). Medical devices are classified into four classes based on their risk level. For Class A and B devices, manufacturers are required to submit a "self-declaration" to the CDSCO. For Class C and D devices, manufacturers must submit a registration application and undergo a review process that includes an evaluation of the device's safety and effectiveness.

12.3 Key Standards

Most key standards such as the ISO have four main key elements:

1. Management responsibility;
2. Resource management;
3. Product realization;
4. Measurement, analysis, and improvement.

12.3.1 *ISO 13485*

ISO 13485 is an international standard [4] that sets out the requirements for a quality management system (QMS) for medical devices. It is specifically designed to ensure that medical device manufacturers establish and maintain effective processes and controls to consistently produce safe and effective products. ISO 13485 is applicable to organizations involved in the entire life cycle of medical devices, including design, development, production, storage, distribution, installation, and servicing.

The primary objective of ISO 13485 is to facilitate compliance with regulatory requirements and enhance customer satisfaction by demonstrating the ability to consistently meet customer and regulatory requirements. It establishes a framework for organizations to establish and maintain a quality management system that encompasses all aspects of the product life cycle, from design and development to post-market surveillance.

The standard outlines various requirements that organizations must fulfill to achieve ISO 13485 certification. These requirements cover the following areas:

Management responsibility: Top management must demonstrate commitment to the QMS, establish quality policies and objectives, and ensure adequate resources are available.

Resource management: Organizations must determine and provide the necessary resources, including competent personnel, infrastructure, and a suitable work environment.

Product realization: This includes design and development processes, purchasing and supplier control, production and service provision, and control of monitoring and measuring equipment.

Measurement, analysis, and improvement: Organizations are required to establish processes for monitoring and measuring product quality, conducting internal audits, addressing customer feedback and complaints, and implementing corrective and preventive actions.

Compliance with ISO 13485 demonstrates an organization's commitment to quality and compliance with applicable regulatory requirements. It can help organizations gain access to international markets and enhance their reputation among customers, regulators, and stakeholders. ISO 13485 certification is often a prerequisite for selling medical devices in many countries.

It is important to note that ISO 13485 is harmonized with other key regulatory frameworks, such as the European Medical Devices Regulation (MDR) and the Canadian Medical Devices Regulations (CMDR). This alignment simplifies compliance with multiple regulatory requirements and supports organizations in their efforts to meet both ISO 13485 and relevant regional regulations.

Organizations seeking ISO 13485 certification should engage in a comprehensive implementation process that includes establishing and documenting processes, conducting internal audits, and undergoing external assessments by accredited certification bodies to verify compliance with the standard's requirements.

12.3.2 *ISO 10993*

ISO 10993 is a series of international standards [5] developed by the International Organization for Standardization (ISO) that provides guidance on the biological evaluation of medical devices. These standards outline the principles and procedures for assessing the potential risks associated with medical devices and their interactions with the human body.

The ISO 10993 series covers various aspects of biological evaluation, including the selection and testing of materials, sample preparation, and test methods for evaluating the biocompatibility of medical devices. The ultimate goal of these standards is to ensure the safety and compatibility of medical devices with the intended biological environment.

The series consists of several individual parts, each addressing specific aspects of biocompatibility testing:

ISO 10993-1: Introduction and overview of the biological evaluation of medical devices.

ISO 10993-2: Animal welfare requirements and guidance on the use of animals in testing medical devices.

ISO 10993-3: Tests for genotoxicity, carcinogenicity, and reproductive toxicity.

ISO 10993-4: Selection of tests for interactions with blood.

ISO 10993-5: Tests for *in vitro* cytotoxicity.

ISO 10993-6: Tests for local effects after implantation.

ISO 10993-7: Ethylene oxide sterilization residuals.

ISO 10993-10: Tests for irritation and skin sensitization.

ISO 10993-11: Tests for systemic toxicity.

ISO 10993-12: Sample preparation and reference materials.

ISO 10993-13: Identification and quantification of degradation products from medical devices.

ISO 10993-14: Identification and quantification of metals and alloys released from medical devices.

ISO 10993-17: Establishment of allowable limits for leachable substances.

ISO 10993-18: Chemical characterization of materials.

It is important to note that compliance with the ISO 10993 series is typically required by regulatory authorities as part of the medical device approval process. Manufacturers are expected to conduct bio-compatibility evaluations based on the specific device, its intended use, and the duration and nature of patient contact.

When performing biological evaluations, manufacturers often follow a risk-based approach, considering factors such as device classification, material composition, intended use, and existing scientific literature. Testing may involve a combination of *in vitro* assays, animal studies, and clinical evaluations to assess the potential adverse effects of the medical device on human health.

ISO 10993 standards provide a systematic framework for manufacturers to assess the biocompatibility of medical devices, mitigate risks, and ensure patient safety. They also help in establishing harmonized practices across the industry, facilitating communication between manufacturers, regulatory authorities, and other stakeholders involved in the evaluation and approval of medical devices.

Table 12.3 may help identify what type of tests need to be carried out. The type of tests will depend on the different applications and the different categories. A surface device will need a fewer number of tests as compared to an implantable device.

12.4   Best Practices to get Product Registration Approval Quicker

There are some best practices that companies can follow to streamline the process and potentially expedite approval. The following are a few examples:

Preparation and Organization: One of the key factors in expediting the registration process is being well prepared and organized. This means having all of the necessary documentation and data in order, including clinical trial results, product testing data, and manufacturing process information. Companies should also have a clear understanding of the regulatory requirements and standards for the country in which they are seeking approval.

Early Consultation with Regulatory Agencies: Companies can consult with regulatory agencies early in the development process to

Table 12.3. Evaluation tests could be required depending on category and application.

Category	Contact	contact duration A – limited (≤ 24 h) B – prolonged (> 24 h to 30 d) C – permanent (> 30 d)	Cytotoxicity	Sensitization	Irritation or intracutaneous reactivity	Systemic toxicity (acute)	Subchronic toxicity (subacute toxicity)	Genotoxicity	Implantation	Haemocompatibility
Surface device		A	X [a]	X	X					
		B	X	X	X					
		C	X	X	X					
	Mucosal membrane	A	X	X	X					
		B	X	X	X					
		C	X	X	X		X	X		
	Breached or compromised surface	A	X	X	X					
		B	X	X	X					
		C	X	X	X		X	X		
External communicating device	Blood path, indirect	A	X	X	X	X				X
		B	X	X	X	X				X
		C	X	X		X	X	X		X
	Tissue/bone/dentin	A	X	X	X					
		B	X	X	X	X	X	X	X	
		C	X	X	X	X	X	X	X	
	Circulating blood	A	X	X	X	X				X
		B	X	X	X	X	X	X	X	X
		C	X	X	X	X	X	X	X	X
Implant device	Tissue/bone	A	X	X	X					
		B	X	X	X	X	X	X	X	
		C	X	X	X	X	X	X	X	
	Blood	A	X	X	X	X	X		X	X
		B	X	X	X	X	X	X	X	X
		C	X	X	X	X	X	X	X	X

[a] The crosses indicate data endpoints that can be necessary for a biological safety evaluation, based on a risk analysis. Where existing data are adequate, additional testing is not required.

ensure that their products are designed to meet regulatory requirements and standards. This can help to identify potential issues early on and avoid delays during the approval process.

Participation in Expedited Approval Programs: Some countries offer expedited approval programs for certain types of medical devices, such as devices for rare diseases or devices that address an unmet medical need. Companies can explore these programs to potentially expedite the approval process.

Non-regulated Markets: Companies may also consider launching products in markets without mandatory medical device regulation yet, e.g., Hong Kong, New Zealand, and Chile.

Markets that are linked together: It is interesting to aware if your product is launched in Hong Kong and you will be eligible to launch in Greater Bay Area in China after another simple approval process.

Collaboration with Contract Research Organizations (CROs): Companies can work with CROs to conduct clinical trials and prepare regulatory submissions. CROs can provide expertise in navigating the regulatory process and help companies meet the necessary requirements and standards.

Engage with Local Regulatory Consultants: Many countries have unique regulatory requirements and standards that can be challenging for foreign companies to navigate. Engaging with local regulatory consultants can help companies understand these requirements and expedite the approval process.

It is important to note that while these best practices can potentially expedite the approval process, regulatory approval is ultimately based on a rigorous evaluation of the safety and effectiveness of the device. Companies should prioritize safety and efficacy above all else, and work closely with regulatory agencies to ensure that their products meet the necessary standards.

12.4.1 *Risk Classifications of Medical Devices*

There are three classes of risk classifications for medical devices as described in the following:

Class I: Low-risk devices are not intended for use in supporting or sustaining life (e.g., elastic bandages, examination gloves, and handheld surgical instruments).

Class II: Medium-risk devices are intended for more serious medical conditions (e.g., powered wheelchairs, infusion pumps, scaffolds, and surgical drapes). In some regions like the European Union and Australia, this class is subdivided into Class IIa and IIb:

Class IIa (Low-Medium Risk, e.g., catheters) and Class IIb (Medium-High Risk, e.g., scaffolds for bone tissue engineering).

Class III: High-risk devices support or sustain human life (e.g., pacemakers, external defibrillators, hip implants, and heart valves).

12.4.2 *Clinical Trials*

Clinical trials must comply with Good Clinical Practice regulations. Clinical trials are biomedical or health-related research studies in

Table 12.4. Clinical trial summaries.

I	II	III	IV
Small group of people (**20-80**) for the **first time** to **evaluate** its safety, **determine** a safe dosage range, and **identify** side effects.	Larger group of people (**100-300**) to see if it is effective and to **further evaluate** its safety.	Larger groups of people (**1,000-3,000**) to **confirm** its effectiveness, **monitor** side effects, **compare** it to commonly used treatments, and **collect** information that will allow the experimental drug or treatment to be used safely.	Post marketing studies delineate **additional information** including the drug's risks, benefits, and optimal use.

humans that follow a predefined protocol. Table 12.4 illustrates the various clinical trial categories.

12.5 Case Studies

12.5.1 *Registration of a Class 1 Medical Device in the United States (Listing)-Product: Disposable Surgical Gloves as shown in Figure 12.1*

Overview:

A medical device manufacturer based in the United States has developed a line of disposable surgical gloves and intends to register it with the U.S. Food and Drug Administration (FDA) for marketing and distribution.

Process:

Regulatory Research:

The manufacturer conducts thorough research on the FDA's regulatory requirements for Class 1 medical devices. The company reviews the relevant guidance documents, regulations, and resources provided by the FDA to understand the registration process.

Product Classification:

Determine Device Classification: Confirm that your medical device falls under Class 1 according to the FDA's classification system, which includes low-risk devices that are generally exempt from pre-market notification (510(k)) or pre-market approval (PMA) requirements.

Quality Management System (QMS):

The manufacturer establishes and implements a robust quality management system (QMS) that complies with FDA regulations. It ensures processes are in place to maintain product consistency, quality, and safety, including adherence to good manufacturing practices (GMP).

FDA Listing:

Establish an Account in the FDA's FURLS: Create an account in the FDA Unified Registration and Listing System (FURLS) by visiting the FDA website. FURLS is an online portal used for device registration and listing.

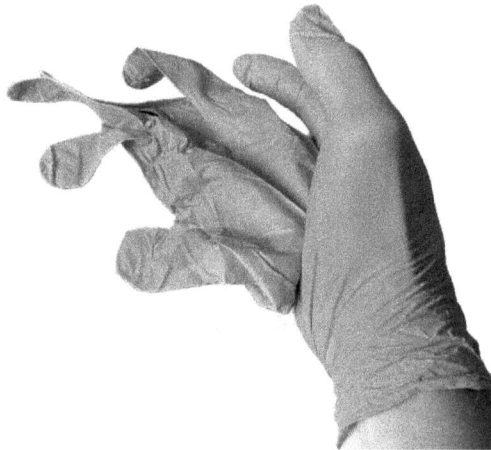

Figure 12.1. Disposable surgical gloves.

Log in to Device Registration and Listing Module: After creating an account, log in to the Device Registration and Listing (DRLM) module within FURLS to access the registration and listing features.

Provide Company and Establishment Information: Enter the necessary details about your company and the manufacturing establishment responsible for producing the Class 1 medical device.

Enter Device Information: Submit the relevant information about the Class 1 medical device, including its intended use, product code, description, and any applicable regulatory information.

Pay User Fee (if applicable): Some Class 1 devices may require a user fee for registration and listing. Check the FDA's Medical Device User Fee webpage to determine if your device is subject to fees and to find information about the current fee schedule.

Review and Confirm Submission: Review all the entered information to ensure accuracy and completeness. Once you are satisfied with the submission, confirm the listing.

Obtain FDA Listing Number: After successful submission and verification by the FDA, you will receive an FDA listing number for your Class 1 medical device. This listing number confirms that your device has been voluntarily listed with the FDA.

Post-Market Responsibilities:

Following clearance, the manufacturer is responsible for post-market activities, such as compliance with medical device reporting (MDR) requirements, post-market surveillance, and maintaining a quality management system (QMS). It must also address any adverse events, conduct post-market studies if necessary, and comply with ongoing FDA regulations.

12.5.2 Registration of a Class 2 Medical Device in the United States (510k)-Product: Automated External Defibrillator (AED) as shown in Figure 12.2

Overview:

A medical device manufacturer based in the United States has developed an Automated External Defibrillator (AED) and intends to

obtain market clearance from the U.S. Food and Drug Administration (FDA) for commercialization and distribution.
Process:

Regulatory Research:

The manufacturer conducts extensive research on the FDA's regulatory requirements for Class 2 medical devices. The company reviews the applicable guidance documents, regulations, and resources provided by the FDA.

Product Classification:

The manufacturer determines the appropriate classification for its AED based on the FDA's classification guidelines. Class 2 medical devices are considered moderate-risk devices and require pre-market clearance through the 510(k) pathway.

Predicate Device Identification:

The manufacturer identifies a suitable predicate device, an already FDA-cleared AED with similar intended use and technological characteristics, to establish substantial equivalence. This predicate device serves as a benchmark for demonstrating the safety and effectiveness of the new AED.

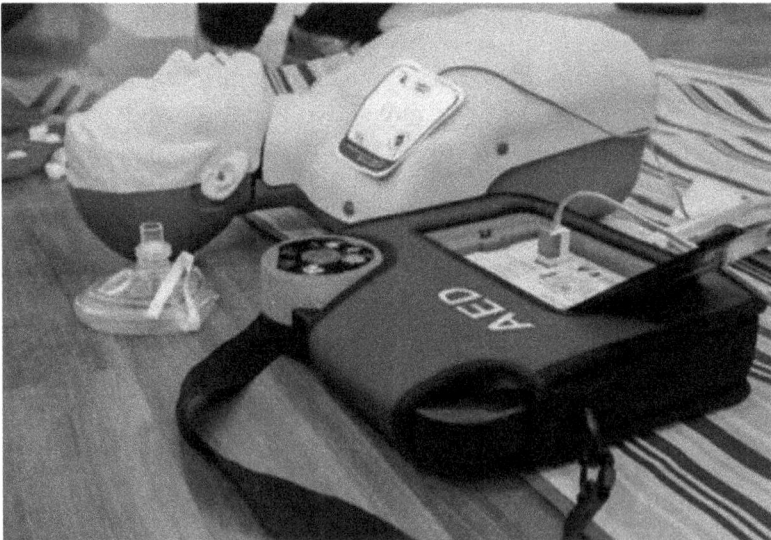

Figure 12.2. Automated external defibrillator (AED).

Preparation of 510(k) Submission:

The manufacturer prepares a comprehensive 510(k) submission, including a detailed description of the new AED, its intended use, design specifications, and performance data. It compiles information on the substantial equivalence of the new device to the predicate device.

Performance Testing:

The manufacturer conducts performance testing and collects relevant data to demonstrate that the AED meets the required safety and performance standards. This may involve electrical safety testing, functional testing, and usability studies.

Risk Management:

The manufacturer performs a thorough risk assessment and develops a comprehensive risk management plan for the AED. It identifies potential hazards, assesses risks, and implements mitigation strategies to minimize any potential harm to users.

510(k) Submission and Review:

The manufacturer submits the completed 510(k) application to the FDA, paying the required user fees. The FDA reviews the submission, evaluating the supporting data, performance testing results, and risk management documentation. It assesses the substantial equivalence of the new AED to the predicate device.

FDA Clearance:

Upon successful review, if the FDA determines that the new AED is substantially equivalent to the predicate device and meets the necessary regulatory requirements, it will grant clearance through the issuance of a 510(k) clearance letter. This clearance allows the manufacturer to market and distribute the AED in the United States.

Post-Market Responsibilities:

Following clearance, the manufacturer is responsible for post-market activities, such as compliance with medical device reporting (MDR) requirements, post-market surveillance, and maintaining a quality management system (QMS). It must also address any adverse events, conduct post-market studies if necessary, and comply with ongoing FDA regulations.

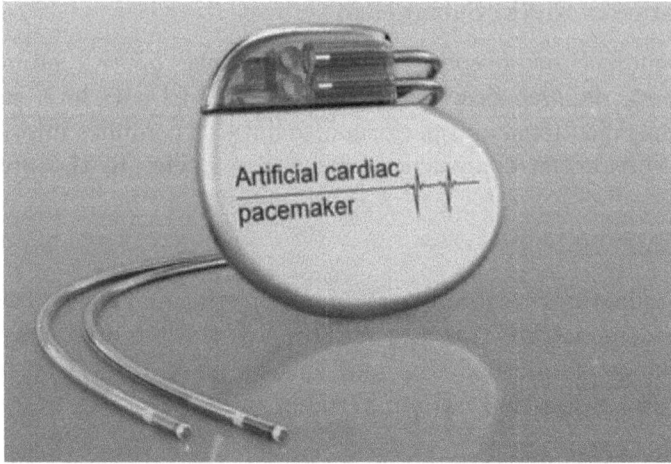

Figure 12.3. An implantable cardiac pacemaker.

This case study outlines the general process for registering a Class 2 medical device in the United States through the FDA's 510(k) pathway. It is essential for manufacturers to consult the FDA's guidance and regulations, as well as engage with the agency throughout the process to ensure compliance with specific requirements and obtain accurate and up-to-date information.

12.5.3 *Registration of a Class 3 Medical Device in the United States (PMA)-Product: Implantable Cardiac Pacemaker as shown in Figure 12.3*

Overview:

A medical device manufacturer based in the United States has developed an implantable cardiac pacemaker with advanced features and capabilities. The company intends to seek approval from the U.S. Food and Drug Administration (FDA) for marketing and commercialization of the device.

Process:

Regulatory Research:

The manufacturer conducts extensive research on the FDA's regulatory requirements for Class 3 medical devices. It reviews the relevant guidance documents, regulations, and resources provided by the FDA, particularly those related to pre-market approval (PMA) applications.

Product Classification:

The manufacturer determines the appropriate classification for its implantable cardiac pacemaker based on the FDA's classification guidelines. Class 3 medical devices are considered high-risk devices that require pre-market approval through the PMA pathway.

Clinical Trial Planning and Execution:

Recognizing the requirement for clinical data, the manufacturer designs and initiates clinical trials to gather safety and effectiveness data for the pacemaker. The company works closely with investigators, obtains necessary approvals, and conducts well-controlled studies on patients to generate robust clinical evidence.

Preparing the PMA Application:

The manufacturer compiles a comprehensive PMA application, which includes detailed information about the pacemaker's design, technology, intended use, manufacturing processes, and clinical trial results. It also addresses device performance, risk assessment, and mitigation strategies.

Risk Management and Quality System:

The manufacturer establishes a thorough risk management plan, identifying potential hazards associated with the pacemaker and implementing appropriate mitigation measures. It also ensures the implementation of a robust quality management system (QMS) that complies with FDA regulations, such as adherence to good manufacturing practices (GMP).

PMA Submission and Review:

The manufacturer submits the PMA application to the FDA, paying the requisite user fees. The FDA reviews the submission, thoroughly assessing the clinical data, preclinical testing results, risk management documentation, and overall safety and effectiveness of the pacemaker. It evaluates whether the benefits of the device outweigh the risks.

FDA Approval:

If the FDA determines that the pacemaker's safety and effectiveness have been adequately demonstrated and the device meets the required regulatory standards, it will grant approval through the issuance of a PMA approval letter. This approval allows the manufacturer to market and distribute the implantable cardiac pacemaker in the United States.

Post-Market Responsibilities:

After approval, the manufacturer fulfills post-market obligations, including adherence to post-market surveillance requirements, reporting of adverse events through the FDA's Medical Device Reporting (MDR) system, and compliance with any post-approval study commitments. It continues to monitor the pacemaker's performance, address any emerging safety concerns, and maintain compliance with FDA regulations.

This case study highlights the general process for registering a Class 3 medical device in the United States through the FDA's PMA pathway. It is crucial for manufacturers to consult the FDA's specific guidance and regulations, engage with the agency throughout the process, and fulfill all requirements to ensure compliance and obtain accurate and up-to-date information.

References

[1] J. Wong and R. Tong, *Medical Regulatory Affairs: An International Handbook for Medical Devices and Healthcare Products Hardcover*, (New York, Jenny Stanford Publishing, 2022).

[2] Asia Regulatory Professionals Association: www.ARPAedu.com.

[3] RA course - https://courses.arpaedu.com/.

[4] ISO13485:2016(E), Medical devices quality management systems-requirements for regulatory purposes. ISO copyright office, Ch. de Blandonnet 8 • CP 401, CH-1214 Vernier, Geneva, Switzerland.

[5] ISO 10993-1:2018, Biological evaluation of medical devices, ISO copyright office, Ch. de Blandonnet 8 • CP 401, CH-1214 Vernier, Geneva, Switzerland.

Chapter 13

Laser Processing for Medical Devices

Zhekun Chen[*], **Xiaohan Xing**[†], **Yuchen Yang**[‡],
and Minghui Hong[§]

*Pen-Tung Sah Institute of Micro-Nano Science and Technology,
Xiamen University, China 361005, China*
[*] *chenzk@stu.xmu.edu.cn*
[†] *xingxiaohan330@stu.xmu.edu.cn*
[‡] *yang_yu_chen_1999@163.com*
[§] *elehmh@xmu.edu.cn*

Laser usage in medicine opens up a new field for life sciences and the clinical diagnoses and treatment of diseases. This chapter discusses what lasers bring to biomedicine from the foundational principles to clinical applications. Different types of lasers and their interactions with various materials are introduced. This chapter is an enlightening voyage in which lasers meet biomedicine.

13.1 Introduction

In the modern medical field, lasers stand as proof of the remarkable discipline of physics and biology. They have tools in biomedicine. This chapter aims to captivate the intersection of lasers and life sciences, revealing their applications in diagnostics, therapy become indispensable, and research.

The core lies in the extraordinary nature of laser light itself. "Laser" is an acronym for Light Amplification by Stimulated Emission of Radiation. Unlike conventional light sources, lasers produce highly coherent and high-intensity monochromatic beams with unique properties that lend themselves to precision and control. Lasers have a wide range of uses in medicine.

In 1961, Charles Campbell of the Eye Research Institute of Columbia Presbyterian Medical Center in the USA used the laser to weld the detached retina in the world's first eye surgery, which marked the beginning of the clinical medical applications of lasers. The applications of lasers in the medical field have the advantages of precision, minimal invasiveness, reduced bleeding, sterility, versatility, enhanced healing, and reduced pain and discomfort. Increasing evidence suggests that lasers have unique advantages in the fabrication of responsive biomaterial surfaces due to their non-contact processes, reduced surface contamination, and negligible mechanical damage to biomaterial surfaces.

Lasers in medicine comprise a new research field, which includes using laser technology to study, diagnose, prevent, and treat diseases. Lasers have been used in internal medicine, surgery, gynecology, pediatrics, ophthalmology, otolaryngology, stomatology, dermatology, oncology, acupuncture, physiotherapy, and other clinical departments. The use of lasers not only opens up a new research field for life sciences and the development of diseases but also provides a new means for clinical diagnoses and treatment of diseases.

13.2   Laser Sources

The development of medical lasers is divided into three stages: Ruby laser and neodymium glass laser pioneered the laser treatment of ocular fundus diseases and skin diseases. Since the 1970s, continuous-wave (CW) lasers, such as CO_2 lasers, He-Ne lasers, and Ar^+ lasers, have become the main lasers for medical applications. In the 1980s, medical lasers were promoted after years of efforts to successfully develop semiconductor lasers.

According to wavelength, lasers can be divided into ultraviolet (UV), visible, and infrared (IR) lasers. According to their energy output modes, lasers can be divided into CW and pulsed lasers. In the interdisciplinary research of biomedical and laser engineering, it is essential to understand the sources and properties of lasers. In this section, different medical laser sources are introduced by different wavelengths and output modes.

13.2.1 *IR, Visible, and UV Lasers*

Laser sources can be divided into the UV, visible, and IR categories according to their spectra as shown in Figure 13.1. Wavelength is inversely correlated with photon energy. In addition, one wavelength can be transformed into another by using frequency conversion crystals. For instance, the Nd: YAG laser has its main wavelength at 1064 nm but also has a frequency-doubled wavelength at 532 nm and a frequency-tripled one at 355 nm.

Several commonly used lasers with their medical applications are listed in Table 13.1. The IR laser is widely used in the biomedical field. It penetrates deep into tissues without damage due to its long wavelength. This property makes it process good results in the treatment of arthritis, tendinitis, and certain neurological diseases. IR lasers also have unique advantages for tissue repair due to their specific absorption properties. Carbon dioxide (CO_2) and fiber lasers are common IR laser sources. The CO_2 laser is one of the highest-power

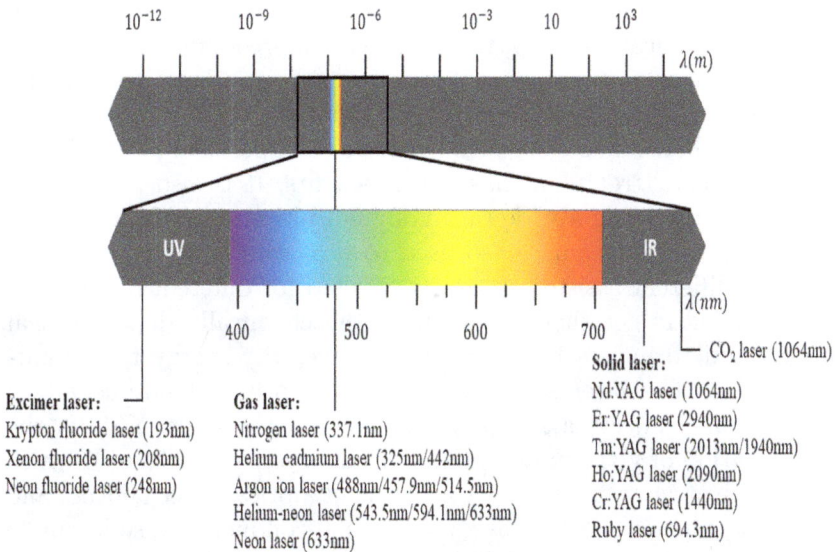

Excimer laser:
Krypton fluoride laser (193nm)
Xenon fluoride laser (208nm)
Neon fluoride laser (248nm)

Gas laser:
Nitrogen laser (337.1nm)
Helium cadmium laser (325nm/442nm)
Argon ion laser (488nm/457.9nm/514.5nm)
Helium-neon laser (543.5nm/594.1nm/633nm)
Neon laser (633nm)

CO_2 laser (1064nm)
Solid laser:
Nd:YAG laser (1064nm)
Er:YAG laser (2940nm)
Tm:YAG laser (2013nm/1940nm)
Ho:YAG laser (2090nm)
Cr:YAG laser (1440nm)
Ruby laser (694.3nm)

Figure 13.1. Typical laser sources and corresponding wavelengths.

Table 13.1.   Types of laser sources for medical applications.

Category	Wavelength (nm)	Medium	Medical Applications
UV	193~400 nm	Excimer: ArF N_2	Laser-assisted In-situ Keratomileusis Coronary sclerosis
Visible	400~700 nm	He-Ne Ar^+ Ruby	Skin Burns, High Blood Pressure Fundus Hemorrhage Glaucoma, Iridectomy
IR	700 nm~29.4μm	YAG CO_2	Acupuncture, Physical Therapy, Operation, Lithotripsy Operation, Aesthetic Surgery

continuous-wave lasers at a wavelength of 10.6 μm. It is usually used for cautery, cutting, and vaporization, working in the far-infrared spectrum. The CO_2 molecules are excited to generate a coherent beam of light at a specific wavelength. Its principle involves the following: The resonator is a cylindrical glass tube filled with carbon dioxide, nitrogen, and helium. The gas is ionized by an electric field which causes the nitrogen molecules to become energized. The electrons of CO_2 molecules move to a higher energy level via energy transfer. The electrons fall back to a lower energy level with the molecules emitting photons.

In the medical industry, the CO_2 laser is predominantly used for skin treatment in a process called carbon dioxide laser resurfacing. CO_2 laser treatment encompasses a number of surgical and dermatological methods. The laser beam removes a superficial layer of skin. The CO_2 laser treatment has many benefits. It is also popular for cutting and welding a wide range of medical materials from steel to fabric. The laser beam is also used to heat materials. To complete cutting, different assisted gases are selected for different materials.

Fiber lasers get their names from the chemically doped optical fibers used to induce the lasing and deliver the energy to the cutting point. The laser source starts with a primer laser, usually a diode, which injects a low-power beam into the fiber. YAG is the abbreviation of yttrium aluminum garnet crystal ($Y_3Al_5O_{12}$), which is a kind of laser medium with excellent optical, mechanical, and thermal properties. YAG has good thermal conductivity, so it can be made into pulsed lasers at a high repetition rate and can be operated at room temperature over a prolonged period. The Nd: YAG laser is one of the most widely used solid-state lasers, which has a high beam quality. It emits a wavelength in the near-infrared spectrum, around 1.06 μm. It can be transmitted by optical fibers, which are often combined with an endoscope to intracavitarily treat tumors, polyps, and bleeding. It is also widely used in material processing, holography, target indication, surgery, etc. The optical fiber to amplify the beam is usually doped with rare earth elements, such as erbium (Er), holmium (Ho), or thulium (Tm). Doping induces the fiber to act as a gain medium, amplifying the laser beam by cascading excitation/emission, as shown in Figure 13.2.

The Er: YAG laser emits a wavelength of 2.94 μm at the highest absorption peak of water. It can heat superficial skin rapidly to vaporize and separate tissues accurately with minimal thermal damage ranging in 30~50 μm. The research on skin rejuvenation using the Er: YAG laser has made great progress. It is safe, reliable, and user-friendly, which is fully in line with the provisions of medical equipment. In Ho: YAG lasers, the laser medium is yttrium aluminum garnet crystals doped with holmium ions. Ho: YAG emits a near-infrared laser produced by activating holmium atoms embedded inside YAG crystals at a wavelength of 2.14 μm, within the absorption range of water. Hence, the main energy is concentrated on tissue

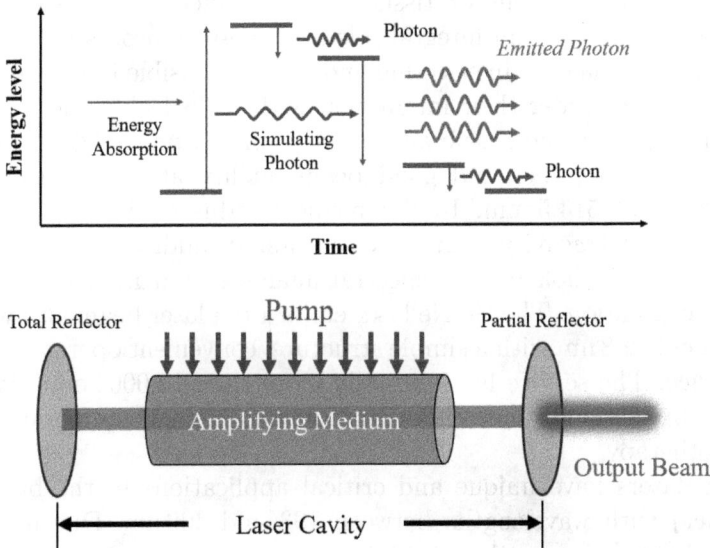

Figure 13.2. Basic principles of laser production.

surface layers, endowing the Ho: YAG laser with excellent cutting ability. The blood vessels can be hemostatic during tissue cutting. The laser beam can be transmitted through quartz fibers with a diameter of 200~1000 μm, which are suitable for various intracavity surgeries. In addition, the Ho: YAG laser also has excellent lithotripsy function and can vaporize stones into fine particles, which are later discharged from the human body [1]. The water contained on the surface and inside the stone is highly vaporized and expanded in an instant, resulting in numerous continuous micro-explosions and secondary shock waves. The stones immediately disintegrate layer by layer from the surface to the interior under a double microburst. Based on these advantages, the Ho: YAG laser is used in urinary surgery, ophthalmology and otorhinolaryngology, dermatology, gynecology, and other branches. Ho: YAG laser technology is currently the gold standard for urological operation. The Tm: YAG laser is a new technology being investigated as an alternative to the Ho: YAG laser.

A visible laser beam is visible to the human eye at a wavelength from 400 to 700 nm. The unique wavelength makes it a significant advantage in multiple medical procedures, such as ophthalmic surgery. The use of low-cost visible lasers to ablate biological tissues effectively has replaced high-cost ophthalmic surgery. Due to its high transparency to tissues, visible lasers are able to accurately illuminate specific cells or tissues without affecting the surroundings. They also play an integral role in diagnostic processes, such as fluorescence imaging. In selecting and applying visible lasers, specialists usually consider their interaction with biological tissues, ensuring that they are both safe and effective in treatment [2]. The Ar^+ laser has high power and good beam quality at the wavelengths of 488.0 and 514.5 nm. In the medical industry, it is used as a "knife" for intracavity tumor treatments. In addition, it has wide applications in holography, spectral analyses, and interstitial laser photocoagulation. The He-Ne laser emits a red laser beam at a wavelength of 632.8 nm with a simple structure, convenient operation, and low price. The service life is usually more than 10,000 hours. It has many applications in anti-inflammation, analgesia, acupuncture, and physiotherapy.

UV lasers have unique and critical applications in the biomedical field with wavelengths between 193 and 400 nm. Due to their high photon energy, they lead to the photochemical reactions of biomolecules, especially DNA and RNA. They have high value in the treatment of skin diseases, disinfection, and sterilization. UV lasers also play a crucial role in biomedical imaging, such as confocal microscopy. Special caution is required to ensure that no harm is done to the surrounding tissues when using UV lasers. In practical applications, the precise control of the affected area and exposure time is essential.

13.2.2 *CW and Pulsed Lasers*

The laser output modes, CW lasers and pulsed lasers, influence their applications and effectiveness in therapy, imaging, and other biomedical industries. Their fundamental difference is reflected in temporal continuity, which provides a variety of treatments and solutions. In this section, the basic principles of these two laser modes and their important applications in the biomedical field are described.

Unlike pulsed lasers that emit high-intensity light in short bursts, CW lasers emit a steady stream of light at a constant power output. This makes them suitable for applications that require continuous and uninterrupted laser energy, such as laser cutting, engraving, laser therapy [3], and scientific research. By maintaining a steady input of energy and continuously circulating the light through the gain medium and optical cavity, the CW laser can produce a continuous and stable beam of light. High-power CW Yb^{3-}-doped fiber lasers operating around $1\,\mu m$ occupy the largest market share of laser material processing. The CW laser is convenient in applications because of its compact structure and complete enclosure. In terms of treatment, both CW and pulsed modes of laser radiation are used to treat various soft tissues and neurologic disorders in the red-to-near infra-red optical region as a nondestructive method [4]. In terms of diagnoses, the optical heterodyne detection-based coherent detection imaging system is a useful method for laser computed tomography (CT) in biomedicine using CW and single-frequency lasers as light sources [5]. The treatment of glaucoma is also an application of continuous lasers. Continuous-wave cyclophotocoagulation (CW-CPC) is often preferred for medical and surgical treatment for managing refractory glaucoma [6].

Five major pulsed lasers are commonly utilized: (1) Q-switched, (2) Gain-switched, (3) Mode-locked, (4) Super-pulsed, and (5) Chopped or gated lasers. Each utilizes a different mechanism to generate light in a pulsed mode and varies in terms of pulse repetition rate, energy, and pulse duration. The concept of super-pulsing was originally developed for the CO_2 laser used in high-power tissue ablative procedures. By generating relatively short pulses (milli-second), the laser media could be excited to higher levels than those normally allowed in the CW mode where heat dissipation constraints limit the maximum amounts of energy that can be used to excite the lasing media. With the original CO_2 super-pulsed lasers, the short pulses confine the thermal energy in tissues (by making the pulse duration shorter than the thermal diffusion time), reducing collateral thermal damage to normal tissues. Q-switching technology can control the output of a pulsed laser by changing the loss in the laser resonator and regulating the process of energy accumulation and release in the excitation medium. The Q-switched 694-nm ruby laser, Q-switched 755-nm alexandrite laser, and 1.064-μm and 532-nm Nd: YAG lasers are commonly used to remove tattoos [7]. Pump modulation is used to modulate the pumping source of the laser (such as laser diode or laser flash) to change the size and time window of pumping energy and to regulate the output characteristics of laser pulses. The sub-nanosecond laser pulse is applied for effective non-invasive diagnostics of gastrointestinal oncological diseases [8]. By changing the phase of a laser pulse, the modulation and interference of the pulse can be controlled. Optical coherence tomography (OCT) technology uses these laser sources [9].

Ultrafast lasers $(10^{-12} \sim 10^{-19}\,\mathrm{s})$ can achieve a stable train of picosecond, femtosecond, and attosecond pulses. Ultrafast lasers have the characteristics of narrow pulse width, high peak power, and a low ablation threshold. The pulses of ultrafast lasers release highly concentrated energy in a very short period of time. Nonlinear effects occur when matter interacts with a laser beam, resulting in a series of unique phenomena. For example, ultrafast lasers can remove tiny areas of matter precisely without significantly heating or damaging the surrounding tissues. This ability is mainly attributed to their extremely short pulse duration, which allows the thermal effect to be virtually eliminated, enabling cold processing.

The main method to generate an ultrafast laser pulse output is mode-locking. Mode-locking lasers usually adopt diode-pumped passively Q-switched technology to produce high repetition rate and high peak power laser pulses [10]. The peak power of the mode-locked fiber laser is high, and the interaction of dispersion and non-linear effect in the fiber can effectively improve the output pulse characteristics, such as beam quality and pulse energy. There are two types of mode-locking technologies: active and passive mode-locking. Active mode-locked fiber lasers introduce an active modulator into the resonator [11]. Active mode-locking mainly refers to the active modulator in the laser cavity, which uses external means to periodically modulate light. Active mode-locked fiber lasers can be used for frequency sweeping. Since active mode-locking requires introducing an external modulating element in the cavity, the structure is generally more complex and the output pulse duration is wider than that of passive mode-locking. Passive mode-locking refers to the modulation of laser pulses by the saturable absorption characteristics of passive devices. The saturable absorber (SA) is a material which absorption or loss varies with input light intensity. It can be used to compress the pulse and eliminate the noise pulse. The saturated absorber can act several times on the laser circulating in the cavity to obtain a stable pulse train output and achieve the mode-locking.

In the biomedical field, ultrafast lasers have become a powerful tool for many applications. Ultrafast lasers can change the states and properties of materials through interactions with them and they can be used to control the materials' processing from the micrometer scale down to the nanometer scale. At present, the applications of ultrafast lasers mainly involve ophthalmology, soft tissue ablation outside of ophthalmology, and hard tissue ablation [12]. A most notable example is ophthalmologic operation, particularly laser-assisted *in situ* keratomileusis (LASIK) surgery. In this application, femtosecond lasers are used to precisely process cornea and corneal flap without significant thermal damage or adverse reactions. In addition, ultrafast lasers have shown excellent capabilities in orthopedic surgery to perform fine bone cutting and removal. Their potential applications in cancer cell therapy, precision drug delivery, and bioimaging are being explored [13].

The size, cost, robustness, and speed of ultrafast laser systems have all improved significantly since their invention, particularly in the case of fiber lasers. The current ultrafast laser systems typically provide pulse repetition rates in the hundreds of kiloHertz to single megaHertz range, enabling faster surgical cutting and imaging. As technology advances, their applications can be expected to cover more treatment options and better therapeutic effects for patients.

13.3 Light–Matter Interactions

The interactions between light and matter take three forms: absorption, scattering, and nonlinearity. The light intensity inside biological samples decreases with depth during the absorption. Relative phenomena include fluorescence, thermal incubation, ultrasonic generation, photoelectricity, and modification, corresponding to optical, photothermic, acoustic, photoelectric, and photochemical effects. When the light passes through the tissues, the momentum and energy of light are changed. This phenomenon is termed light scattering and is classified into two types: elastic and inelastic scatter. Elastic scatter includes reflection, refraction, Rayleigh scattering, and Mie scattering. Inelastic scatter involves Raman scattering, Brillouin scattering, and Doppler shift. The intensity of scattered light depends on the composition and index of tissues and light wavelength. In addition, the material properties change more rapidly when the light interacts with matter at a high power. This leads to nonlinear effects, such as the third-order nonlinear optical responses of organic molecules.

The interaction of lasers with tissues or medical materials is of great significance for laser treatment and surgery in the field of biomedicine. The mechanism is complex and often involves multiple optical effects. A full understanding of these processes can help to provide appropriate laser technology for different medical applications, the mechanism of laser–matter interaction is introduced according to the category of materials.

13.3.1 *Tissues*

The applications of laser technology in medical treatment are mainly attributed to its induced biological effects, which could be divided into five types: laser thermal, photochemical, photo-pressure, electromagnetic, and biostimulation effects. There is no clear boundary among the variety of effects, which is mainly determined by laser and tissue types. The interaction relates to the absorption of laser energy by tissue or by chromophores within the tissue. Chromophores are molecules, such as hemoglobin in blood or melanin in skin, which can absorb light at specific wavelengths. For example, the Er: YAG laser emits a wavelength of 2.94 μm, which is absorbed primarily by water molecules in tissue. The absorption causes water molecules to be heated up and can potentially destroy the tissue. The Nd: YAG laser at a wavelength of 1.064 μm is absorbed primarily by melanin or hemoglobin, which is suitable for hair removal or vascular lesion treatment. The interaction also depends on additional factors, such as laser power and pulse duration, tissue structure, and even skin color. Overall, it relies on the ability to target specific chromophores within the tissue and induce biological responses by laser. The distinction between soft and hard tissues is important in medical fields, which helps in understanding different properties, functions, and vulnerabilities. It also guides our choice of appropriate technique or method for treatments or diagnoses.

Soft tissue makes up most of the human body, including muscles, tendons, ligaments, fat, nerves, blood vessels, and organs like the liver, spleen, and heart. It is often composed of cells, fibers, and extracellular matrix materials like collagen and elastin. Soft tissue has high water content and low mineral content with more flexible, pliable, and deformable properties, providing support, structure, and function to our human bodies. Laser therapy is used in various medical fields to treat soft tissue injuries, alleviate pain, and promote healing. The laser beams reach and act on target tissue accurately. The interaction with soft tissue is mainly attributed to the photochemical and photothermal effects. The lasers stimulate various biochemical and physiological processes at the cellular level. When the laser energy is absorbed by chromophores, such as hemoglobin, myoglobin, and cytochrome, the photochemical effect triggers a series of cellular reactions, including the release of nitric oxide, adenosine triphosphate (ATP), and various growth factors. These effects promote cell proliferation, angiogenesis, and tissue repair. The photothermal effect leads to the temperature increase of the target tissue, which may cause thermal damage. Heat generation is determined by laser processing parameters and the optical properties of biological tissue, mainly referring to irradiation intensity, irradiation time, and absorption coefficient. At a specific wavelength and power intensity, the laser induces controlled thermal effects that selectively act on damaged or abnormal cells, such as cancer cells or scar tissue. Shortened pulse duration is a typical method to control heat accumulation. This process is known as laser ablation or photodynamic therapy. It requires that certain molecules inside tissue, such as hemoglobin and melanin, have a high absorption capability of laser energy over a narrow range of wavelengths. The effect ultimately depends on the type and temperature of biological tissue. The photothermal effects of lasers have been successfully used in certain therapeutic modalities, such as laser hair removal, scar therapy, and tumor hyperthermia. Due to the complexity and inhomogeneity of soft tissue, laser beams are scattered inside the tissue. The scattering affects the optical path and limits the laser penetration depth. However, it could be exploited to increase the interaction of lasers with living tissue, such as in photodynamic therapy.

The water content of the soft tissue also absorbs laser energy, especially in the infrared region. Most soft tissues contain a lot of water. The wetness or moisture is an important factor in determining the effect of laser interaction with tissue. Water absorption requires special attention for tissue mainly composed of water, such as the cornea, to avoid excessive heating and damage. The laser energy absorbed by water is used to many medical treatment, such as laser thermocoagulation. The moisture influences light scattering, which highly determines the penetration depth. In addition, the photoacoustic effect may be obvious when the laser interacts with tissue rich in water. This effect converts light into acoustic waves, providing the basis for photoacoustic imaging. When using lasers for biomedical treatment, the wetness of the tissue must be considered with regard to the effectiveness and safety of the treatment.

Overall, the principle of laser interaction with soft tissue involves using lasers to stimulate or inhibit various cellular processes. The study of laser interaction with soft tissue ensures the safety and effectiveness of the laser treatment.

Laser interaction with hard tissue, mainly including bones and teeth, also depends on laser wavelength. The laser absorption and scattering of the hard tissue are significantly different compared to the soft tissue, due to its inherent mineralization. Some laser energy is reflected since hard tissue has a high reflectivity. It reduces the penetration depth inside the tissue. Appropriate laser processing parameters, such as wavelength and pulse duration, are critical to ensure effectiveness and safety in hard tissue treatment. Calcium phosphate in bone and teeth mainly absorbs laser energy in the middle infrared band. Local heating leads to the demineralization of the tissue, which enables precise cutting in orthopedic surgery and dental treatment. In addition, weak acoustic waves are generated by the photoacoustic effect. It is applied to photoacoustic imaging to provide a non-invasive diagnostic technology for dentistry.

In dentistry, lasers are commonly used for various procedures, such as cavity preparation, gum disease treatment, and teeth whitening. When a laser beam interacts with hard dental tissue, such as enamel and dentin, several mechanisms come into play. In orthopedics, lasers are utilized for procedures such as bone remodeling, fracture healing, and cartilage repair. Laser energy can directly interact with the mineralized components of bone and cartilage, promoting the stimulation of osteoblasts and chondrocytes, which are responsible for bone and cartilage formation, respectively. Figure 13.3 shows the calculated isotherms superimposed on an optical micrograph of a laser-processed area of bone [14]. These mechanisms can provide precise and effective treatment for dental and orthopedic conditions while minimizing damage to surrounding healthy tissue. The interaction between laser and hard tissue involves many effects. Laser applications in the medical field bring new possibilities for hard tissue therapy.

13.3.2 *Medical Materials*

Laser technology is also widely used to treat and process various medical materials. Medical materials can be classified based on various criteria, referring to their compositions and applications. Several laser technologies are applied in the following categories: (1) Biomaterials are compatible with living systems and can be further classified as follows: Metals are used in orthopedic implants, such as stainless steel, titanium, and cobalt-chromium alloys. Polymers are used in various medical devices and implants, such as silicone, polyethylene, and polyurethane. They are implanted into the body for long-term use, such as pacemaker leads, artificial heart valves, and cochlear implants. Ceramic materials are used in dental and orthopedic implants, such as alumina, zirconia, and hydroxyapatite.

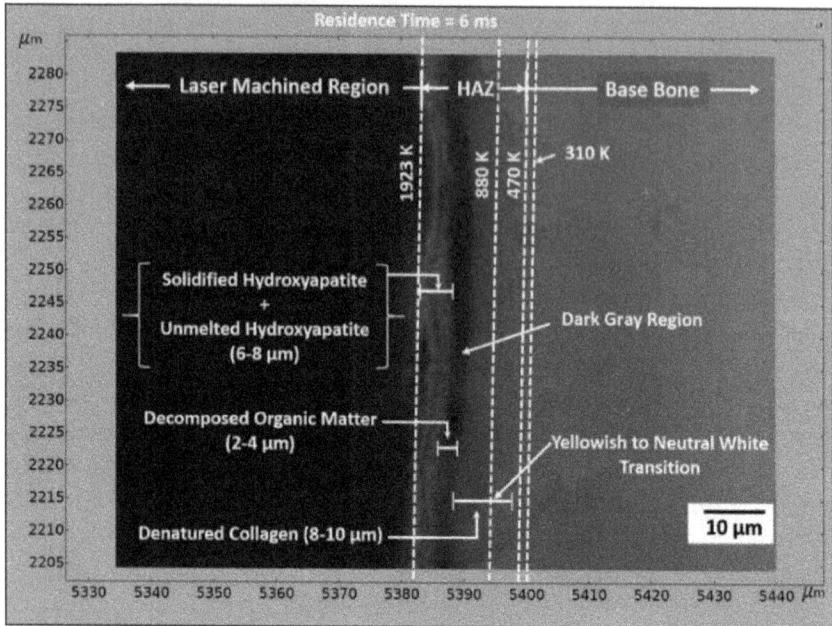

Figure 13.3. Computationally predicted isotherms superimposed on the optical micrograph of a laser-machined region [14] Copyright 2020 by the American Chemical Society.

(2) Drug delivery materials are designed to control the release of drugs or therapeutic agents and are in the form of nanoparticles, films, or hydrogels. (3) Diagnostic materials are used in medical detection, which may involve more composite materials, including metals and nonmetals. In general, the mechanism of interaction between laser and medical materials could be mainly considered for metals and non-metals.

The mechanism of interaction between metals and lasers is an important research topic in many fields. The processes involve heating, melting, and vaporizing metal surfaces. The optical response of a metal surface depends on light reflection, absorption, and heat conduction when it is irradiated. Metals usually have high reflectivity in the visible range. They may cause trouble in some medical applications because they limit energy penetration. Metals are also an ideal choice for protective materials. For example, metals are used as coating for goggles during surgery to protect the operator. When the appropriate laser wavelength is chosen, the metal surface absorbs laser energy effectively. The absorbed energy is quickly converted into heat, leading to a high surface temperature. Due to the high thermal conductivity, energy quickly conducts inside the metal, causing the temperature of the entire metal to rise. When the laser beam is focused, the energy is concentrated on a small area. Metals are modified depending on their physical properties and laser processing parameters. At a low laser power, the metal may experience surface heating and melting. At a high laser power, the metals rapidly reach a melting point, resulting in the melting of the targeted area, as shown in Figure 13.4 [15]. This molten material can be expelled by gas under a high-pressure air stream, creating a cut or a hole in the metal. The laser beam selectively removes materials from the metal surface. This technology is known as laser cutting or drilling. It is commonly used for precise and efficient metal fabrication. The interaction between metal and laser also generates plasma. When a metal is illuminated by a high-intensity laser, electrons on the surface are stripped away, forming plasma. The plasma further absorbs laser energy and affects laser ablation.

The choice of laser parameters, such as wavelength, power, pulse duration, and beam shape, can be optimized for different metals,

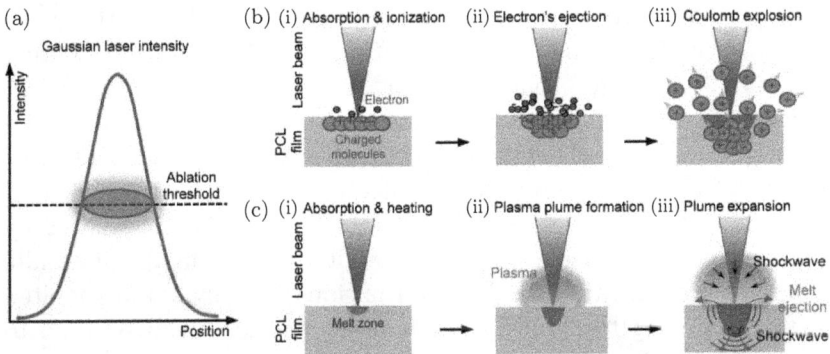

Figure 13.4. Mechanism of interaction between polycaprolactone and femtosecond laser. (a) Schematic diagram illustrating femtosecond laser intensity following Gaussian distribution. Both (b) photochemical and (c) photothermal processes of laser-matter interaciton (i, ii, and iii represent the temporal stages of a femtosecond laser pulse. [15]) Copyright 2015 by the American Chemical Society.

thicknesses, and desired shapes. A deep understanding of this interaction is conducive to processing medical metal materials effectively.

When interacting with lasers, the response of non-metals is different from metals. However, the effects also depend on laser wavelength
and material properties. Non-metals typically have a high absorption
capability in a narrow wavelength range. Scattering in non-metals
also requires more attention, since their internal microstructure is
complex. The incident laser may be scattered many times, resulting in energy dispersion. The thermal conductivity of non-metals is
lower and anisotropic compared to metals. It may lead to cracks or
breakage.

Medical non-metal materials are mainly divided into two categories: polymer and ceramic. Common polymer materials in
medicine are polytetrafluoroethylene, polyimide, polydimethylsilox-
ane, polyethylene terephthalate, polymethyl methacrylate, and more.
The polymer has a high absorption for UV lasers, but the absorption
is relatively low in the IR range. The absorbed energy causes the
local temperature to rise due to the low thermal conductivity, further leading to melting, oxidization, or vaporization. In this process,
both photochemistry and photothermal ablations are contributed.
After photothermal ablation occurs, gaseous molecules form a plasma
plume above the polymer surface. It continuously absorbs the energy
and finally expands to generate shock waves. These shock waves
rapidly decay into acoustic waves and propagate within the polymer to eject the melted molecules from the ablated area. Melting
causes a heat-affected zone, as well as redeposition due to expulsion,
cracks, and non-uniformity. A shorter pulse duration results in more
vaporization and less melting. More vaporization leads to the formation of a plasma plume which affects the quality of the ablated
features. A large heat-affected zone is generated when irradiated by
a laser with long pulse durations. The high molecular weight results
in a low ablation rate due to the formation of highly viscous molten
materials during the ablation. A femtosecond laser can be used to
avoid the thermal effect. A multi-photon absorption effect may be
involved. Biomedical ceramics, referred to bioceramics, is a class of
ceramics specially designed for medical purposes. It is an important
branch of biological materials, which is used for the diagnosis, treatment, or regeneration of human pathological tissues and organs of
inorganic non-metallic materials. As a rapidly developing additive

manufacturing technology, laser 3D printing has significant advantages in the production of complex precision ceramic parts: no mold needed, high precision, fast response, and short cycle. It can realize the flexible deployment of ceramic parts.

13.4 Laser Technologies

13.4.1 *Laser Cutting*

Laser cutting in medicine is a versatile and precise technique used for various applications. Laser cutting is employed in some common areas as follows: (1) In surgical procedures, lasers are used to cut tissues with high precision and minimal bleeding. The laser energy can coagulate blood vessels during the cutting. In ophthalmology, lasers are frequently used for procedures like laser-assisted in-situ keratomileusis (LASIK) for vision correction. (2) In dental applications, lasers are employed to cut soft tissues, such as gum contouring or removing lesions, and shape hard tissues like teeth and bones. (3) In medical device manufacturing, laser cutting is used to precisely cut and shape stents used in vascular or cardiac interventions. It is also employed in manufacturing various medical implants, such as orthopedic implants and dental prosthetics. (4) In diagnostic techniques, laser cutting is utilized in microdissection, where specific cells or tissues are targeted for analyses. (5) In skin resurfacing, the laser is employed to break down tattoo pigments for removal.

Laser cutting in medicine offers several advantages, including precision, reduced bleeding, and minimal damage to surrounding tissues. It requires specialized equipment, training, and careful consideration of safety measures. The choice of laser type (e.g., CO_2, diode, and erbium) depends on the specific medical applications. In this section, we will introduce laser cutting technology with examples according to materials categories and applications.

Precision is a key factor for surgical tools or medical equipment. Lasers can cut metals in a highly precise manner, which is especially critical in manufacturing medical devices. Stainless steel and some special medical alloys are the first choices in the medical field. For example, stainless steel is a corrosion-resistant metal with high strength and biocompatibility, suitable for the manufacture of surgical instruments, surgical forceps, blades, and more. Titanium has excellent biocompatibility and low density, making it ideal for manufacturing bone implants. Ti-6Al-4V is a common titanium alloy used in the manufacture of hip joints. Cobalt-chromium alloys have high strength and corrosion resistance, and are commonly used in heart stents, artificial heart valves, and other implants. Nickel titanium alloy, also known as nitinol, has shape memory and is widely used to make vascular stents and other devices that require shape changes. Its excellent corrosion resistance, strength, and biocompatibility makes it ideal for use in the manufacture of implants or surgical instruments. Laser cutting can maintain the superior properties of these materials. Precious metals can also be used in some special medical devices, such as pacemakers and other electronic equipment connection parts. Laser cutting provides extremely high accuracy on precious metal surfaces, which is essential for these devices that require fine machining. A relatively small heat-affected zone reduces the risk of material deformation or damage, which is important to maintain the original nature and appearance of the precious metals. In addition to the properties of the material, the quality of laser cutting also depends on the process. Various parameters and auxiliary methods are studied to improve the effectiveness and efficiency of laser cutting. Laser parameters are usually the first to be regulated, including laser power, repetition rate, and scanning speed. For example, different cut-edge microstructures and surface roughness are obtained when using a CO_2 laser to cut titanium alloy Ti-6Al-4V. Laser power, scanning speed, and assisted gas pressure have influences on the integrity of cutting areas in high-energy CO_2 laser cutting. The objective is to optimize the surface roughness of the cut edge to improve performance. When using a CO_2 laser to cut materials that are easily oxidized, a reactive cutting process is generally adopted. The laser beam heats a localized area with a high-pressure stream of oxygen. The oxygen stream causes the metal to oxidize and burn, then the material is removed [16].

An optimized scanning path contributes to enhancing the laser ablation rate and decreasing debris. The path alteration leads to a wide kerf line, enabling the assisted air to efficiently remove the debris deposited on the kerf bottom. By employing ultrafast lasers, the production of heat-affected zones and the accumulation of thermal energy can be decreased in medical device applications. Hence, laser cutting becomes a powerful fabrication technique to form alloy materials exhibiting superelastic and shape memory properties. Developments in laser micromachining drive medical device technology substantially, such as self-expanding stents [17]. High-precision profile cutting with minimum post-processing is widely desirable in medical device fabrication, especially in coronary stents. Nd: YAG lasers are usually used to profile thin tubular metallic materials and cut stents. Water flow can be introduced in the tubes to prevent back wall damage. Heat-affected zone, kerf width, surface roughness, and debris deposition can be improved compared with dry cutting [18]. Surgical instruments usually require extremely high precision to ensure the precise operation of surgeons. The diameter of a laser beam is small, usually at the tens of micron to sub-millimeter scale. It means that manufacturing features are on the microscopic scale, which is critical for the performance and safety of medical devices. The cut edge is smooth without additional surface treatment. The smoothness and surface quality of the device surface directly affect its performance in surgery, reducing potential trauma and wear. Smooth surfaces reduce the possibility of bacterial growth, which is essential for maintaining biocompatibility. Medical implants, such as artificial joints and intervertebral discs, require an exact match with human tissue. Laser cutting enables the precise texturing of these implants, ensuring that their shape meets medical needs and reduces risks.

High precision and flexibility make customized and personalized medical devices more feasible. Laser cutting can be used to create customized implants to fit the anatomy of an individual patient. Minimally invasive surgery requires smaller and more elaborate tools to minimally invade the patient's body. Laser cutting technology can be used to make micro-instruments, providing the tools needed to perform fine operations at the microscopic level. For example, high-performance multifunctional minimally invasive medical tools of small size can be fabricated by laser micro-fabrication on cylindrical substrates. A NiTi shape memory alloy tube has been fabricated by spiral cutting with a femtosecond laser. A silicone rubber tube covers the outside of the processed NiTi shape memory alloy to constitute a small-diameter active bending catheter, which is used for intravascular minimally invasive diagnostics and therapy. The active catheter is effective for insertion into the branches of blood vessels that diverge at acute angles where it is difficult to proceed [19]. In the development of medical devices, laser cutting technology provides the possibility for rapid design validation and product improvement. For example, silicone rubber and platinum foil are patterned by the Nd: YAG laser to fabricate microelectrode arrays. arrays. The minimal achievable feature size of laser cutting is about $30\,\mu$m. Laser cutting does not require expensive clean room facilities and offers an extremely short design-to-prototype time of less than 1 day [20]. In addition, laser cutting is a non-contact processing method, which means that no external contaminants are introduced during the cutting process. It reduces the risk of extra contamination compared to conventional mechanical cutting, ensuring the surface cleanliness of medical devices. It does not require post-treatment and cleaning. In the medical field, this helps to ensure that products meet strict hygiene standards. Laser cutting technology applied in the medical field not only improves production efficiency but also ensures the quality and precision of medical devices, providing reliable support for medical progress.

Laser glass cutting also has various applications in medical fields. Glass microfluidic devices are used in medical diagnostics and research. Laser cutting is employed to create precise channels and chambers on glass chips, enabling the manipulation and analyses of small fluid volumes for applications, such as blood analyses, DNA sequencing, and drug discovery. Some medical implants are made of glass, such as bioactive glass for bone repair and dental applications. Laser cutting can be used to shape and customize these implants for specific patient needs. Laser cutting is chosen for these applications because it provides high precision and minimal thermal stress to the glass material. This accuracy is vital in medical and scientific contexts where exact measurements and reproducibility are paramount. Additionally, laser cutting allows for the creation of intricate and customized designs, making it a valuable tool for glass-based medical and research applications.

Precise glass cutting usually requires a high-quality edge and no significant cracks, which is a high-challenge task for laser microfabrication. It is difficult for nanosecond lasers to directly process glass due to the low absorption. Stress-induced microcracks are generated by heat accumulation during the laser ablation. The pocket scanning technique is proposed to meet this challenge. It leads to high-quality glass cutting with a low-energy nanosecond laser. Pocket scanning involves scanning the laser beam parallel to the overlapped paths with the last path along the structure edge. The cracks formed around the edges are reduced significantly compared to direct scanning, whose size can be minimized to less than $10\,\mu$m. The ablation depth is also enhanced linearly with laser fluence and scanning loop [21].

Water-jet-guided laser processing is a technology in which the laser beam is guided inside the water jet by total internal reflection at the water/air interface. The water jet hits the sample, which is machined by the laser beam. The water jet functions not only similarly to optical fibers but also cools the materials and removes the cut debris during the processing. Compared with direct laser processing, the water-jet-guided laser has advantages in the reduction of the heat-affected zone and burr formation material deposition. Such a technique has demonstrated significant precise cut edges, which is one of the most important features of glass cutting. This technique is mainly applied to cutting metals and semiconductor wafers. The main disadvantage is that the resolution is limited by the water jet diameter, typically between 50 and $200\,\mu$m [22]. Cutting transparent materials, such as sapphire and glass, has also been developed now. For example, sapphire of up to 3 mm thickness exhibits parallel walls with a roughness of $<0.5\,\mu$m and a kerf width of $<100\,\mu$m [23]. In terms of efficiency, one study demonstrated that the cutting speed of a water-jet-guided laser is improved by 40% over abrasive sawing while maintaining a high cut quality without damage and contamination to the substrates [24]. Another study on water-assisted femtosecond laser processing shows that the ablation threshold of fused silica is reduced from 2.22 to $1.02\,\text{J/cm}^2$ with the assistance of distilled water [25].

Most laser cutting processes are based on laser-induced ablation, including the two techniques mentioned earlier. The laser energy interacts with the substrate directly and leads to the removal of substrate materials. The absorption of laser energy by the substrate materials determines the efficiency of the cutting process. However, the high transparency of glass usually prevents light from being absorbed efficiently. Some indirect methods have been proposed to meet this requirement, such as laser-induced plasma-assisted ablation (LIPAA) and laser-induced backside wet etching (LIBWE). Figure 13.5 demonstrates the LIPAA process. Plasmas are generated from the interaction between laser and a target, which applies

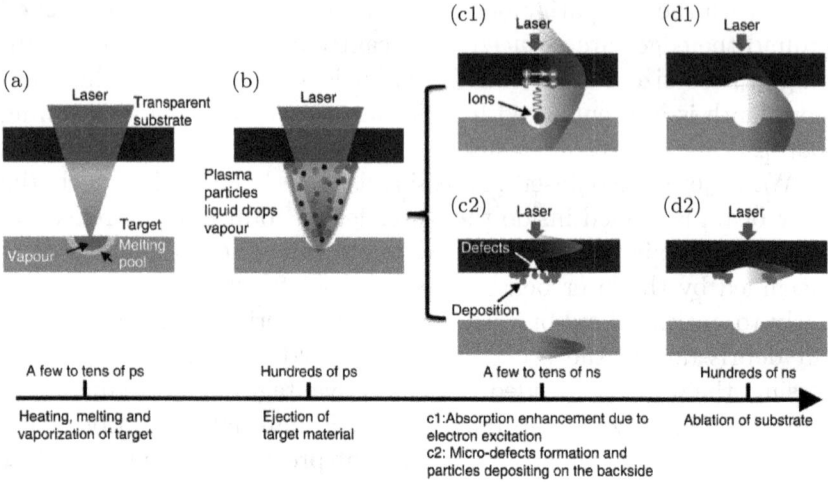

Figure 13.5. Schematic illustration of LIPAA process. (a) Heating effect of the laser irradiation causes localized melting and vaporization. (b) The laser-induced melting and vaporization lead to the ejection of target materials. (c1, d1) Case 1: There is an overlap between the later part of the pulse and the time for absorption enhancement originating from the laser-induced plasma. Laser ablation occurs due to strong absorption enhancement at the rear surface. (c2, d2) Case 2: There is no overlap between the laser pulse and the absorption enhancement. The absorption enhancement from the micro-defects and deposition results in the ablation by subsequent pulses [29] Copyright 2021, Springer Nature.

to all transparent materials. The laser beam passes through the glass and then irradiates the target, which is located behind the glass at a distance. For actual applications, the distance depends on the laser processing parameters and target materials, typically a few hundred micrometers. The laser fluence is below the ablation threshold of glass, which does not process it directly. The target has a high absorption of laser energy. A high-temperature and high-pressure plasma is induced when laser irradiates on the target surface. Then, the plasma flies forward to the rear surface of the glass at a high speed. LIPAA is a complicated and highly dynamic process on a time scale of nanoseconds, including laser–target interaction, plasma generation, and interactions among plasma, laser, and substrate. The process starts with heating and photoionization of the irradiated area by the laser beam. Subsequently, the plasma is induced from the target by releasing solid particles, vapors, and liquid drops. LIPAA technology has unique advantages in glass micromachining. First, this technique is capable of cutting glass effectively using conventional visible or IR lasers. Absorption depends on the property of the target rather than glass. Second, LIPAA can reduce the risk of microcrack formation owing to less heat accumulation due to the assistance of the plasma. Third, the laser process's efficiency and productivity can be improved. A comparative study shows that processing time of LIPAA is reduced by up to 84% compared to direct laser ablation [26]. LIPAA has been extensively studied for the fabrications of microstructures and micro-patterns on a variety of glasses. Metal materials are usually used as the target, including copper, silver, and aluminum. Nanosecond lasers are commonly applied to the LIPAA process with wavelength range from deep UV to IR. The surface roughness generated by nanosecond laser LIPAA is around 100 nm [27]. The use of femtosecond lasers in LIPAA has recently been of interest for micro/nano-processing of transparent materials [28]. Femtosecond lasers deliver more advantages to achieve higher quality and lower roughness in microstructure fabrication. A much lower surface roughness can be realized, down to 18.1 nm. This high-quality LIPAA method has been used in various practical applications, including glass precise scribing and cutting. It can enhance the advanced manufacturing of next-generation functional medical devices on glass.

LIBWE is another hybrid laser micromachining technique, which can be used for high-quality glass cutting. Because it is difficult for nanosecond lasers to directly process glass, additional absorptive liquid is introduced to enhance the laser energy absorption and reduce the ablation threshold fluence as shown in Figure 13.6. A highly absorptive liquid is in contact with one side of the glass to enhance the absorption. The laser irradiates from the other side, passes through the glass, and then focuses on the solid–liquid interface. The temperature at the interface increases rapidly due to the high absorption of the liquid, which leads to a significant reduction of the ablation threshold. Similar to the LIPAA process, nanosecond lasers are widely used in LIBWE with lower cost and higher reliability compared to ultrafast lasers. Similar to the LIPAA process, nanosecond lasers are widely used in LIBWE with lower cost and higher reliability. Ultrafast lasers are used for smaller heat affected zone, higher resolution, and higher surface quality [30]. A two-step

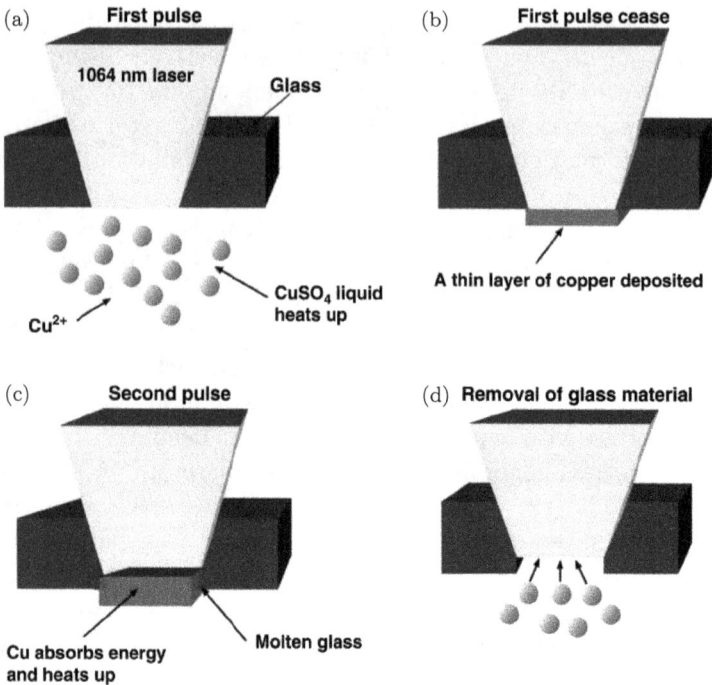

Figure 13.6. Proposed mechanism of LIBWE using 1064-nm laser and CuSO$_4$ solution as the liquid absorber. (a) Laser irradiates from the top. (b) Copper deposition on the backside of the glass. (c) The deposited copper absorbs the laser energy and heats the immediate glass region. (d) Removal of the molten substrate [29] Copyright 2021 Springer Nature.

model was proposed to describe the etching mechanism. For example, aqueous copper sulfate (CuSO$_4$) solution is used as an absorber [31]. The first step is the deposition of copper on the glass surface due to a photochemical process upon the laser irradiation. In the second step, the laser energy is absorbed by the deposited copper, resulting in the melting and removal of the glass materials. LIBWE technology allows the well-defined microstructuring of glass at a relatively low laser fluence. For practical applications, it is important to precisely control the etching rate to achieve high surface quality. Many factors and parameters are involved in the LIBWE process, including liquid properties, solution concentration, and laser fluence. For example, a short-wavelength laser has a high etch rate due to the high absorption coefficient of the liquid [32]. The etch rate with $\lambda = 266$ nm is approximately 5 times higher than $\lambda = 355\,\text{nm}$ at the same condition. LIBWE has been used in a broad range of applications relating to the micro-processing of glass, including precise cutting. For example, a 1-mm-thick glass slide can be cut through by a 1.064-μm laser using $CuSO_4$ solution as an absorber [31]. Various shapes are diced out from the glass slides by the LIBWE without significant cracking. Optimization of the laser processing parameters leads to the precise cutting of glass with a high etching rate and high surface quality to meet the requirements of medical devices.

13.4.2 *Laser Drilling*

Laser drilling is a common type of laser application. This method offers certain advantages over traditional mechanical drilling methods, including precision, reduced thermal damage, and the potential for minimally invasive procedures. The following are the key aspects of the laser methods in bone drilling: (1) Reduced thermal damage: Laser drilling generates less heat compared to traditional mechanical drills, reducing the risk of thermal necrosis in surrounding tissues. This is particularly important in preserving the structural integrity of bone and minimizing damage to adjacent soft tissues. (2) Contactless ablation: Laser drilling is a contactless process, meaning there is no direct physical contact between the laser device and the bone. This characteristic minimizes the risk of contamination and reduces the need for frequent tool sterilization. (3) Coagulation and sterilization: Laser energy can have coagulative effects, helping to control bleeding during the surgery. Additionally, the high temperatures during the laser ablation contribute to sterilization. These effects can enhance the overall safety of the surgical procedure. (4) Versatility: Laser systems can be adapted for various types of bone procedures, which allow their use in a wide range of orthopedic applications, from joint surgeries to spinal procedures.

13.4.3 *Laser Texturing*

Micro/nanostructures on the surface of metals, polymers, ceramics, and glasses have many important applications in the medical and biological fields. Surface texturing, involving the creation of patterns on material surfaces, provides particular functionality

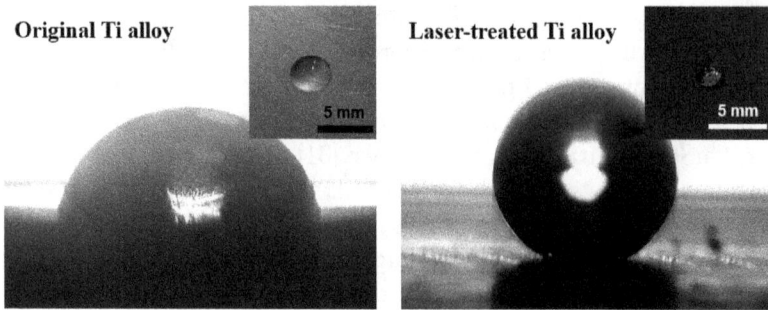

Figure 13.7. Wettability transformation on Ti alloy by laser texturing.

for special medical purposes. For example, laser texturing produces superhydrophilic surfaces on metals, which could later turn superhydrophobic after the surface treatment as shown in Figure 13.7. The developed superhydrophobic surfaces could be employed for anti-biofouling. Laser surface texturing is a potential method and has been widely used in different fields due to its high efficiency, controllability, accuracy, and environment friendliness. Laser processing allows the manufacturing of surface structures with dimensions from the nanometer to micrometer scale, which can realize tailored surface functionalization combined with modified chemical properties. In comparison to other texturing techniques employed to create micro/nano-features, such as micro-milling, ion-beam etching, lithography, hot embossing, and electrochemical machining, laser texturing has advantages such as a one-step non-contact process at low cost. When a laser beam focuses on the target surfaces, the ablation process occurs. The mechanism is mainly divided into two types: pyrolytic and photolytic processes. In the case of the pyrolytic process, laser energy is converted into heat, which leads to the melting and vaporization of materials. In the photolytic process, a chemical reaction is induced by the absorption of a photon, and the binding energy of the material is overcome [33]. Laser texturing is applied to various materials like ceramics, metals, alloys, and polymers. Combined with a galvanometer or stage, various patterns like micro-grooves or micro-cones can be created. To obtain the desired surface patterns, the laser source and parameters must be reasonably selected according to the material properties. The laser fluence on the target and the number of laser pulses, as well as the processing strategy, are decisive for the processing results. The laser wavelength should be selected to match the optical absorption property of the materials. In addition, the ultrafast laser has become a prominent technique for generating functional surfaces, which has proved to be ideal for producing structures with dimensions down to the nanometer scale. Ultrashort laser pulses enable nonlinear absorption, by which transparent materials can also be processed. The quality and processing rate strongly depend on the correct choice of parameters. Laser surface texturing can be processed under different environments. As compared to laser ablation in air, employing liquids or inert gases as media provides higher accuracy and more uniformity by limiting the heat-affected zone and other undesired defects to a large extent.

With the development of laser sources and different processes, laser texturing offers great possibilities in medical and biomedical applications. The rapid development of high-repetition-rate laser sources and novel beam delivery technology provides a clear tendency toward higher processing speeds in the future. In the past 20 years, the average output power of ultrafast lasers has followed a type of Moore's law that doubles every two to three years. Shortly, cheaper and more stable devices on an industrial scale will be suitable for applications in the medical field. This will improve medical technology, therapeutics, and biological research, which will lead to innovations and advancements.

13.5 Conclusions

Lasers open new possibilities in the development of modern medicine. Although the mechanism of interaction of light with matter needs to be further explored, this innovative micro/nano-fabrication technique has been successfully used for diagnoses, therapies, and surgical procedures. This chapter introduces what lasers bring to biomedicine from the foundational principles to the practical applications. The distinctive characteristics of flexible, high-energy-density, and short duration offer the potential to change materials and tissues which are not achievable normally by traditional methods. Laser cutting and texturing have high impact on traditional surgical procedures and device manufacturing. From laser-assisted surgeries to diagnostic procedures, lasers have become invaluable tools in clinical operations, offering patients safer and more effective treatments.

The outlook for lasers in biomedicine is filled with promise and potential. Emerging trends and technologies promote the innovation of nanomedicine, personalized medicine, and artificial intelligence combined with laser technologies. The next frontier in diagnostics would well see the integration of laser-based diagnoses with artificial intelligence, serving precision and efficiency in healthcare. The therapies are combined with diagnostics and guided by real-time data and advanced imaging technologies. The convergence of lasers with nanomedicine also holds immense potential, which brings the promise of precision in targeting diseases at the molecular level. With ongoing developments of laser sources, the applications and markets of devices using laser technologies will be expanded, offering new solutions to personalized medicine tailored to individual profiles.

References

[1] P. Kronenberg and B. Somani, Advances in lasers for the treatment of stones-a systematic review, *Current Urology Reports*, 2018, 19(6):45.

[2] M.B. Totonchy and M.W. Chiu, UV-based therapy. *Dermatologic Clinics*, 2014, 32(3):399–413.

[3] O. Tekeli and H.C. Kose, Comparison of aqueous flare values after micropulse transscleral laser treatment and continuous wave transscleral cyclophotocoagulation, *Ocular Immunology and Inflammation*, 2023, 31(3):541–549.

[4] T.I. Karu, Cellular and molecular mechanisms of photobiomodulation (Low-Power Laser Therapy). *IEEE Journal of Selected Topics in Quantum Electronics*, 2014, 20(2):143–148.

[5] B. Devaraj, M. Usa, K.P. Chan, *et al.*, Recent advances in coherent detection imaging (CDI) in biomedicine: Laser tomography of human tissues *in Vivo* and *in Vitro*. *IEEE Journal of Selected Topics in Quantum Electronics*, 1996, 2(4):1008–1016.

[6] S. Souissi, Y. Le Mer, F. Metge, *et al.*, An update on continuous-wave cyclophotocoagulation (CW-CPC) and micropulse transscleral laser treatment (MP-TLT) for adult and paediatric refractory glaucoma, *Acta Ophthalmologica*, 2021, 99(5):E621–E653.

[7] K.M. Kent and E.M. Graber, Laser tattoo removal: A review, *Dermatologic Surgery*, 2012, 38(1):1–13.

[8] K. Fedin, M. Inochkin, L. Khloponin, *et al.*, Subnanosecond 1 J laser for medicine and technolog, *Optical and Quantum Electronics*, 2017, 49(5):178.

[9] B.E. Bouma, G.J. Tearney, I.P. Bilinsky, *et al.*, Self-phase-modulated Kerr-lens mode-locked Cr:forsterite laser source for optical coherence Tomography, *Optics Letters*, 1996, 21(22):1839–1841.

[10] F. Chen, X. Yu, X. Li, *et al.*, High power diode-pumped passively Q-switched and mode-locking Nd:GdVO$_4$ laser at 912 nm. *Optics Communications*, 2011. 284(2):635–639.

[11] Y.D. Gong, P. Shum, M.K. Rao, *et al.*, Novel cavity length feedback and stable operation of actively mode locked fiber ring laser, in *3rd International Conference on Microwave and Millimeter Wave Technology*, Beijing, China, 2002, pp. 1079–1082.

[12] K. Sugioka, Progress in ultrafast laser processing and future prospects, *Nanophotonics*, 2017, 6(2):393–413.

[13] F. Sima and K. Sugioka, Ultrafast laser manufacturing of nanofluidic systems, *Nanophotonics*, 2021, 10(9):2389–2406.

[14] M.V. Pantawane, Y.-H. Ho, W.B. Robertson, *et al.*, Thermal assessment of ex vivo laser ablation of cortical bone, *ACS Biomaterials Science & Engineering*, 2020, 6(4):2415–2426.

[15] Z. Wang, Z. Du, J.K.Y. Chan, *et al.*, Direct laser microperforation of bioresponsive surface-patterned films with through-hole arrays for vascular tissue-engineering application. *ACS Biomaterials Science & Engineering*, 2015. 1(12):1239–1249.

[16] B. El Aoud, M. Boujelbene, A. Boudjemline, *et al.*, Investigation of cut edge microstructure and surface roughness obtained by laser cutting of titanium alloy Ti-6Al-4V, in *11th International Conference on Materials, Processing and Characterization (ICMPC)*, Indore, India, 2020, pp. 2775–2780.

[17] C.-H. Hung, F.-Y. Chang, T.-L. Chang, *et al.*, Micromachining NiTi tubes for use in medical devices by using a femtosecond laser, *Optics and Lasers in Engineering*, 2015, 66:34–40.

[18] N. Muhammad, D. Whitehead, A. Boor, *et al.*, Comparison of dry and wet fibre laser profile cutting of thin 316L stainless steel tubes for medical device applications, *Journal of Materials Processing Technology*, 2010, 210(15):2261–2267.

[19] Y. Haga, Y. Muyari, S. Goto, *et al.*, Development of minimally invasive medical tools using laser processing on cylindrical substrates, *Electrical Engineering in Japan*, 2011, 176(1):65–74.

[20] M. Schuettler, S. Stiess, B.V. King, *et al.*, fabrication of implantable microelectrode arrays by laser cutting of silicone rubber and platinum foil, *Journal of Neural Engineering*, 2005, 2(1):S121–S128.

[21] B. Lan, M.H. Hong, K.D. Ye, *et al.*, Laser microfabrication of glass substrates by pocket scanning, in *4th International Symposium on Laser Precision Microfabrication*, Munich, Germany, 2003 pp. 133–136.

[22] B. Richerzhagen, M. Kutsuna, H. Okada, *et al.*, Water-jet-guided laser processing, in LAMP 2002:*International Congress on Laser Advanced Materials Processing*, Osaka, Japan, 2003, pp. 91–94.

[23] A. Richmann, Y. Kuzminykh, B. Richerzhagen, *et al.*, Laser microjet© cutting of up to 3 mm thick sapphire, in *International Congress on Applications of Lasers & Electro-Optics*, Orlando, USA, 2014, pp. 1139–1143.

[24] S. Green and D. Perrottet, Damage-free dicing of SiC wafers by water jet-guided laser, in *CS MANTECH Conference*, Vancouver, Canada, 2006, pp. 145–146.

[25] X. Sun, J. Yu, Y. Hu, *et al.*, Study on ablation threshold of fused silica by liquid-assisted femtosecond laser processing, *Applied Optics*, 2019, 58(33):9027–9032.

[26] R. Malhotra, I. Saxena, K. Ehmann, *et al.*, Laser-induced Plasma Micro-machining (LIPMM) for enhanced productivity and flexibility in laser-based Micro-machining processes, *CIRP Annals-Manufacturing Technology*, 2013, 62(1):211–214.

[27] H. Jaber, A. Binder, and D. Ashkenasi, High-efficiency micro structuring of VUV window materials by laser-induced plasma-assisted ablation (LIPAA) with a KrF excimer laser, in *Conference on Photon Processing in Microelectronics and Photonics III*. San Jose, USA, 2004, pp. 557–567.

[28] Y. Li, H. Liu, and M. Hong, High-quality sapphire microprocessing by dual-beam laser induced plasma assisted ablation, *Optics Express*, 2020, 28(5):6242–6250.

[29] H. Liu, W. Lin, and M. Hong, Hybrid laser precision engineering of transparent hard materials: Challenges, solutions and applications, *Light: Science & Applications*, 2021, 10(1):162.

[30] M. Ehrhardt, G. Raciukaitis, P. Gecys, *et al.*, Microstructuring of fused silica by laser-induced backside wet etching using picosecond laser pulses, *Applied Surface Science*, 2010, 256(23):7222–7227.

[31] Z.Q. Huang, M.H. Hong, T.B.M. Do, *et al.*, Laser etching of glass substrates by 1064 nm laser irradiation, *Applied Physics A-Materials Science & Processing*, 2008, 93(1):159–163.

[32] G. Kopitkovas, T. Lippert, C. David, *et al.*, Fabrication of micro-optical elements in quartz by laser induced backside wet etching, *Microelectronic Engineering*, 2003, 67-8:438–444.

[33] D. Bhaduri, A. Batal, S.S. Dimov, *et al.*, On design and tribological behaviour of laser textured surfaces, *Procedia CIRP*, 2017, 60:20–25.

Index